Resistance to Targeted Anti-Cancer Therapeutics

Volume 20

Series Editor:
Benjamin Bonavida

More information about this series at http://www.springer.com/series/11727

Myron R. Szewczuk • Bessi Qorri
Manpreet Sambi

Editors

Current Applications for Overcoming Resistance to Targeted Therapies

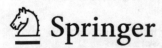 Springer

Editors
Myron R. Szewczuk
Department of Biomedical and Molecular
Sciences
Queen's University
Kingston, ON, Canada

Bessi Qorri
Department of Biomedical and Molecular
Sciences
Queen's University
Kingston, ON, Canada

Manpreet Sambi
Department of Biomedical and Molecular
Sciences
Queen's University
Kingston, ON, Canada

ISSN 2196-5501 ISSN 2196-551X (electronic)
Resistance to Targeted Anti-Cancer Therapeutics
ISBN 978-3-030-21479-1 ISBN 978-3-030-21477-7 (eBook)
https://doi.org/10.1007/978-3-030-21477-7

This Springer imprint is published by the registered company Springer Nature Switzerland AG
The registered company address is: Gewerbestrasse 11, 6330 Cham, Switzerland

Aims and Scope

For several decades, treatment of cancer consisted of chemotherapeutic drugs, radiation, and hormonal therapies. Those were not tumor specific and exhibited several toxicities. During the last several years, targeted cancer therapies (molecularly targeted drugs) have been developed and consisting of immunotherapies (cell mediated and antibody) drugs or biologicals that can block the growth and spread of cancer by interfering with surface receptors and with specific dysregulated gene products that control tumor cell growth and progression. These include several FDA-approved drugs/antibodies/inhibitors that interfere with cell growth signaling or tumor blood vessel development, promote the cell death of cancer cells, stimulate the immune system to destroy specific cancer cells, and deliver toxic drugs to cancer cells. Targeted cancer therapies are being used alone or in combination with conventional drugs and other targeted therapies.

One of the major problems that arise following treatment with both conventional therapies and targeted cancer therapies is the development of resistance, preexisting in a subset of cancer cells or cancer stem cells and/or induced by the treatments. Tumor cell resistance to targeted therapies remains a major hurdle, and, therefore, several strategies are being considered in delineating the underlining molecular mechanisms of resistance and the development of novel drugs to reverse both the innate and acquired resistance to various targeted therapeutic regimens.

The new series *Resistance of Targeted Anti-Cancer Therapeutics* was inaugurated and focuses on the clinical application of targeted cancer therapies (either approved by the FDA or in clinical trials) and the resistance observed by these therapies. Each book will consist of updated reviews on a specific target therapeutic and strategies to overcome resistance at the biochemical, molecular, and both genetic and epigenetic levels. This new series is timely and should be of significant interest to clinicians, scientists, trainees, students, and pharmaceutical companies.

Benjamin Bonavida
David Geffen School of Medicine
University of California Los Angeles
Los Angeles, CA, USA

Series Editor Biography

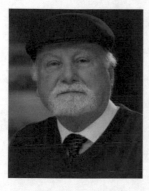

Benjamin Bonavida, Ph.D. (Series Editor) is currently Distinguished Research Professor at the University of California, Los Angeles (UCLA). His research career, thus far, has focused on basic immunochemistry and cancer immunobiology. His research investigations have ranged from the mechanisms of cell-mediated killing, sensitization of resistant tumor cells to chemo-/immunotherapy, characterization of resistant factors in cancer cells, cell-signaling pathways mediated by therapeutic anticancer antibodies, and characterization of a dysregulated NF-κB/Snail/YY1/RKIP/PTEN loop in many cancers that regulates cell survival, proliferation, invasion, metastasis, and resistance. He has also investigated the role of nitric oxide in cancer and its potential antitumor activity. Many of the above studies are centered on the clinical challenging features of cancer patients' failure to respond to both conventional and targeted therapies. The development and activity of various targeting agents, their modes of action, and resistance are highlighted in many refereed publications.

Acknowledgment

The Series Editor acknowledges the various assistants who have diligently worked in both the editing and formatting of the various manuscripts in each volume. They are Inesa Navasardyan and Kaiya Kozuma.

Preface

The book *Current Applications for Overcoming Resistance to Targeted Therapies* is designed to provide a comprehensive review of the key mechanisms by which resistance to targeted therapy develops and highlight recent advancements for overcoming or circumventing this resistance.

We now have significantly more therapeutic options for cancer than even just a decade ago. Targeted therapies have been attractive alternatives to traditional cancer therapies such as chemotherapy to avoid systemic toxicity. Despite initial favorable results, resistance to targeted therapy invariably develops, rendering treatment ineffective. Thus, the failure of targeted therapy as a result of the development of resistance presents as a major clinical challenge in cancer treatment. The development of resistance can include molecular alterations such as mutations in the drug target or interaction with the tumor cells. The extensive interactions within the tumor microenvironment add another layer of complexity in our attempt to overcome resistance to targeted therapy. In attempts to enhance our understanding of these processes, we have divided this book into ten chapters, each with a distinct focus. However, given the intricate landscape of the tumor microenvironment, the chapters are inextricably linked.

This book is intended for researchers, research students, and cancer research practitioners. This book is also of interest to researchers and clinicians within the realm of cancer and drug discovery and delivery. The contents of this book will highlight the transdisciplinary approach that will be necessary for the future of cancer treatment. We have aimed to cover the breadth and depth of the development of resistance to targeted therapies to the best of our ability. Thus, the contents of this book will be of interest to a broader audience.

The chapter authors were selected based on their expertise and their research breakthroughs that have had significant impacts on overcoming resistance to targeted therapy. We would like to convey our sincerest appreciation to all of the chapter contributors. Without their expertise, hard work, and cooperation during the writing and editing process, this book would not have been possible. Our special thanks to Dr. Benjamin Bonavida and Mr. Murugesan Tamilselvan from Springer Nature Series for their continuous, kind support and great efforts in bringing the book to fruition.

Kingston, ON, Canada   Bessi Qorri
                                                                Manpreet Sambi
                                                              Myron R. Szewczuk

Contents

Contributors

Sirin A. Adham Department of Biology, College of Science, Sultan Qaboos University, Muscat, Oman

Noura Al-Zeheimi Department of Biology, College of Science, Sultan Qaboos University, Muscat, Oman

Bangxing Hong Department of Neurosurgery, McGovern Medical School, University of Texas Health Science Center at Houston, Houston, TX, USA

Balveen Kaur Department of Neurosurgery, McGovern Medical School, University of Texas Health Science Center at Houston, Houston, TX, USA

Vineet Kumar Department of Physiology, National University of Singapore, Singapore, Singapore

Jenny H. Lee Faculty of Medicine and Health Sciences, Macquarie University, Sydney, NSW, Australia

Melanoma Institute Australia, Sydney, NSW, Australia

Cole T. Lewis Department of Neurosurgery, McGovern Medical School, University of Texas Health Science Center at Houston, Houston, TX, USA

Cecile Malardier-Jugroot Department of Chemistry and Chemical Engineering, Royal Military College of Canada, Kingston, ON, Canada

Ryan M. McCormack Department of Neurosurgery, McGovern Medical School, University of Texas Health Science Center at Houston, Houston, TX, USA

Matt McTaggart Department of Chemistry and Chemical Engineering, Royal Military College of Canada, Kingston, ON, Canada

W. Hans Meisen Cell and Gene Therapy Group, Amgen Inc., South San Francisco, CA, USA

Rita Nahta Department of Pharmacology, Emory University School of Medicine, Atlanta, GA, USA

Department of Hematology and Medical Oncology, Emory University School of Medicine, Atlanta, GA, USA

Winship Cancer Institute, Emory University, Atlanta, GA, USA

Molecular and Systems Pharmacology Program, Graduate Division of Biological and Biomedical Sciences, Emory University, Atlanta, GA, USA

Somaira Nowsheen Mayo Clinic Medical Scientist Training Program, Mayo Clinic Alix School of Medicine and Mayo Clinic Graduate School of Biomedical Sciences, Mayo Clinic, Rochester, MN, USA

Andreia V. Pinho Faculty of Medicine and Health Sciences, Macquarie University, Sydney, NSW, Australia

Melanoma Institute Australia, Sydney, NSW, Australia

Bessi Qorri Department of Biomedical and Molecular Sciences, Queen's University, Kingston, ON, Canada

John Markus Rieth Department of Internal Medicine, Carver College of Medicine, Iowa City, IA, USA

Helen Rizos Faculty of Medicine and Health Sciences, Macquarie University, Sydney, NSW, Australia

Melanoma Institute Australia , Sydney, NSW, Australia

Manpreet Sambi Department of Biomedical and Molecular Sciences, Queen's University, Kingston, ON, Canada

Subbaya Subramanian Department of Surgery, University of Minnesota Medical School, Minneapolis, MN, USA

Masonic Cancer Center, University of Minnesota, Minneapolis, MN, USA

Jessica Swanner Department of Neurosurgery, McGovern Medical School, University of Texas Health Science Center at Houston, Houston, TX, USA

Myron R. Szewczuk Department of Biomedical and Molecular Sciences, Queen's University, Kingston, ON, Canada

Mukesh Verma Methods and Technologies Branch, Epidemiology and Genomics Research Program, Division of Cancer Control and Population Sciences, National Cancer Institute, National Institutes of Health, Bethesda, MD, USA

Dechen Wangmo Department of Surgery, University of Minnesota Medical School, Minneapolis, MN, USA

Fen Xia Department of Radiation Oncology, University of Arkansas for Medical Sciences, Little Rock, AR, USA

Ce Yuan Department of Surgery, University of Minnesota Medical School, Minneapolis, MN, USA

Xianda Zhao Department of Surgery, University of Minnesota Medical School, Minneapolis, MN, USA

About the Editors

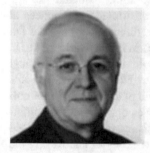

Myron R. Szewczuk, Ph.D. is currently Professor of Immunology and Medicine in the Department of Biomedical and Molecular Sciences and Medicine, Queen's University, Kingston, Ontario, Canada, for the past 38 years. He received his B.Sc. in Chemistry (University of Guelph), M.Sc. in Biochemistry (Guelph), Ph.D. in Immunochemistry (University of Windsor), and postdoctoral training with Gregory Siskind, M.D. in Cellular Immunology at Cornell University Medical College, New York City. Dr. Szewczuk's recent research has focused on the role of glycosylation in receptor activation with a particular focus on Toll-like, nerve growth factor Trk, EGFR, and insulin receptors. He has discovered a novel receptor-signaling platform and its targeted translation in multistage tumorigenesis and metabolic syndrome. He is now in the development of engineered drug delivery systems.

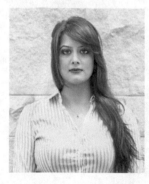

Manpreet Sambi is currently a Ph.D. candidate in the Department of Biomedical and Molecular Sciences, Queen's University, Kingston, Ontario, Canada. She is under the direct supervision of Dr. Myron R. Szewczuk (co-editor of this volume) and is co-supervised by Dr. William Harless, M.D., Ph.D., certified Medical Oncologist and CEO of Encyt Technologies, Inc., Sydney, Nova Scotia. She received her B.Sc. in Integrative Biology and her M.Sc. in Physiology from the University of Toronto. Her Masters research focused on regenerative medicine, directed differentiation of stem cells, and tissue regeneration. Manpreet's doctoral research focuses on therapeutic targeting cancer stem cells (CSC). To do this, she is working toward understanding the mechanisms of cancer stem cell activation and proliferation with an emphasis on the influence of key inflammatory cytokines in modulating these processes. She is also exploring therapeutic avenues to target this population of cancer cells by coupling nanomedicine with multimodal therapeutic approaches for more effective targeting of cancer stem cells. Collectively, this knowledge will improve the potency of conventional treatment options and improve patient survival.

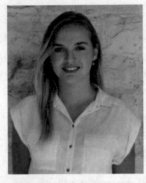

Bessi Qorri is currently a Ph.D. student in the Department of Biomedical and Molecular Sciences at Queen's University, under the direct supervision of Dr. Myron R. Szewczuk and Dr. William Harless, M.D., Ph.D., certified Medical Oncologist and CEO of Encyt Technologies, Inc., Sydney, Nova Scotia. Bessi's research interests lie in the field of cancer and immunology. Her doctoral work involves optimizing the combination of a drug cocktail consisting of drugs repurposed as anticancer agents. She is working on uncovering the overlapping mechanisms of action of the combination of aspirin, metformin and oseltamivir phosphate in targeting multistage tumorigenesis in pancreatic cancer via a novel signaling paradigm identified by Dr. Myron R. Szewczuk.

Chapter 1
Introduction to the Acquisition of Resistance to Targeted Therapy

Manpreet Sambi and Myron R. Szewczuk

Abstract The complex process of cancer development and tumorigenesis involves several critical events that take place concurrently or build upon each other, ultimately manifesting as a malignancy with therapeutically targetable components. Given the broad and unspecific cytotoxic effects of chemotherapy, supplementing conventional therapeutic options with targeted therapies initially showed promise in the clinic, particularly in cases where oncogenic addiction (i.e. the dependence on one pathway to maintain tumorigenesis) was a factor. A combination of one or more of these targeted therapeutic options has also shown promise. However, the underlying challenge of treating cancer is its uncanny ability to seamlessly adapt and resist the therapeutic effects of these targeted agents, rendering them ineffective. Other mechanisms can include relying on alternative pathways to sustain their growth. This introduction provides a comprehensive overview of the mechanisms of acquired resistance as they pertain to targeted therapies and indicate in which chapters specific topics will be addressed in more detail. Collectively, this book aims to provide current advancements in the therapeutic arms race between cancer and clinicians and scientists alike to overcome resistance to targeted therapies. We provide a comprehensive overview of the challenges and solutions to resistance to several conventional targeted therapies in addition to providing a discussion on broad topics including targeting components of the tumor microenvironment, emerging therapeutic options, and novel areas to be explored concerning nanotechnology and the epigenome.

Keywords Acquisition of resistance · Targeted therapy · Compensatory pathways · Receptor tyrosine kinases · Hallmarks of cancer · Transdifferentiation · Dedifferentiation · Cancer stem cells · Epigenetics · Vascular mimicry

M. Sambi · M. R. Szewczuk (✉)
Department of Biomedical and Molecular Sciences, Queen's University,
Kingston, ON, Canada
e-mail: m.sambi@queensu.ca; szewczuk@queensu.ca

© Springer Nature Switzerland AG 2019

M. R. Szewczuk et al. (eds.), *Current Applications for Overcoming Resistance to Targeted Therapies*, Resistance to Targeted Anti-Cancer Therapeutics 20, https://doi.org/10.1007/978-3-030-21477-7_1

Abbreviations

ABC	ATP-binding cassette
AKT	Protein kinase B
BCL-2	B-cell lymphoma-2
BCR-ABL	Breakpoint cluster region protein—Abelson murine leukemia viral oncogene homolog 1
Bv-8	Bombina variegate peptide 8
CAF	Cancer-associated fibroblasts
c-FLIP	cellular FLICE (FADD-like IL-1β-converting enzyme)-inhibitory protein
CpG	Cytosine and guanine-rich sequences
CSC	Cancer stem cell
DNMT	DNA methyltransferase
ECM	Extracellular matrix
EGFR	Epidermal growth factor receptor
EMT	Epithelial-to-mesenchymal transition
ERK	Extracellular signal-regulated kinase
FGF	Fibroblast growth factor
HAT	Histone acetyltransferase
HER	Human epidermal growth factor receptor
HIF-1 α	Hypoxia-inducible factor-1α
JAK	Janus kinase
Klf-4	Kruppel Like Factor 4
mAb	Monoclonal antibody
MAPK	Mitogen-activated protein kinase
MDR1	Multidrug resistance protein 1
MEK	Mitogen activated protein kinase kinase
MET	Mesenchymal-to-epithelial transition
miRNA	Micro-RNA
mTOR	Mammalian target of rapamycin
NF-κB	Nuclear factor kappa-light-chain-enhancer of activated B cells
NP1	Neuropilin
NSCLC	Non-small cell lung cancer
OCT-1	Organic-cation transporter-1
Oct-4	Octamer-binding transcription factor 4
OP	Oseltamivir phosphate
PARP	Poly ADP-ribose polymerase
PDGF	Platelet-derived growth factor
PI3K	Phosphoinositide 3-kinase
PIGF	Placental growth factor
RTKs	Receptor tyrosine kinases
STAT3	Signal transducer and activator of transcription 3
TAM	Tumor-associated macrophage

TGF-α   Transforming growth factor alpha
TKI   Tyrosine kinase inhibitors
TME   Tumor microenvironment
VEGF   Vascular endothelial growth factor

1.1 Introduction

The main objective of targeted therapies involves inhibiting one or more hallmark features of cancer, including those that were classified by Hanahan and Weinberg [1] as emerging and enabling characteristics. Concerning the proposed molecular events leading to the development of cancer, several driver mutations result in the activation of oncoproteins that are required for tumor growth and progression including *ALK, BCR-ABL, BRAF, EGFR,* and *RAS*, to name a few [2]. Genomic analyses on cancer progression and development led to the discovery of several oncogenic pathways that are required for tumor survival and growth. These pathways represent a form of "oncogenic addiction," where a tumor's dependency on one or more critical oncogenic pathways is required for its survival [2, 3]. The discovery of these pathways was the predecessor to the development of targeted therapies which presented as viable therapeutic options. Unfortunately, it is rare that a cancer type is exclusively dependent on one critical pathway. Nevertheless, some clinical success has been observed in therapies targeting epidermal growth factor receptor (EGFR), BRAF-mutant cancers and human epidermal growth factor-2 (HER-2) [2–4]. However, difficulties in targeting all important oncogenic pathways, many of which are intertwined in complex interactions and crosstalk, is one of the contributors to treatment failure in the clinic. This clinical failure has translated into the development of other targeted therapies including vascular endothelial growth factor (VEGF), exploitation of mutations such as defects in critical DNA repair processes using poly ADP-ribose polymerase (PARP) inhibitors and recruiting immune cells to invade or reactivate in tumor tissues using immunotherapy. The intention of supplementing chemotherapy with one or a combination of these targeted therapies was to improve the overall response rate in addition to overcoming resistance and enhance sensitivity to chemotherapy. However, the development of resistance to targeted therapies has led to an additional complication in the treatment of cancer.

The term "resistance" is an umbrella definition that incorporates circumstances when drugs are rendered ineffective and no longer exert their therapeutic effects. The causes of resistance range from the drug target being mutated to the acquisition of a resistant variant that prevents the drug from acting on its target. These events can be intrinsic, where the cancer is innately unresponsive to the drugs prior to treatment, or acquired, where cancer becomes unresponsive post-treatment [2, 5].

Due to the overlapping mechanisms of action and the broadly applicable consequences of resistance to targeted therapy, this introductory chapter is divided into two subparts. The first part aims to provide a thorough overview of genetic and cellular events (Sects 1.2 and 1.3, respectively) that contribute to the development of resistance to targeted therapies. The second part (Sect. 1.4) discusses the development of resistance to select classes/specific types of targeted therapies and the known or proposed mechanisms contributing to this resistance.

1.2   Molecular Events Leading to the Acquisition of Resistance to Targeted Therapy

Mechanisms of acquired resistance will be the primary focus of this book, particularly as they relate to various targeted therapies that are available for the treatment of cancer. Methods to overcome resistance to once-promising targeted therapies is critical for the continued efficacy of treatment options for cancer. In general, the genomic mechanisms of developing resistance to targeted therapies can be broadly grouped into four main categories [2, 4–6]:

1. Alterations of drug target expression to prevent therapeutic action.
2. Activation of the compensatory pathway(s) parallel or downstream of the inhibited pathway.
3. Activation of alternative survival pathways.

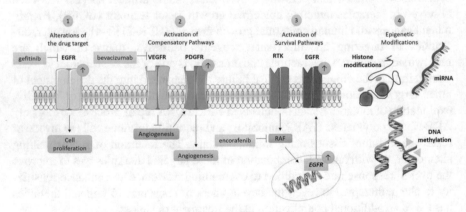

Fig. 1.1 Genetic Mechanisms of Resistance. Genetic mechanisms that lead to the development of resistance include alterations to the drug target, activation of compensatory pathways, activation of survival pathways and epigenetic mechanisms. For example, (1) The effects of gefitinib mediated inhibition of the epidermal growth factor receptor are overcome by several methods, but as depicted here, this mechanism involves amplification of the drug target, in this case, EGFR. (2) Inhibition of angiogenesis through the action of bevacizumab is overcome by activation of other pro-angiogenic pathways such as PDGFR (3) inhibition of a key oncogenic pathway as shown here leads to the activation of a second oncogenic pathway (i.e. EGFR) in order to maintain tumorigenesis. (4) Lastly, epigenetic mechanisms that can potentially contribute to the development of resistance include DNA methylation, histone modifications and microRNA related alterations to the drug target. *EGFR* epidermal growth factor receptor; *PDGFR* platelet-derived growth factor receptor

4. Epigenetic regulation of the development of resistance.

The first three categories are well developed and represent genetic events; however, the epigenetic events that confer resistance have recently gained attention due to the broad consequences of their activity and have been included as an essential category to explore. A summary of these molecular events is presented in Fig. 1.1.

1.2.1   Alterations in Drug Target Expression to Prevent Therapeutic Action

Perhaps the most convenient and effective method to counter or override the therapeutic effects of a drug is to alter the target itself, rendering the therapy ineffective. This method can be applied to drugs including those that target proteins such as cell surface receptors as well as driver gene mutations such as *BRAF* [2, 3]. Driver gene mutations are defined as critical mutations and are a hallmark of cancer. These mutations have been attributed to several processes that sustain cancer growth, progression, and survival. Therapies that can target these genes have a transient effect after which point therapeutic resistance develops. The mechanism of action involves upregulating the expression of the driver gene so that any inhibition is dampened by the overwhelming increased expression of the driver gene being targeted [7]. Alterations to the drug target can include mutation of the target, amplification of a driver oncogene to dampen the effectiveness of the drug, receptor downregulation in order to reduce the available targets and alternative splice variants that the drug cannot recognize [2, 5].

Mutations of Drug Target Mutations of the drug target essentially prevent the drug from recognizing and binding to the target of interest rendering the therapy ineffective. Mutations can include those that target the kinase domain, thereby preventing the drug from targeting the receptor, ultimately leading to the development of resistance [2, 8]. These mutations typically occur following exposure to the treatment of a specific target, as has been the case for receptor tyrosine inhibitors (RTKs) and monoclonal antibodies (mAb) [8]. For example, in patients that develop resistance to EGFR-TK inhibitors, EGFR mutations have been documented in 50% of patients that develop resistance. The mutation occurs on the T790 M allele and is further amplified in order to overcome EGFR-TK inhibitors. This will be discussed in more detail in Sect. 1.4.

Amplification of Drug Target Amplification of the drug target is a process by which the target of interest is overexpressed or there is an increase in gene copy, which leads to the target continuing to carry out its functions in the presence of the drug. Ultimately, this leads to enhanced activation of the signaling pathway. Furthermore, hyperactivation of the target could lead to the "on-state" being the preferred state of activity, resulting in decreased binding affinity for therapeutic agents [9]. For example, colorectal cancers with *KRAS* or *BRAF* mutations have demonstrated dependency on the mitogen-activated protein kinase (MAPK) pathway as a result of these two mutations [2, 9]. The substrates of RAF kinases are mitogen-activated protein kinase kinase 1/2 (MEK1/2) which phosphorylates extracellular signal-related kinase (ERK). Although these all represent possible therapeutic targets, colorectal cancer cell lines treated with MEK1/2 inhibitors have gained resistance by amplifying their driver oncogene, that being *KRAS* or *BRAF*. This amplification leads to an increase in activated MEK, which in turn decreases the lethality of MEK inhibitors and increases the baseline ERK levels required for continued functionality [9].

Alternative RNA Splicing of Drug Target Alternative splicing represents a post-transcriptional modification that leads to alternative mRNA transcripts which can produce variants of proteins of interest that cannot be recognized by therapeutic agents designed for non-spliced variants, rendering therapy ineffective [10]. This is a form of acquired resistance as this generally takes place in response to initial treatment. Splicing can also confer protection against cytotoxicity, leading to an indirect method of resistance. This is true of caspase-2 which, when spliced to its *CASP-2S* form, inhibits apoptosis and protects cancer cells from cytotoxic agents [11]. Alternative splicing has many other mechanisms of action that are critical to cancer progression in general, and while such details are beyond the scope of this introduction, Wang and Lee provide an eloquent discussion on RNA splicing [10].

Downregulation of Drug Target As discussed, downregulating the target of interest leads to resistance to therapy due to the lack of availability of the drug target and represents another form of acquired resistance that develops post-treatment. This can be mediated by fluctuations in the tumor microenvironment such as changes in hypoxic conditions [12]. For example, upon oxygen deprivation, pro-apoptotic proteins Bid and Bad were downregulated, and this was mediated by hypoxia-inducible factor 1 (HIF-1) [12].

1.2.2 Activation of Compensatory Pathways

Activation of compensatory pathways is one of the most challenging aspects of acquired resistance because of the seamless transition from dependence on one pathway to another. This is particularly difficult with respect to inhibitors that are designed to target specific pathways of interest. Following inhibition of a pathway, cancer cells can bypass this inhibition and activate a parallel pathway capable of engaging the same processes as the inhibited pathway [2, 5]. The broad mechanism of compensation involves recruiting other signaling pathways that can be maintained to stabilize cellular processes such as cellular proliferation and differentiation in response to the inhibition of other pathways that regulate this activity. For example, the PI3K/mTOR/Akt pathways are highly interconnected, and the inhibition of mTOR is compensated for by PI3K and Akt, thereby maintaining cellular proliferation [13]. Furthermore, the JAK/STAT pathway regulates many cancer-related processes and is activated in response to inhibition of many upstream kinases [14]. Since the receptor tyrosine kinase (RTKs) family is highly interconnected, many compensatory mechanisms are investigated in this family and will be discussed in detail in Sect. 1.4.

1.2.3   Activation of Alternative Pathways to Ensure Survival

Activation of alternative survival pathways can involve the emergence of a second oncogenic driver or an entirely separate oncogenic driver and is defined as "addiction switching" [2, 3]. These pathways can be those that are upstream or downstream of the drug target, such as the RAS pathway or the HER family, including EGFR, PI3K-AKT-mTOR or MYC[1] [2]. For example, mutated *BRAF* inhibition in colorectal cancer cells is ineffective because EGFR is activated leading to a feedback mechanism that recruits alternative pathways in response to *BRAF* inhibition. This is also reported in thyroid cancers with a mutation in *BRAF*, where upregulation of HER-3 leads to *BRAF* inhibition being ineffective through reactivation of MAPK pathway signaling [15]. This method of activating an inhibited kinase through redundant pathways has also been observed following EGFR inhibition, after which the Met pathway is recruited and amplified [3].

Furthermore, aberrations in the apoptotic pathway also present as an alternative survival pathway that can be recruited to resist the effects of targeted therapies. Typically, cancer cells have been characterized to preferentially depend on specific anti-apoptotic proteins that directly confer resistance to the effects of drugs, including BCL-2 family members[2] and flice-like inhibitory protein (c-FLIP), a caspase 8 inhibitor [5]. Amplifications, mutations, and upregulation of genes that transcribe these proteins lead to resistance to targeted therapy as the intended cytotoxic effect of targeted therapies are overridden, allowing for prolonged survival. Resistance to anti-apoptotic inhibitors will be discussed below.

1.2.4   Epigenome: Regulating Acquired Resistance and Modifying Drug Activity

The epigenome comprises several key constituents all of which finetune gene expression in response to various perturbations in the internal and external environment. In recent years, understanding the extent of the epigenome in regulating tumorigenesis has drawn international attention, particularly concerning therapeutically targeting its components to overcome epigenetic-mediated resistance to conventional chemo- and targeted therapies. The role of epigenetics concerning cancer

---

[1] MYC is a proto-oncogene that regulates cell proliferation and growth.

[2] Bcl-2 is a family of proteins that regulate apoptosis.

will be thoroughly discussed in Chap. 9; however, this section will briefly discuss epigenetic regulation.

The epigenome represents an extensive collection of components that can modulate the genome. Unlike genetic mutations, these minute changes in gene activity, though reversible, have been shown to have lasting effects. Modifications to genes occur through the action of DNA methylation, facilitated by DNA methyltransferases (DNMTs), histone modification, facilitated by histone acetyltransferases (HATs) and lastly, non-coding microRNAs (miRNAs) which regulate genes.

Epigenetic Mechanisms Conferring Resistance to Targeted Therapies Epigenetic regulation of drug resistance has recently gained intense interest because these temporary genetic modifications confer resistance to cancer or directly affect activation of the therapeutic agent. Epigenetics is defined as modifications in gene expression that are maintained over the course of cell turnover [16]. These modifications are regulated by alterations of DNA and/or histone proteins through methylation and acetylation events, respectively. Collectively these changes regulate the accessibility of candidate genes to be transcribed and therefore directly control gene expression.

DNA methylation typically occurs at cytosine residues by DNA methyltransferases (DNMTs) and leads to transcription elongation when transcribed locations are methylated or gene silencing when promoter regions are methylated [17, 18]. With respect to cancer, cytosine and guanine-rich sequences (CpG islands) of tumor suppressor genes have been characterized to be hypermethylated [19]. On the other hand, histone modifications are regulated by histone-specific enzymes and include alterations such as acetylation, methylation, butyrylation, and ubiquitylation, to name a few [20]. Collectively these post-translational modifications lead to variations in DNA accessibility for transcription. Typically, acetylation events lead to gene expression as genes are more readily transcribed and deacetylation has the opposite effect.

Concerning the acquisition of drug resistance, varying methylation patterns have been observed on candidate genes that confer resistance such as hypomethylation on the promoter sites of drug efflux genes [21]. In addition to modifying specific genes that contribute to drug resistance, DNA methylation of enzymes can also confer resistance by affecting drug metabolism. This process involves the methylation of enzymes that are typically required to activate drugs [5]. For example, capecitabine, an antimetabolite, requires the activity of thymidine phosphorylase for its active form 5-fluorouracil, however, when the gene coding this enzyme is methylated, thymidine phosphorylase is rendered inactive [22]. To overcome this issue, DNMT inhibitors have been used, and this resistance can be reversed [5].

MicroRNAs and the Acquisition of Resistance MicroRNAs (mRNAs)[3] are small non-coding RNAs that have mRNA modification functionalities [23]. The mode by which miRNAs modify mRNAs is through base pair binding with mRNAs leading to the arrest of translation and potential destabilization of the mRNA transcript [24].

---

[3] MicroRNAs are transcribed by RNA polymerase II and are later processed by endonuclease reactions into miRNAs.

Thorough genomic analyses of miRNAs that are aberrantly active in cancer cells have revealed their wide-ranging regulatory activities, some of which modulate the acquisition of drug resistance to conventional chemotherapeutic agents.

For instance, increased expression of miRNA-21 in breast cancer cells was able to promote resistance of MCF-7 cells to doxorubicin chemotherapy [25]. Although the role of miRNAs conferring resistance to chemotherapies has been an area of intense research focus, its implications in the acquisition of resistance to targeted therapies have just recently gained interest. The specific mechanism of resistance to which miRNAs can contribute to a variety of cancers is thoroughly reviewed elsewhere [8, 26]. In brief, miRNAs are proposed to regulate drug resistance by directly targeting mRNAs that promote drug resistance and upregulate pathways associated with cell survival and apoptosis [23]. Additionally, miRNAs can directly modify drug targets, and enzymes involved in drug metabolism and transport [27]. Together, these events lead to the acquisition of resistance to targeted therapies.

Concerning regulation of specific cellular pathways, miRNAs such as miRNA-21, have been shown to target *PTEN* in several cancers [25, 28]. Furthermore, concerning drug metabolism, miRNAs such as miRNA-27a and miRNA-451, have recently been shown to upregulate multidrug-resistant P-glycoprotein [23]. With respect to targeted therapies, miRNA-214 has been implicated in regulating resistance to gefitinib therapy by regulating the activation of the PTEN/Akt pathway [29]. Although miRNAs have been implicated in other aspects of tumorigenesis, their role in the development of resistance to targeted therapies is a relatively new area of research that requires further investigation.

1.3 Cellular Events Contributing to the Development of Resistance

Unlike the relatively definitive genetic mechanisms that confer resistance, the non-genetic events that lead to resistance to targeted therapy are far more challenging to distinguish from one another. This is primarily a consequence of several complex processes that confer this resistance, including but not limited to, epithelial to mesenchymal transition (EMT), selection of a cancer stem cell/self-renewing subpopulation, quiescence, and differentiation processes. These processes are dynamic and can overlap, and thus are not rigidly defined as unique processes; rather a complex interaction exists between them. Lastly, the tumor microenvironment is an extensively studied component of tumorigenesis, but for this introductory chapter, the primary focus will be on its contribution to drug resistance. Here, we have grouped non-genomic events that lead to resistance into two general categories and have presented them in Fig. 1.2:

1. Transformation, dedifferentiation, and trans-differentiation of phenotypes to overcome the effects of targeted therapies.

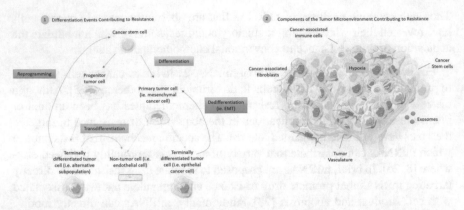

Fig. 1.2 Non-genetic components contributing to the development of resistance. Differentiation events and components of the tumor microenvironment. (1) This simplified sequence of differentiation events can be involved in the development of resistance including dedifferentiation, transdifferentiation and reprogramming of cancer cells. These events typically result following exposure to therapeutic agents in an effort to reconstruct components of the tumor microenvironment that have been targeted by drugs. For example, differentiated tumor cells can transdifferentiate into endothelial cells in response to anti-angiogenic treatment. (2) The tumor microenvironment comprises a large collection of tumor (including cancer stem cells) and supporting stromal cells (such as cancer-associated fibroblasts and tumor-associated immune cells) that contribute to the development of resistance. For example, the development of a hypoxic environment as a result of aberrant tumor vasculature contributes to dedifferentiation processes and the upregulation of pro-survival and self-renewal pathways which collectively overcome the cytotoxic effects of targeted therapies

2. Components of the tumor microenvironment that contribute to the acquisition of resistance.

1.3.1 Transformation/Dedifferentiation Mechanisms and Indirect Resistance to Therapeutic Action

Cellular plasticity is a broad term that describes the ability of cells to undergo phenotype switching in response to environmental stresses in order to acclimatize. However, recent investigations into fate determination have revealed that lineage commitment is far more plastic than previously understood, and has broad, yet challenging implications concerning cancer. In the context of cancer, cellular plasticity through dedifferentiation and transdifferentiation is abnormal and typically has one purpose: survival and evading the effects of conventional therapeutics. However, whether this leads to a resistant phenotype through selective pressures or in response to therapies has not yet been firmly established.

The process of dedifferentiation involves reverting to a progenitor phenotype or a less differentiated phenotype [30]. Alternatively, transdifferentiation refers to a process whereby a differentiated cell can change from one identity to an entirely different cell type. The mechanism of this process can include a dedifferentiation step followed by differentiation to the new cell type, or direct transformation into an entirely different cell type by activating a pathway not involved in normal cell development [30, 31]. Tumor cells have demonstrated the ability to dedifferentiate and transdifferentiate and provide a challenging complication concerning treatment regimens. This is particularly important to consider with respect to the tumor microenvironment, which will be discussed in Sect. 1.3.2.

A commonly studied dedifferentiation phenomenon in cancer is the process of epithelial to mesenchymal transition (EMT), which has been implicated in indirectly contributing to the development of resistance [32, 33]. The acquisition of resistance regarding the mesenchymal phenotype, similar to that of cancer stem cells, arises from the expression of drug efflux channels, which will be thoroughly discussed in Chap. 5, as well as the upregulation of several pathways that induce EMT [34]. The process of EMT involves reversion of epithelial cells, which are normally attached to the basement membrane, to mesenchymal cells, which have migratory capabilities [35]. At the molecular level, cancer cells undergoing EMT typically display a decrease in epithelial genes including E-cadherin with a concomitant increase in mesenchymal genes such as N-cadherin and fibronectin [36]. The signaling events that regulate this process include upregulation of the TGF-β pathway [34]. In this process, the binding of TGF-β leads to the activation of other TGF-β family members (i.e. bone morphogenic proteins; BMPs), after which mesenchymal genes are upregulated through SMAD-dependent and SMAD-independent activity [37]. In the SMAD-dependent pathway, mesenchymal genes are expressed when SMAD2/3 from a complex with SMAD 4 and are translocated to the nucleus, where they transcribe EMT transcription factors such as Snail/Slug and Twist. In contrast, the SMAD-independent pathway involves the induction of EMT alternative pathways such as PI3K and MAPK [38], Notch [39] and NF-κB [40], to name a few. Furthermore, Twist1 has also been reported to regulate EMT by promoting stemness and is overexpressed in cancers that have greater tumorigenic potential [41].

Concerning cancer, EMT has negative connotations as metastatic burden typically results in patients following this process [42]. In normal tissues, this process is relatively well understood and has specific functions, for example regenerating damaged tissues; however, in the context of cancer, EMT is an aberrant process that confers additional, more detrimental abilities, such as upregulation of self-renewal pathways [32]. This allows mesenchymal cells to undergo the reverse process of mesenchymal to epithelial transition (MET) to colonize and establish micrometastases and recapitulate the primary tumor from which the cells originated.

An added layer of complexity is that both of these processes can be triggered by a plethora of factors including perturbations in the tumor microenvironment (i.e. inflammation) and response to drug treatment and other stresses [30]. Specific components of the tumor microenvironment (TME) and their targeting will be thoroughly discussed in Chap. 2; however, for this introduction, the primary focus will be on select features of the TME that contribute to the acquisition of resistance to targeted therapy.

1.3.2 The Tumor Microenvironment and the Development of Resistance to Targeted Therapies

Constructing a microenvironment that is conducive to tumor growth and development is critical. The tumor microenvironment and its establishment are thoroughly reviewed elsewhere [43–45], and the focus of this section will be on its contribution to the development of resistance. The tumor microenvironment is comprised of non-cancer cells including cancer-associated fibroblasts (CAFs), tumor-associated macrophages (TAMs), blood vessels, soluble factors (i.e. growth factors, cytokines, and chemokines), the extracellular matrix (ECM), stromal cells and extracellular vesicles. Collectively, these components function in concert to manifest resistance to targeted therapies and will be discussed with a focus on the genomic and cellular events that contribute to this resistance.

Tumor Vasculature and Indirect Acquisition of Resistance As with any healthy organ requiring an adequate blood supply, the tumor depends on this network of blood vessels in order to continue to grow and metastasize. Consistent with other aspects of the tumor microenvironment, tumor angiogenesis produces abnormal vasculature. The consequences of this aberrant architecture is an unequal distribution of nutrients and oxygenation which ultimately leads to varying local conditions. These variations can contribute to the development of heterogeneous subpopulations within the tumor mass including the selection of cancer stem cells and initiation of metastasis [46, 47]. In particular, uneven distribution of vasculature can lead to the development of hypoxic conditions that can further upregulate the expression of VEGF in a mechanism of positive feedback through the hypoxia-inducible factor-1α (HIF-1 α) [48].

In normal physiological settings, the first steps of development of vasculature begin with vasculogenesis, an early embryonic event that includes differentiation events that produce terminally differentiated endothelial cells, mural cells [49][4] and other vascular associated cells [50]. This eventually leads to angiogenesis where endothelial cells proliferate and begin to form ordered blood vessels, eventually creating a network of blood vessels. Angiogenesis is regulated by several angiogenic pathways that are inhibited or activated for controlled sprouting of blood vessels [50]. In contrast, the development of tumor vasculature is termed neoangiogenesis

---

[4] Mural cells include vascular smooth muscle cells and pericytes which provide stability to blood vessels. These cells are aberrantly organized in tumor blood vessels and lead to leaky and a disorganized network of blood vessels.

or neovascularization because it is a non-embryonic event that defines the process of new blood vessel development [50, 51]. Development of tumor vasculature involves four main steps [51]:

1. Local injury to the basement membrane leading to the development of hypoxia.
2. Pro-angiogenic factors stimulate endothelial cells to proliferate.
3. Proliferating endothelial cells stabilize.
4. Secretion of pro-angiogenic factors continue to drive neoangiogenesis.

Angiogenic factors that are upregulated to promote the growth of blood vessels in order to feed the growing tumor include VEGF [50–52], basic fibroblast growth factor (bFGF), angiogenin, platelet-derived growth factor (PDGF), and TGF-β [51]. Karamysheva thoroughly reviews the specific processes that lead to the development of tumor vasculature [50], but in the remainder of this section, the contribution of vascularization to the development of resistance will be discussed.

At the time of preparing this book, there was no reported relationship between tumor vasculature and the development of resistance to targeted therapy. However, complicated mechanisms that contribute to the acquisition of resistance include the development of a hypoxic environment which leads to the selection of CSCs, a population of cells notoriously drug-resistant and will be discussed below. Several studies have demonstrated that hypoxic environments regulate cancer cell plasticity and can upregulate several transcription factors that regulate self-renewal programs [53–55]. Specifically, the activity of hypoxia-inducible factors (HIFs) modulates several cancer-related processes including pro-angiogenic, pro-glycolysis and self-renewal pathways. HIF-2α has been demonstrated to be the key regulator of the stem cell phenotype [54]. Recent reports have also revealed that hypoxic conditions also regulate epigenetic components such as histone demethylases [56]. As previously discussed, epigenetic regulators contribute to the development of resistance to conventional targeted therapies, and therefore, a hypoxic TME may further exacerbate the development of resistance to targeted therapies.

Cancer Stem Cells and Their Role in Development of Resistance The cancer stem cell hypothesis (CSC), postulates that a core population of cells exists within every tumor and are the driving force of metastatic burden and relapse observed at the clinical level, as they can recapitulate the primary tumor. The origin of this subpopulation of cells is widely debated, and a firm understanding of their potential concerning cancer progression remains to be established. The origins of cancer stem cells, also referred to as tumor-initiating cells, are discussed here [57, 58], and investigations into targeting this elusive population are reviewed here [59–61]. However, the focus of this introduction is their role in the development of resistance. The mechanism by which cancer stem cells are proposed to lead to resistance to convential therapies is attributed to their quiescent state during tumor growth and progression [62], where therapies broadly targeting rapid proliferation cannot ablate this population, leading to indirect therapy resistance through clonal selection.

Alternative models that apply stem cell differentiation to cancer stem cells suggest that cancer stem cells can differentiate into subpopulations that are necessary for survival [31]. Establishing the tumor microenvironment was widely attributed to cancer-mediated recruitment of specific cell populations capable of establishing a pro-tumor niche [31]. However, recent re-evaluations have shown that cancer stems can also differentiate into the non-malignant cells of the TME such as endothelial cells [63] through a VEGF-independent mechanism of action [31]. This suggests that the tumor can reproduce the required vasculature regardless of whether therapies targeting VEGF are being delivered. Additional components include CAFs, inflammatory immune cells and mesenchymal stem cells [31].

Taken collectively, CSCs represent a cellular form of compensation where a differentiation program can be accessed in order to overcome the effects of targeted therapies that ablate specific cells of the tumor microenvironment. This method represents a non-genetic mechanism that renders targeted therapies ineffective. Therefore, targeting this population is particularly important given its seemingly endless potential in overcoming the effects of many conventional therapies. Furthermore, a thorough understanding of the exact potential of CSCs regarding the development of resistance needs to be ascertained so effective targeted therapies can be developed while anticipating CSCs compensating for their therapeutic effects.

Role of Stromal Cells in the Development of Resistance The tumor stroma is an extensive collection of heterogeneous cells including immune cells, CAFs, endothelial cells, and extracellular vesicles, to name a few, which function to maintain a pro-tumor microenvironment and regulate many of the hallmarks of cancer [64]. For instance, immune cells have been implicated in contributing to the sustained proliferation of tumor cells, evasion of growth suppression and non-tumor associated immune cells, mediating metastasis, promoting angiogenesis, and preventing apoptosis [64]. CAFs contribute to all of the hallmarks mentioned above in addition to regulating the metabolic activity of cancer. For this introduction, the primary focus will be on CAFs, tumor-associated immune cells and extracellular vesicles and their contribution to the development of resistance to targeted therapies.

Cancer-associated fibroblasts have recently been implicated in melanoma by releasing factors such as HGF and IGF1 [65] to promote cell survival [64, 66], particularly in the presence of BRAF inhibitors [67]. Concerning IGF, secretion by CAFs was shown to increase IGFR/IR by secreting IGF2, leading to resistance to EGFR inhibitors in cholangiocarcinoma [65]. Furthermore, CAFs also play a critical role in EMT and foster a metastatic microenvironment to promote metastasis, which in turn leads to the development of resistance to the therapeutic effects of various drugs. Although the importance of CAFs in tumor progression and development of chemoresistance has been well reported, its role in conferring resistance to targeted therapies has only recently been uncovered and is an exciting avenue to explore.

Although tumor-associated macrophages (TAMs) and other immune cells are attributed to the development of resistance to immunotherapy (to be discussed in Chap. 4) and oncolytic virotherapy (to be discussed in Chap. 3), they have also been associated with the development of resistance to other forms of therapy, particularly anti-angiogenic therapy. For instance, in response to bevacizumab-mediated hypoxic and reduced angiogenic regions, TAMs play a crucial role in promoting angiogenesis by recruiting more pro-angiogenic macrophages [68]. Furthermore, myeloid-derived suppressor cells (MDSCs) play an important role in the development of metastasis and contribute to angiogenesis [69]. MDSCs contribute to the development of resistance to anti-angiogenic therapy by recruiting additional MDSCs and activate alternative growth factors essential to angiogenesis [70, 71]. The mechanisms of anti-angiogenic therapy will be discussed in more detail in Sect. 1.4.1.

Extracellular vesicles or exosomes have become an area of intense research focus given their broad applications in cancer and role in cell-cell communication. Exosomes typically carry genetic or biochemical materials and have been implicated in the development of chemoresistance [72]. Although their role in the acquisition of resistance to targeted therapies has not yet been explored, it can be speculated that similar mechanisms that confer resistance to chemotherapy apply to targeted therapies. For example, exosomes can carry miRNAs that have been associated with modulating the activity of multidrug resistance efflux transports such as MDR1 [73]. As an extension of this, it is possible that exosomes can theoretically carry miRNAs that regulate responsiveness to targeted therapies. For example, miRNA-21 which leads to widespread resistance in tumors initially sensitive to gefitinib. Additionally, exosomes can also carry proteins; thus, soluble factors that promote cell proliferation, angiogenesis, pro-survival signals can also theoretically be secreted in response to targeted therapy and confer resistance.

The TME presents a very complex collection of components that can all contribute to the development of resistance to targeted therapies and could not all be addressed in this introduction. Unfortunately, the complex signaling pathways and crosstalk make this a challenging area to explore concerning elucidating mechanisms of resistance and requires in-depth research to provide conclusive evidence of mediated resistance programs in cancer cells beyond what is currently known.

1.3.3 The Activity of Drug Efflux Transporters

One of the most well-known perpetrators of drug resistance is multidrug resistant efflux channels. This will be thoroughly reviewed in Chap. 5; however, here we provide a brief overview of their role in the development of resistance to targeted therapies.

The development of resistance to many therapies can be attributed to the activity of drug efflux transporters, which actively remove therapeutic agents from the interior of cells, circumventing the intended therapeutic effect. Although their activity is typically associated with chemoresistance, failure of targeted therapies at the clinic has led researchers to reconsider the action of these transporters as it applies to the acquisition of resistance to targeted therapies. The majority of drug efflux channels are members of the ATP-binding cassette (ABC) superfamily [74]. Members of this family exhibit differential drug efflux capacities. For example, ABCB1, ABCC1, and ABCG2 have all been implicated in eliminating chemotherapeutics and topoisomerases [5]. On the other hand, the multidrug resistance protein 1 (MDR1) has been implicated in eliminating targeted therapies including imatinib, erlotinib and nilotinib [75].

Epigenetic modifications also contribute to drug efflux channel activity in response to drug treatment, although these mechanisms are not well understood. Proposed epigenetic mechanisms that can regulate drug efflux channel activity include increased DNA methylation of genes transcribing drug efflux channels. These events have been observed at the ABCB1 promoter region leading to increased expression [20]. Additionally, upon treatment with histone acetylases at the same promoter region led to increased expression of ABCB1, implicating an essential epigenetic mechanism of action to the acquisition of drug resistance.

1.3.4   Other Considerations of Mechanisms Potentially Contributing to the Acquisition of Resistance

The acquisition of resistance to targeted therapies is a complex process that involves multiple cellular and molecular events which collectively present clinical challenges when treating patients. Although the above mechanisms are currently under investigation, other processes which are not well understood require discussion.

Cellular reprogramming is an experimental process through which differentiated cells are induced to dedifferentiate into other cell types and represents another form a cell lineage plasticity that has been considered to better understand cancer cells [30]. Initially, this experimental process was applied to adult fibroblasts and other cells, where four critical factors, known as the Yamanaka factors,[5] were induced in adult cells which consequently lead to a pluripotent stem cell phenotype being induced [76]. Although these four factors are typically associated with experimental reprogramming of adult cells, cancer cells can exert a similar mechanism to confer cellular plasticity and give rise to aggressive malignant phenotypes. For example,

---

[5] The Yamanaka factors are four critical stem cell transcription factors whose collective expression induces reprogramming of differentiated cells and produced induced pluripotent stem cells. These four factors are Oct-4, Sox-2, c-Myc and Klf-4 (OKSM).

c-Myc, in alliance with *Kras* mutations, can induce EMT and a self-renewing metastatic phenotype in pancreatic cancer [77]. Additionally, tumor suppressor genes such as *TP53* and *PTEN* also play similar reprogramming roles, particularly in response to therapy.

1.4   Specific Mechanisms of Acquired Resistance to Select Targeted Therapies

Currently available targeted therapies range from those that exploit oncogenic addiction characteristic of many cancers to critical components of the TME. Here, we provide a brief overview of select targeted therapies, their mechanism of action, followed by a comprehensive overview of the molecular and cellular mechanisms of resistance.

1.4.1   Mechanisms of Resistance to Anti-Angiogenic Therapy

As outlined in Sect. 1.3.2, the development of a vascular network is a critical event in tumorigenesis and a key component of the tumor microenvironment that contributes to the development of resistance. In light of this, the first inhibitor of angiogenesis, bevacizumab, was approved for metastatic colon cancer based on the success observed in a phase III clinical trial [78, 79]. In this clinical trial, bevacizumab, an anti-VEGF mAb, was administered in combination with conventional chemotherapeutic agents such as fluorouracil. The outcome of this trial showed an increase in overall survival and has since been administered to patients with non-small cell lung cancer (NSCLC) in combination with paclitaxel and platinum-based chemotherapies and lead to a significant benefit in survival outcomes [80]. Anti-angiogenic therapies continue to be administered in conjunction with standard of care chemotherapeutics for NSCLC, breast cancer, and renal cancer.

The mechanism of action of conventional anti-angiogenic therapies is to inhibit vascularization of the tumor, subsequently inhibiting tumor growth and prevent metastasis [52, 81, 82]. Anti-VEGF therapies bind directly to VEGF and prevent VEGF-mediated proliferation, invasion, and migration of endothelial cells, permeabilizing of vasculature, tumor cell proliferation and migration and other pro-angiogenic events [82]. Additional proposed mechanisms of action include inhibiting pro-survival pathways in endothelial cells, restricting blood flow to the tumor, and normalizing existing vasculature [81]. The resulting normalization of tumor vasculature, though widely debated, postulated that anti-angiogenic therapies reestablish a balance between anti- and pro-angiogenic mechanisms, thereby reorganizing the vasculature network to one that reflects the architecture of nonmalignant organs. This, in turn, allows for more effective perfusion of cytotoxic therapies. However, one of the biggest pitfalls of this hypothesis has been the optimal timing and dosing required for this to occur and is currently an emerging concept concerning anti-angiogenic mechanisms of action.

Following the success of bevacizumab, two additional anti-angiogenic agents have been developed that are small molecular inhibitors of targeting VEGFR[6] known as sorafenib [83] and sunitinib [84]. Interestingly, these two VEGFR tyrosine kinase inhibitors (TKIs) exhibit cross-reactivity against PDGFR and FGFR [85]. Additionally, neuropilins (NP1 and NP2) are co-receptors of VEGFRs and increase VEGF binding [86, 87], as such, targeting both VEGF and NP1 has shown greater efficacy than either agent alone [88]. VEGR neutralizing antibodies that target the extracellular region of VEGFR1 have also demonstrated efficacy in reducing tumor growth and preventing metastasis [89].

Although the aforementioned anti-angiogenic therapies initially showed success in the clinic, resistance eventually develops. Alternative pro-angiogenic pathways that can be recruited to resume neovascularization of the tumor include PIGF, angiopoietin [90], Bv-8 [91] and PDGF [91]. PIGF is a member of the VEGF family and can induce proliferation of endothelial cells in addition to tumor cells [92]. Patients treated with anti-VEGF therapies demonstrated increased PIGF activity [93]. Additionally, increased in expression of angiopoietin [94], BV8 [95] and PDGF [96] were observed, suggesting the development of resistance of anti-VEGF therapy. Pre-clinical animal models investigating the effects of the recruitment of these alternative pathways revealed an increase in tumor growth after an initial short-lived response to therapy [82, 97]. A negative consequence of anti-angiogenic therapy is the development of regions of hypoxia upon vascular construction and destruction. Such conditions are conducive to the development of drug resistance and can lead to the selection of cancer stem cells and the upregulation of self-renewal pathways and EMT, all of which lead to an aggressive malignancy.

Additionally, cellular mechanisms of resistance include vascular mimicry and transdifferentiation of stem cells. Vascular mimicry is a mode by which cancer cells can overcome the effects of anti-angiogenic therapy, observed in highly aggressive cancers such as melanoma [98], breast cancer [99], lung cancer [100] and many others [101]. This form of mimicry involves tumor cells forming vessel-like structures in order to promote tumorigenesis and metastasis, a function typical of the angiogenic driven pathway that creates tumor vasculature [98, 101]. Vascular mimicry employs the use of an angiogenic-independent pathway to give rise to vasculature driven by tumor cells [102]. This method essentially provides the same exchange of nutrients and waste typical of blood vessels derived from embryonic vascularization programs [101]. This novel network of vessels interacts with components of the ECM to ensure direct contact with blood flow with the tumor to maintain tumor growth and progression. Although the exact mechanisms contribut-

---

[6]VEGF include five glycoproteins called VEGFA (most well characterized and referred to as VEGF), VEGFB, VEFC, VEGFD and placenta growth factor. VEGF binds to receptor tyrosine kinases VEGFR1, VEGFR2, VEGFR3 leading to downstream signaling that regulates angiogenesis.

ing to vasculogenic mimicry are not well understood, several hypotheses have been proposed; however, the most widely accepted relate to CSC and EMT [103]. The underlying processes include transdifferentiation and dedifferentiation that allows CSCs to form a tube and branch-like structures typical of blood vessel architecture. These tubes then connect and merge with existing blood vessels derived from angiogenesis. Additional conformational studies have shown that vasculogenic mimicry can be initiated by populations expressing CD133, a common CSC marker, in both breast [104] and lung cancer [105] and reveal another differentiation process that can contribute to the indirect development of resistance to therapies targeting the vasculature. Since EMT regulation goes hand in hand with invasiveness and metastasis, vascular mimicry can be promoted by secreting molecules, such a VE-cadherin, conducive to the formation of tube-like structures [41]. The challenge of this form of pseudo-vasculature is that it is not formed by endothelial cells as it originates from transdifferentiated CSCs and may require the application of CSC therapies.

Taken collectively, not only are there genetic events that lead to the acquisition of resistance, but the non-genetic mechanism shed light on a particularly challenging type of resistance which requires further exploration.

1.4.2   Resistance to Tyrosine Kinase Inhibitors

Receptor tyrosine kinases (RTKs) represent a viable drug target in the treatment of cancer as they are typically overactive in cancer cells. They are comprised of 20 classes of receptor families including EGFR, insulin receptor, PDGF, VEGF, and HGF, to name a few [106]. RTKs typically have aberrant mechanisms of activity including bypassing ligand-dependent activation [107]. This bypass method can involve (1) overexpression of RTKs so that homo/heterodimers are stabilized independently of their ligands [108] or (2) mutations in the receptor itself that maintain a stabilized active state [106]. RTKs regulate several tumor progression and maintenance pathways; however, despite their promising therapeutic potential, resistance develops against inhibitors that target single RTKs.

TKIs represent a large class of kinase inhibitors that exploit the overactivity of these kinases and their associated receptors in cancer [109]. Currently available TKIs to treat cancer come in four classes. Type I TKIs recognize active kinase conformations and compete directly with ATP to bind and type II TKIs recognize inactive kinases and stabilize inactive enzymes [109]. The two other classes of TK inhibitor are allosteric inhibitors which bind at a non-ATP binding site and display high selectivity to specific kinases and covalent inhibitors, which form an irreversible bond at the active site of the kinase.

A recent discovery has revealed that resistance to TKIs can largely be attributed to "gatekeeper" mutations [110]. These mutations occur in a conserved residue that is located on the ATP-binding site of kinases [5, 110, 111]. ATP-competitive kinase inhibitors are not able to overcome the enhanced ATP-binding affinity leading to resistance [111]. The proposed alternative option for this resistance is the application of irreversible inhibitors which, rather than competing for the ATP-binding site, covalently bind to the ATP-binding pocket effectively removing themselves from competing with ATP.

TKIs have also been shown to engage alternative pathways that are interconnected in order to maintain activity. For example, following EGFR inhibition, activation of alternative pathways such as the HGF signaling pathway can maintain downstream intracellular signaling [112]. This is because the signaling pathways are interconnected and the ensuing intracellular functionality can continue to be activated by other pathways despite inhibition by a selective in inhibitor of an RTK. Here, we outline specific resistance mechanisms associated with select RTKs; however, the mechanisms of resistance outlined in this section are broadly applicable to the majority of RTKs.

Resistance to HER Pathway Inhibitors Human epidermal growth factor (HER) is a member of RTK family and includes HER-1 (epidermal growth factor receptor; EGFR), HER-2, HER-3 and HER-4 [113]. These receptors (except for HER-2, which is reviewed in Chap. 7) are activated upon ligand binding and lead to homo- or heterodimerization. This dimerization translates to intracellular signaling cascades through PI3K/Akt and RAS/MAPK signaling pathways [113]. For this introduction, HER-1/EGFR will be discussed concerning the development of resistance given the intense research focus on targeting this overexpressed receptor and its subsequent downstream signaling intermediates.

HER-1/EGFR (known hereafter as EGFR) is overexpressed in many cancers including, but not limited to, lung [114], breast [113] and pancreatic cancers [115]. Typically, ligand-dependent activation of EGFR is required, where one of six ligands (including epidermal growth factor; EGF and transforming growth factor alpha; TGF-α) bind to EGFR [116]. This binding leads to a conformational change that facilitates receptor dimerization and phosphorylation of intracellular tyrosine residues and the subsequent activation of signaling pathways including the Ras/Raf/Erk, PI3K/Akt and STAT. This signaling ultimately leads to several processes involved in multistage tumorigenesis including cell proliferation (regulated by ERK1/2), angiogenesis and metastasis [114].

Given that EGFR is overexpressed in many cancers, targeting this proto-oncogene was of clinical relevance, particularly in the case of NSCLC [117] and melanoma. Currently, available EGFR therapies include EGFR TKIs such as erlotinib, gefitinib, osimertinib and monoclonal antibodies such as cetuximab [118]. The anti-EGFR TKIs exert their therapeutic action through reversible binding to the ATP-binding site, thereby preventing homodimerization and phosphorylation of tyrosine residues which are required for downstream signal transduction [119]. Conversely, cetuximab, which been approved for treatment of metastatic colorectal cancer [120], NSCLC and head and neck cancer [121], exerts its therapeutic effects by binding to the extracellular region of EGFR and preventing its ligand from binding and activating downstream signal transduction [121]. Regardless of the mechanism of therapeutic action, sensitivity and clinical success of anti-EGFR inhibitors were due to the exploitation of specific mutations in specific cancers. For example, patients with NSCLC with activating point mutations in the *EGFR* gene were more sensitive to anti-EGFR therapy [122, 123]. Additionally, cetuximab efficacy is similarly dictated by the *KRAS* mutational status of patients receiving this form of anti-EGFR therapy, where only wild type *KRAS* tumors respond [124]. Though initially effective, acquired resistance to EGFR therapies eventually leads to unresponsiveness in the clinic.

The proposed genetic mechanisms of action that contribute to the development of resistance are:

1. Gene amplification of EGFR.
2. Mutations at the ATP-binding site.
3. Activation of parallel or associated pathways such as the recruitment of other RTKs to reactivate EGFR activity.
4. Activation of alternative survival pathways.

Due to the highly adaptive nature of cancer cells, activation of EGFR can also be ligand-independent or a result of overexpression of EGFR. For example, HER-2 receptor amplification can lead to ligand-independent activation of EGFR [108], a process that contributes to the development of resistance to EGFR-therapies [108]. Additionally, recent investigations into genetic events that lead to resistance have determined that a second mutation in the threonine 790 residue (T790 M), the gatekeeper of EGFRs, leads to increased ATP-binding affinity, specifically in NSCLCs [111, 125]. Typically, small molecular TKIs are efficacious when treating cancers such as NSCLC, owing to an initial mutation which renders EGFRs susceptible to gefitinib and erlotinib because of reduced affinity to ATP in mutants. However, the second mutation returns ATP-affinity to that of wild type, leading to increased ATP-affinity which contributes to resistance to anti-EGFR therapy. An alternative method of resistance is the recruitment of IGFR-1 to form a heterodimer with EGFR which facilitates the activation of the downstream effectors in the presence of EGFR inhibitors [126]. Finally, activation of alternative signaling pathways is an especially challenging mechanism of resistance exhibited in response to EGFR inhibition. For instance, upon EGFR inhibition, activation of the PI3K/Akt pathway, as well as MET amplification, contributes to survival and continued growth and proliferation of tumor cells [124].

Although the mechanism contributing to the development of resistance to anti-EGFR therapy is an area of intense research focus primarily due to its initial clinical efficacy, the underlying contributors to the acquisition of resistance to this targeted therapy continue to remain an enigma.

Resistance Mechanisms of BCR-ABL Tyrosine Kinase Inhibitor The oncogene BCR-ABL is the result of a fusion between the BCR gene, and the ABL tyrosine kinase gene characteristic of chronic myelogenous leukemia (CML) and is a critical molecular event that takes place to induce a malignant phenotype [127]. Currently available BCR-ABL therapies include tyrosine kinase inhibitors such as imatinib and nilotinib both of which are type II TKIs and dasatinib, which is a type I TKI [128]. Although this targeted therapy has shown clinical efficacy, 20% of patients eventually develop resistance [10]. The proposed genetic mechanisms of action that contribute to the development of resistance include point mutations of the ATP binding pocket [91], activation of alternative survival pathways [128], alternative splicing events [10], and amplification of the *BCR-ABL* gene [3].

Concerning point mutations in the ATP binding pocket, this proposed mechanism of resistance follows a similar method in increasing ATP binding affinity to overcome the action of imatinib. This point mutation occurs in the ATP-binding loop as well as the aspartate-phenylalanine-glycine motif [128]. Alternative splicing events that lead to resistance to BCR-ABL targeted therapies produce *BCR-ABL35INS* which is associated with minimal response to TKIs [129]. However, the exact mechanism of drug resistance of this splice variant is unknown. Activation of survival pathways such as STAT3 [130] and PI3K/Akt/mTOR [131] have all been shown to be upregulated in response to imatinib-treated patients. Amplification of the BCR-ABL gene, though not well understood, is another proposed mechanism of acquired resistance. However, overexpression of this oncoprotein has been correlated with the advanced form of CML and is one of the first molecular events that eventually leads to kinase domain point mutations [132].

Additionally, the proposed non-genetic mechanisms of action that confer resistance to anti-BCR-ABL therapy include the activity of cancer stem cells, which are proposed to render BCR-ABL therapies ineffective due to their lack of responsiveness due to their quiescent state [133]. The activity of drug influx/efflux pumps has also been associated with resistance to BCR-ABL inhibitors. Although ABC transporters are typically associated with resistance due to their efflux abilities, in the case of imatinib, drug influx activity has demonstrated variations in the activity of this inhibitor [128]. Expression levels of organic-cation transporter-1 (OCT-1) are directly related to how readily imatinib is taken up and whether patients respond favorably [134, 135].

Theoretically, a useful treatment option would be one that can broadly target several critical oncogenic pathways at once so that it is difficult to engage the processes involved in the acquisition of resistance. Our group has reported on a novel mechanism of action of oseltamivir phosphate (OP), which is a structural analog of α-2,3-sialic acid residues located on RTKs [136–138]. These residues are present on the majority of RTKs and thus represent a method to broadly target multistage tumorigenesis and prevent the development of resistance. Our group has gone to apply this agent in novel applications including nanomedicine [139–141] and three-dimensional tumor spheroid models [142, 143]. We are currently assessing the downstream effects of the inhibition of RTK activity; however, thus far data from our laboratory have demonstrated decreased tumor volume, diminished neovascularization, reversal of EMT and prevention of metastatic disease.

Furthermore, because RTKs are overexpressed on cancer cells, participate in crosstalk and have heavily interconnected intracellular signaling, broadly targeting these receptors with OP presents as a promising therapeutic avenue to overcome the acquisition of resistance by preventing engagement of the previously discussed modes of developing resistance. Additionally, given the broad resistance mechanisms of action that cancer possesses in its repertoire, our group is also assessing novel multimodal approaches repurposing other therapeutic agents [144]. Additional applications of this novel therapy will be discussed in Chap. 2.

1.4.3 Resistance to Anti-Apoptosis Inhibitors

As briefly discussed, inhibiting the activity of apoptosis is a critical hallmark of cancer cells that render them to unresponsive to the cytotoxic effects of chemo- and radiotherapy [1]. Members of the BLC-2 family of oncoproteins are critical regulators of apoptotic events [145]. BCL-2 is a mitochondrial protein and includes pro-apoptotic proteins Bax and Bak which are only activated by BH3 proteins and are inhibited by BCL-2 and BCL-Xi [146]. Although the pro-survival mechanisms of action are controversial, they are thoroughly reviewed here [145], however, it is proposed that BCL-2 interacts with Bax, in order to override the apoptosis and allowed cancer cells to continue to proliferate in the presence of therapeutic agents [147, 148].

As such, therapeutically targeting this hallmark has been thoroughly investigated; however, as with other targeted therapies, resistance ultimately develops. The proposed genetic mechanisms of action that contribute to the development of resistance are (1) recruitment of other members of the BCL-2 family, (2) downregulation of drug targets, and (3) epigenetic modifications. Currently available inhibitors of apoptosis include ABT-263, commercially known as navitoclax, and ABT-737, both of which target the BCL-2 family of proteins [5]. When administered in combination with chemo- and/or radiation therapy, cytotoxicity is observed. The development of resistance to this targeted therapy involves the binding of ABT-737 to another member of the BCL-2 family, MCL1 [149]. Downregulation of the drug target can be modulated by the TME and can lead to reduced availability of BCL-2 in order to inhibit its antiapoptotic activity [12]. Concerning epigenetic modifications, both DNA methylation patterns [150] and histone modifications [151] contribute to resistance to apoptosis. Therefore, although anti-apoptotic inhibitors may initially function to reactivate apoptosis pathways, hyperactivated anti-apoptosis pathways as regulated by epigenetic modifications can theoretically confer resistance to these inhibitors.

1.5 Future Directions of Targeted Therapy

As outlined in this introductory chapter, targeted therapies were developed as not only a mode to exploit the hallmarks of cancer but also as a method to overcome chemoresistance by supplementing conventional therapeutic regimens with targeted therapies. However, the development of resistance to these combinatorial approaches has led to the reassessment of currently available therapeutic options to overcome resistance to targeted therapy. A key component of overcoming resistance to several promising targeted therapies is to understand the underlying mechanism that contributes to resistance and targeting these processes.

The goal of this book is to provide an overview of the therapeutic options currently being explored to overcome resistance to select targeted therapies. The chapters are arranged based on four general groupings:

1. Cancer and the development of resistance (Chap. 2).
2. Resistance to widely applicable therapeutic options (Chaps. 3–5).
3. Resistance to specific targeted therapies (Chaps. 6 and 7).
4. Emerging therapies and novel approaches to overcome resistance to targeted therapies (Chaps. 8–10).

Physiologically *Homo sapiens* are one of the most complex organisms, and this complexity is a monument to the cycles of evolution that produced an entity capable of adapting to a plethora of environmental challenges. This is equally true at the cellular level because cancer cells originate from healthy cells which have evolved to survive by any means necessary. As such, cancer cells retain this primal capacity to survive and evolve under a constant assault of radiation, chemotherapy, targeted therapies, and surgery, all of which select and/or confer a resistant phenotype to ensure survival. The mistake in treating this disease, therefore, is not entirely due to the gaps in our understanding of cancer biology, but rather, a failure to appreciate the underlying evolutionary mechanisms that allow cancer cells to evade and resist many conventional therapies. That being said, in order to develop a therapy capable of successfully targeting and ablating cancer, drug design needs to appreciate and pay homage to survival mechanisms deeply rooted in malignant and non-malignant cells and to employ any means necessary to survive another day.

This book aims to provide a comprehensive overview of the robust research currently underway to overcome resistance to targeted therapy by acknowledging the processes above and providing the most up-to-date advancements to improve patient outcome and progression-free survival.

References

1. Hanahan D, Weinberg RA. Hallmarks of cancer: the next generation. Cell. 2011;144(5):646–74. https://doi.org/10.1016/j.cell.2011.02.013.
2. Groenendijk FH, Bernards R. Drug resistance to targeted therapies: deja vu all over again. Mol Oncol. 2014;8(6):1067–83. https://doi.org/10.1016/j.molonc.2014.05.004.
3. Lackner MR, Wilson TR, Settleman J. Mechanisms of acquired resistance to targeted cancer therapies. Future Oncol. 2012;8(8):999–1014. https://doi.org/10.2217/fon.12.86.
4. Redmond KL, Papafili A, Lawler M, Van Schaeybroeck S. Overcoming resistance to targeted therapies in cancer. Semin Oncol. 2015;42(6):896–908. https://doi.org/10.1053/j.seminoncol.2015.09.028.
5. Holohan C, Van Schaeybroeck S, Longley DB, Johnston PG. Cancer drug resistance: an evolving paradigm. Nat Rev Cancer. 2013;13(10):714–26. https://doi.org/10.1038/nrc3599.
6. Neel DS, Bivona TG. Resistance is futile: overcoming resistance to targeted therapies in lung adenocarcinoma. NPJ Precis Oncol. 2017;1:3. https://doi.org/10.1038/s41698-017-0007-0.
7. Mohd Sharial MS, Crown J, Hennessy BT. Overcoming resistance and restoring sensitivity to HER2-targeted therapies in breast cancer. Ann Oncol. 2012;23(12):3007–16. https://doi.org/10.1093/annonc/mds200.
8. Migliore C, Giordano S. Resistance to targeted therapies: a role for microRNAs? Trends Mol Med. 2013;19(10):633–42. https://doi.org/10.1016/j.molmed.2013.08.002.
9. Corcoran RB, Dias-Santagata D, Bergethon K, Iafrate AJ, Settleman J, Engelman JA. BRAF gene amplification can promote acquired resistance to MEK inhibitors in cancer cells harboring the BRAF V600E mutation. Sci Signal. 2010;3(149):ra84. https://doi.org/10.1126/scisignal.2001148.
10. Wang BD, Lee NH. Aberrant RNA splicing in cancer and drug resistance. Cancers (Basel). 2018;10(11). https://doi.org/10.3390/cancers10110458.
11. Solier S, Logette E, Desoche L, Solary E, Corcos L. Nonsense-mediated mRNA decay among human caspases: the caspase-2S putative protein is encoded by an extremely short-lived mRNA. Cell Death Differ. 2005;12(6):687–9. https://doi.org/10.1038/sj.cdd.4401594.
12. Erler JT, Cawthorne CJ, Williams KJ, Koritzinsky M, Wouters BG, Wilson C, et al. Hypoxia-mediated down-regulation of Bid and Bax in tumors occurs via hypoxia-inducible factor 1-dependent and -independent mechanisms and contributes to drug resistance. Mol Cell Biol. 2004;24(7):2875–89.
13. Chandarlapaty S. Negative feedback and adaptive resistance to the targeted therapy of cancer. Cancer Discov. 2012;2(4):311–9. https://doi.org/10.1158/2159-8290.CD-12-0018.
14. von Manstein V, Yang CM, Richter D, Delis N, Vafaizadeh V, Groner B. Resistance of cancer cells to targeted therapies through the activation of compensating signaling loops. Curr Signal Transduct Ther. 2013;8(3):193–202. https://doi.org/10.2174/1574362409666114020621931.
15. Montero-Conde C, Ruiz-Llorente S, Dominguez JM, Knauf JA, Viale A, Sherman EJ, et al. Relief of feedback inhibition of HER3 transcription by RAF and MEK inhibitors attenuates their antitumor effects in BRAF-mutant thyroid carcinomas. Cancer Discov. 2013;3(5):520–33. https://doi.org/10.1158/2159-8290.CD-12-0531.
16. Chang HH, Hemberg M, Barahona M, Ingber DE, Huang S. Transcriptome-wide noise controls lineage choice in mammalian progenitor cells. Nature. 2008;453(7194):544–7. https://doi.org/10.1038/nature06965.
17. Cedar H, Bergman Y. Epigenetics of haematopoietic cell development. Nat Rev Immunol. 2011;11(7):478–88. https://doi.org/10.1038/nri2991.
18. Maunakea AK, Nagarajan RP, Bilenky M, Ballinger TJ, D'Souza C, Fouse SD, et al. Conserved role of intragenic DNA methylation in regulating alternative promoters. Nature. 2010;466(7303):253–7. https://doi.org/10.1038/nature09165.

19. De Smet C, Lurquin C, Lethe B, Martelange V, Boon T. DNA methylation is the primary silencing mechanism for a set of germ line- and tumor-specific genes with a CpG-rich promoter. Mol Cell Biol. 1999;19(11):7327–35.
20. Cohen I, Poreba E, Kamieniarz K, Schneider R. Histone modifiers in cancer: friends or foes? Genes Cancer. 2011;2(6):631–47. https://doi.org/10.1177/1947601911417176.
21. Wilting RH, Dannenberg JH. Epigenetic mechanisms in tumorigenesis, tumor cell heterogeneity and drug resistance. Drug Resist Updat. 2012;15(1–2):21–38. https://doi.org/10.1016/j.drup.2012.01.008.
22. Kosuri KV, Wu X, Wang L, Villalona-Calero MA, Otterson GA. An epigenetic mechanism for capecitabine resistance in mesothelioma. Biochem Biophys Res Commun. 2010;391(3):1465–70. https://doi.org/10.1016/j.bbrc.2009.12.095.
23. Zheng T, Wang J, Chen X, Liu L. Role of microRNA in anticancer drug resistance. Int J Cancer. 2010;126(1):2–10. https://doi.org/10.1002/ijc.24782.
24. Sood P, Krek A, Zavolan M, Macino G, Rajewsky N. Cell-type-specific signatures of microRNAs on target mRNA expression. Proc Natl Acad Sci U S A. 2006;103(8):2746–51. https://doi.org/10.1073/pnas.0511045103.
25. Wang ZX, Lu BB, Wang H, Cheng ZX, Yin YM. MicroRNA-21 modulates chemosensitivity of breast cancer cells to doxorubicin by targeting PTEN. Arch Med Res. 2011;42(4):281–90. https://doi.org/10.1016/j.arcmed.2011.06.008.
26. Si W, Shen J, Zheng H, Fan W. The role and mechanisms of action of microRNAs in cancer drug resistance. Clin Epigenetics. 2019;11(1):25. https://doi.org/10.1186/s13148-018-0587-8.
27. Giovannetti E, Erozenci A, Smit J, Danesi R, Peters GJ. Molecular mechanisms underlying the role of microRNAs (miRNAs) in anticancer drug resistance and implications for clinical practice. Crit Rev Oncol Hematol. 2012;81(2):103–22. https://doi.org/10.1016/j.critrevonc.2011.03.010.
28. Eto K, Iwatsuki M, Watanabe M, Ida S, Ishimoto T, Iwagami S, et al. The microRNA-21/PTEN pathway regulates the sensitivity of HER2-positive gastric cancer cells to trastuzumab. Ann Surg Oncol. 2014;21(1):343–50. https://doi.org/10.1245/s10434-013-3325-7.
29. Wang YS, Wang YH, Xia HP, Zhou SW, Schmid-Bindert G, Zhou CC. MicroRNA-214 regulates the acquired resistance to gefitinib via the PTEN/AKT pathway in EGFR-mutant cell lines. Asian Pac J Cancer Prev. 2012;13(1):255–60.
30. Le Magnen C, Shen MM, Abate-Shen C. Lineage plasticity in cancer progression and treatment. Annu Rev Cancer Biol. 2018;2:271–89. https://doi.org/10.1146/annurev-cancerbio-030617-050224.
31. Huang Z, Wu T, Liu AY, Ouyang G. Differentiation and transdifferentiation potentials of cancer stem cells. Oncotarget. 2015;6(37):39550–63. https://doi.org/10.18632/oncotarget.6098.
32. Shibue T, Weinberg RA. EMT, CSCs, and drug resistance: the mechanistic link and clinical implications. Nat Rev Clin Oncol. 2017;14(10):611–29. https://doi.org/10.1038/nrclinonc.2017.44.
33. Sui H, Zhu L, Deng W, Li Q. Epithelial-mesenchymal transition and drug resistance: role, molecular mechanisms, and therapeutic strategies. Oncol Res Treat. 2014;37(10):584–9. https://doi.org/10.1159/000367802.
34. Du B, Shim JS. Targeting epithelial-mesenchymal transition (EMT) to overcome drug resistance in cancer. Molecules. 2016;21(7). https://doi.org/10.3390/molecules21070965.
35. Hay ED. An overview of epithelio-mesenchymal transformation. Acta Anat (Basel). 1995;154(1):8–20.
36. Lamouille S, Xu J, Derynck R. Molecular mechanisms of epithelial-mesenchymal transition. Nat Rev Mol Cell Biol. 2014;15(3):178–96. https://doi.org/10.1038/nrm3758.
37. Kaimori A, Potter J, Kaimori JY, Wang C, Mezey E, Koteish A. Transforming growth factor-beta1 induces an epithelial-to-mesenchymal transition state in mouse hepatocytes in vitro. J Biol Chem. 2007;282(30):22089–101. https://doi.org/10.1074/jbc.M700998200.

38. Moustakas A, Heldin CH. Non-Smad TGF-beta signals. J Cell Sci. 2005;118(Pt 16):3573–84. https://doi.org/10.1242/jcs.02554.
39. Timmerman LA, Grego-Bessa J, Raya A, Bertran E, Perez-Pomares JM, Diez J, et al. Notch promotes epithelial-mesenchymal transition during cardiac development and oncogenic transformation. Genes Dev. 2004;18(1):99–115. https://doi.org/10.1101/gad.276304.
40. Kim HJ, Litzenburger BC, Cui X, Delgado DA, Grabiner BC, Lin X, et al. Constitutively active type I insulin-like growth factor receptor causes transformation and xenograft growth of immortalized mammary epithelial cells and is accompanied by an epithelial-to-mesenchymal transition mediated by NF-kappaB and snail. Mol Cell Biol. 2007;27(8):3165–75. https://doi.org/10.1128/MCB.01315-06.
41. Mani SA, Guo W, Liao MJ, Eaton EN, Ayyanan A, Zhou AY, et al. The epithelial-mesenchymal transition generates cells with properties of stem cells. Cell. 2008;133(4):704–15. https://doi.org/10.1016/j.cell.2008.03.027.
42. Chaffer CL, San Juan BP, Lim E, Weinberg RA. EMT, cell plasticity and metastasis. Cancer Metastasis Rev. 2016;35(4):645–54. https://doi.org/10.1007/s10555-016-9648-7.
43. Park CC, Bissell MJ, Barcellos-Hoff MH. The influence of the microenvironment on the malignant phenotype. Mol Med Today. 2000;6(8):324–9.
44. Quail DF, Joyce JA. Microenvironmental regulation of tumor progression and metastasis. Nat Med. 2013;19(11):1423–37. https://doi.org/10.1038/nm.3394.
45. Farrow B, Albo D, Berger DH. The role of the tumor microenvironment in the progression of pancreatic cancer. J Surg Res. 2008;149(2):319–28. https://doi.org/10.1016/j.jss.2007.12.757.
46. Fukumura D, Jain RK. Tumor microvasculature and microenvironment: targets for anti-angiogenesis and normalization. Microvasc Res. 2007;74(2–3):72–84. https://doi.org/10.1016/j.mvr.2007.05.003.
47. Huang G, Chen L. Tumor vasculature and microenvironment normalization: a possible mechanism of antiangiogenesis therapy. Cancer Biother Radiopharm. 2008;23(5):661–7. https://doi.org/10.1089/cbr.2008.0492.
48. Bottaro DP, Cancer LLA. Out of air is not out of action. Nature. 2003;423(6940):593–5. https://doi.org/10.1038/423593a.
49. Stratman AN, Pezoa SA, Farrelly OM, Castranova D, Dye LE III, Butler MG, et al. Interactions between mural cells and endothelial cells stabilize the developing zebrafish dorsal aorta. Development. 2017;144(1):115–27. https://doi.org/10.1242/dev.143131.
50. Karamysheva AF. Mechanisms of angiogenesis. Biochemistry (Mosc). 2008;73(7):751–62.
51. Nishida N, Yano H, Nishida T, Kamura T, Kojiro M. Angiogenesis in cancer. Vasc Health Risk Manag. 2006;2(3):213–9.
52. Tugues S, Koch S, Gualandi L, Li X, Claesson-Welsh L. Vascular endothelial growth factors and receptors: anti-angiogenic therapy in the treatment of cancer. Mol Asp Med. 2011;32(2):88–111. https://doi.org/10.1016/j.mam.2011.04.004.
53. Heddleston JM, Li Z, McLendon RE, Hjelmeland AB, Rich JN. The hypoxic microenvironment maintains glioblastoma stem cells and promotes reprogramming towards a cancer stem cell phenotype. Cell Cycle. 2009;8(20):3274–84. https://doi.org/10.4161/cc.8.20.9701.
54. Heddleston JM, Li Z, Lathia JD, Bao S, Hjelmeland AB, Rich JN. Hypoxia inducible factors in cancer stem cells. Br J Cancer. 2010;102(5):789–95. https://doi.org/10.1038/sj.bjc.6605551.
55. Schoning JP, Monteiro M, Gu W. Drug resistance and cancer stem cells: the shared but distinct roles of hypoxia-inducible factors HIF1alpha and HIF2alpha. Clin Exp Pharmacol Physiol. 2017;44(2):153–61. https://doi.org/10.1111/1440-1681.12693.
56. Xia X, Lemieux ME, Li W, Carroll JS, Brown M, Liu XS, et al. Integrative analysis of HIF binding and transactivation reveals its role in maintaining histone methylation homeostasis. Proc Natl Acad Sci U S A. 2009;106(11):4260–5. https://doi.org/10.1073/pnas.0810067106.
57. Zhou J, Chen Q, Zou Y, Zheng S, Chen Y. Stem cells and cellular origins of mammary gland: updates in rationale, controversies, and cancer relevance. Stem Cells Int. 2019;2019:4247168. https://doi.org/10.1155/2019/4247168.
58. Zheng S, Xin L, Liang A, Fu Y. Cancer stem cell hypothesis: a brief summary and two proposals. Cytotechnology. 2013;65(4):505–12. https://doi.org/10.1007/s10616-012-9517-3.

59. Allegra A, Alonci A, Penna G, Innao V, Gerace D, Rotondo F, et al. The cancer stem cell hypothesis: a guide to potential molecular targets. Cancer Investig. 2014;32(9):470–95. https://doi.org/10.3109/07357907.2014.958231.

60. Turdo A, Veschi V, Gaggianesi M, Chinnici A, Bianca P, Todaro M, et al. Meeting the challenge of targeting cancer stem cells. Front Cell Dev Biol. 2019;7:16. https://doi.org/10.3389/fcell.2019.00016.

61. Zhao Y, Dong Q, Li J, Zhang K, Qin J, Zhao J, et al. Targeting cancer stem cells and their niche: perspectives for future therapeutic targets and strategies. Semin Cancer Biol. 2018;53:139–55. https://doi.org/10.1016/j.semcancer.2018.08.002.

62. Talukdar S, Bhoopathi P, Emdad L, Das S, Sarkar D, Fisher PB. Dormancy and cancer stem cells: An enigma for cancer therapeutic targeting. Adv Cancer Res. 2019;141:43–84. https://doi.org/10.1016/bs.acr.2018.12.002.

63. Bussolati B, Bruno S, Grange C, Ferrando U, Camussi G. Identification of a tumor-initiating stem cell population in human renal carcinomas. FASEB J. 2008;22(10):3696–705. https://doi.org/10.1096/fj.08-102590.

64. Hanahan D, Coussens LM. Accessories to the crime: functions of cells recruited to the tumor microenvironment. Cancer Cell. 2012;21(3):309–22. https://doi.org/10.1016/j.ccr.2012.02.022.

65. Vaquero J, Lobe C, Tahraoui S, Claperon A, Mergey M, Merabtene F, et al. The IGF2/IR/IGF1R pathway in tumor cells and myofibroblasts mediates resistance to EGFR inhibition in cholangiocarcinoma. Clin Cancer Res. 2018;24(17):4282–96. https://doi.org/10.1158/1078-0432.CCR-17-3725.

66. Almeida FV, Douglass SM, Fane ME, Weeraratna AT. Bad company: Microenvironmentally mediated resistance to targeted therapy in melanoma. Pigment Cell Melanoma Res. 2019;32(2):237–47. https://doi.org/10.1111/pcmr.12736.

67. Hirata E, Girotti MR, Viros A, Hooper S, Spencer-Dene B, Matsuda M, et al. Intravital imaging reveals how BRAF inhibition generates drug-tolerant microenvironments with high integrin beta1/FAK signaling. Cancer Cell. 2015;27(4):574–88. https://doi.org/10.1016/j.ccell.2015.03.008.

68. Castro BA, Flanigan P, Jahangiri A, Hoffman D, Chen W, Kuang R, et al. Macrophage migration inhibitory factor downregulation: a novel mechanism of resistance to anti-angiogenic therapy. Oncogene. 2017;36(26):3749–59. https://doi.org/10.1038/onc.2017.1.

69. Safarzadeh E, Orangi M, Mohammadi H, Babaie F, Baradaran B. Myeloid-derived suppressor cells: Important contributors to tumor progression and metastasis. J Cell Physiol. 2018;233(4):3024–36. https://doi.org/10.1002/jcp.26075.

70. Finke J, Ko J, Rini B, Rayman P, Ireland J, Cohen P. MDSC as a mechanism of tumor escape from sunitinib mediated anti-angiogenic therapy. Int Immunopharmacol. 2011;11(7):856–61. https://doi.org/10.1016/j.intimp.2011.01.030.

71. Rivera LB, Meyronet D, Hervieu V, Frederick MJ, Bergsland E, Bergers G. Intratumoral myeloid cells regulate responsiveness and resistance to antiangiogenic therapy. Cell Rep. 2015;11(4):577–91. https://doi.org/10.1016/j.celrep.2015.03.055.

72. Yousafzai NA, Wang H, Wang Z, Zhu Y, Zhu L, Jin H, et al. Exosome mediated multidrug resistance in cancer. Am J Cancer Res. 2018;8(11):2210–26.

73. Corcoran C, Rani S, O'Brien K, O'Neill A, Prencipe M, Sheikh R, et al. Docetaxel-resistance in prostate cancer: evaluating associated phenotypic changes and potential for resistance transfer via exosomes. PLoS One. 2012;7(12):e50999. https://doi.org/10.1371/journal.pone.0050999.

74. Dean M. ABC transporters, drug resistance, and cancer stem cells. J Mammary Gland Biol Neoplasia. 2009;14(1):3–9. https://doi.org/10.1007/s10911-009-9109-9.

75. Shukla S, Chen ZS, Ambudkar SV. Tyrosine kinase inhibitors as modulators of ABC transporter-mediated drug resistance. Drug Resist Updat. 2012;15(1–2):70–80. https://doi.org/10.1016/j.drup.2012.01.005.

76. Takahashi K, Tanabe K, Ohnuki M, Narita M, Ichisaka T, Tomoda K, et al. Induction of plu-
    ripotent stem cells from adult human fibroblasts by defined factors. Cell. 2007;131(5):861–
    72. https://doi.org/10.1016/j.cell.2007.11.019.
77. Ischenko I, Zhi J, Moll UM, Nemajerova A, Petrenko O. Direct reprogramming by oncogenic
    Ras and Myc. Proc Natl Acad Sci U S A. 2013;110(10):3937–42. https://doi.org/10.1073/
    pnas.1219592110.
78. Ferrara N, Hillan KJ, Gerber HP, Novotny W. Discovery and development of bevacizumab, an
    anti-VEGF antibody for treating cancer. Nat Rev Drug Discov. 2004;3(5):391–400. https://
    doi.org/10.1038/nrd1381.
79. Berretta M, Lleshi A, Zanet E, Bearz A, Simonelli C, Fisichella R, et al. Bevacizumab plus
    irinotecan-, fluorouracil-, and leucovorin-based chemotherapy with concomitant HAART
    in an HIV-positive patient with metastatic colorectal cancer. Onkologie. 2008;31(7):394–7.
    https://doi.org/10.1159/000132360.
80. Sandler A, Gray R, Perry MC, Brahmer J, Schiller JH, Dowlati A, et al. Paclitaxel-carboplatin
    alone or with bevacizumab for non-small-cell lung cancer. N Engl J Med. 2006;355(24):2542–
    50. https://doi.org/10.1056/NEJMoa061884.
81. Jain RK. Antiangiogenic therapy for cancer: current and emerging concepts. Oncology
    (Williston Park). 2005;19(4 Suppl 3):7–16.
82. Ellis LM, Hicklin DJ. VEGF-targeted therapy: mechanisms of anti-tumour activity. Nat Rev
    Cancer. 2008;8(8):579–91. https://doi.org/10.1038/nrc2403.
83. Kane RC, Farrell AT, Saber H, Tang S, Williams G, Jee JM, et al. Sorafenib for the treat-
    ment of advanced renal cell carcinoma. Clin Cancer Res. 2006;12(24):7271–8. https://doi.
    org/10.1158/1078-0432.CCR-06-1249.
84. Goodman VL, Rock EP, Dagher R, Ramchandani RP, Abraham S, Gobburu JV, et al. Approval
    summary: sunitinib for the treatment of imatinib refractory or intolerant gastrointestinal
    stromal tumors and advanced renal cell carcinoma. Clin Cancer Res. 2007;13(5):1367–73.
    https://doi.org/10.1158/1078-0432.CCR-06-2328.
85. Zhang J, Gold KA, Kim E. Sorafenib in non-small cell lung cancer. Expert Opin Investig
    Drugs. 2012;21(9):1417–26. https://doi.org/10.1517/13543784.2012.699039.
86. Klagsbrun M, Takashima S, Mamluk R. The role of neuropilin in vascular and tumor biology.
    Adv Exp Med Biol. 2002;515:33–48.
87. Halder JB, Zhao X, Soker S, Paria BC, Klagsbrun M, Das SK, et al. Differential expression
    of VEGF isoforms and VEGF (164)-specific receptor neuropilin-1 in the mouse uterus sug-
    gests a role for VEGF (164) in vascular permeability and angiogenesis during implantation.
    Genesis. 2000;26(3):213–24.
88. Batchelor TT, Sorensen AG, di Tomaso E, Zhang WT, Duda DG, Cohen KS, et al. AZD2171,
    a pan-VEGF receptor tyrosine kinase inhibitor, normalizes tumor vasculature and alleviates
    edema in glioblastoma patients. Cancer Cell. 2007;11(1):83–95. https://doi.org/10.1016/j.
    ccr.2006.11.021.
89. Bae DG, Kim TD, Li G, Yoon WH, Chae CB. Anti-flt1 peptide, a vascular endothelial growth
    factor receptor 1-specific hexapeptide, inhibits tumor growth and metastasis. Clin Cancer
    Res. 2005;11(7):2651–61. https://doi.org/10.1158/1078-0432.CCR-04-1564.
90. Bergers G, Hanahan D. Modes of resistance to anti-angiogenic therapy. Nat Rev Cancer.
    2008;8(8):592–603. https://doi.org/10.1038/nrc2442.
91. Ellis LM, Hicklin DJ. Resistance to targeted therapies: refining anticancer therapy in the era
    of molecular oncology. Clin Cancer Res. 2009;15(24):7471–8. https://doi.org/10.1158/1078-
    0432.CCR-09-1070.
92. Park JE, Chen HH, Winer J, Houck KA, Ferrara N. Placenta growth factor. Potentiation of
    vascular endothelial growth factor bioactivity, in vitro and in vivo, and high affinity binding
    to Flt-1 but not to Flk-1/KDR. J Biol Chem. 1994;269(41):25646–54.
93. Kopetz S, Hoff PM, Morris JS, Wolff RA, Eng C, Glover KY, et al. Phase II trial of infu-
    sional fluorouracil, irinotecan, and bevacizumab for metastatic colorectal cancer: efficacy

and circulating angiogenic biomarkers associated with therapeutic resistance. J Clin Oncol. 2010;28(3):453–9. https://doi.org/10.1200/JCO.2009.24.8252.

94. Sfiligoi C, de Luca A, Cascone I, Sorbello V, Fuso L, Ponzone R, et al. Angiopoietin-2 expression in breast cancer correlates with lymph node invasion and short survival. Int J Cancer. 2003;103(4):466–74. https://doi.org/10.1002/ijc.10851.
95. Shojaei F, Wu X, Zhong C, Yu L, Liang XH, Yao J, et al. Bv8 regulates myeloid-cell-dependent tumour angiogenesis. Nature. 2007;450(7171):825–31. https://doi.org/10.1038/nature06348.
96. Crawford Y, Kasman I, Yu L, Zhong C, Wu X, Modrusan Z, et al. PDGF-C mediates the angiogenic and tumorigenic properties of fibroblasts associated with tumors refractory to anti-VEGF treatment. Cancer Cell. 2009;15(1):21–34. https://doi.org/10.1016/j.ccr.2008.12.004.
97. Itatani Y, Kawada K, Yamamoto T, Sakai Y. Resistance to anti-angiogenic therapy in cancer-alterations to anti-VEGF pathway. Int J Mol Sci. 2018;19(4). https://doi.org/10.3390/ijms19041232.
98. Maniotis AJ, Folberg R, Hess A, Seftor EA, Gardner LM, Pe'er J, et al. Vascular channel formation by human melanoma cells in vivo and in vitro: vasculogenic mimicry. Am J Pathol. 1999;155(3):739–52. https://doi.org/10.1016/S0002-9440(10)65173-5.
99. Wagenblast E, Soto M, Gutierrez-Angel S, Hartl CA, Gable AL, Maceli AR, et al. A model of breast cancer heterogeneity reveals vascular mimicry as a driver of metastasis. Nature. 2015;520(7547):358–62. https://doi.org/10.1038/nature14403.
100. Williamson SC, Metcalf RL, Trapani F, Mohan S, Antonello J, Abbott B, et al. Vasculogenic mimicry in small cell lung cancer. Nat Commun. 2016;7:13322. https://doi.org/10.1038/ncomms13322.
101. Ge H, Luo H. Overview of advances in vasculogenic mimicry—a potential target for tumor therapy. Cancer Manag Res. 2018;10:2429–37. https://doi.org/10.2147/CMAR.S164675.
102. Shen R, Ye Y, Chen L, Yan Q, Barsky SH, Gao JX. Precancerous stem cells can serve as tumor vasculogenic progenitors. PLoS One. 2008;3(2):e1652. https://doi.org/10.1371/journal.pone.0001652.
103. Liu Q, Qiao L, Liang N, Xie J, Zhang J, Deng G, et al. The relationship between vasculogenic mimicry and epithelial-mesenchymal transitions. J Cell Mol Med. 2016;20(9):1761–9. https://doi.org/10.1111/jcmm.12851.
104. Liu TJ, Sun BC, Zhao XL, Zhao XM, Sun T, Gu Q, et al. CD133+ cells with cancer stem cell characteristics associates with vasculogenic mimicry in triple-negative breast cancer. Oncogene. 2013;32(5):544–53. https://doi.org/10.1038/onc.2012.85.
105. Wu S, Yu L, Wang D, Zhou L, Cheng Z, Chai D, et al. Aberrant expression of CD133 in non-small cell lung cancer and its relationship to vasculogenic mimicry. BMC Cancer. 2012;12:535. https://doi.org/10.1186/1471-2407-12-535.
106. Segaliny AI, Tellez-Gabriel M, Heymann MF, Heymann D. Receptor tyrosine kinases: Characterisation, mechanism of action and therapeutic interests for bone cancers. J Bone Oncol. 2015;4(1):1–12. https://doi.org/10.1016/j.jbo.2015.01.001.
107. Sierra JR, Cepero V, Giordano S. Molecular mechanisms of acquired resistance to tyrosine kinase targeted therapy. Mol Cancer. 2010;9:75. https://doi.org/10.1186/1476-4598-9-75.
108. Worthylake R, Opresko LK, Wiley HS. ErbB-2 amplification inhibits down-regulation and induces constitutive activation of both ErbB-2 and epidermal growth factor receptors. J Biol Chem. 1999;274(13):8865–74.
109. Zhang J, Yang PL, Gray NS. Targeting cancer with small molecule kinase inhibitors. Nat Rev Cancer. 2009;9(1):28–39. https://doi.org/10.1038/nrc2559.
110. Mondal J, Tiwary P, Berne BJ. How a kinase inhibitor withstands gatekeeper residue mutations. J Am Chem Soc. 2016;138(13):4608–15. https://doi.org/10.1021/jacs.6b01232.
111. Yun CH, Mengwasser KE, Toms AV, Woo MS, Greulich H, Wong KK, et al. The T790M mutation in EGFR kinase causes drug resistance by increasing the affinity for ATP. Proc Natl Acad Sci U S A. 2008;105(6):2070–5. https://doi.org/10.1073/pnas.0709662105.

112. Engelman JA, Zejnullahu K, Mitsudomi T, Song Y, Hyland C, Park JO, et al. MET amplification leads to gefitinib resistance in lung cancer by activating ERBB3 signaling. Science. 2007;316(5827):1039–43. https://doi.org/10.1126/science.1141478.
113. Rimawi MF, De Angelis C, Schiff R. Resistance to anti-HER2 therapies in breast cancer. Am Soc Clin Oncol Educ Book. 2015;2015:e157–64. https://doi.org/10.14694/EdBook_AM.2015.35.e157.
114. Tsui DWY, Murtaza M, Wong ASC, Rueda OM, Smith CG, Chandrananda D, et al. Dynamics of multiple resistance mechanisms in plasma DNA during EGFR-targeted therapies in non-small cell lung cancer. EMBO Mol Med. 2018;10(6). https://doi.org/10.15252/emmm.201707945.
115. Gilmour AM, Abdulkhalek S, Cheng TS, Alghamdi F, Jayanth P, O'Shea LK, et al. A novel epidermal growth factor receptor-signaling platform and its targeted translation in pancreatic cancer. Cell Signal. 2013;25(12):2587–603. https://doi.org/10.1016/j.cellsig.2013.08.008.
116. Scaltriti M, Baselga J. The epidermal growth factor receptor pathway: a model for targeted therapy. Clin Cancer Res. 2006;12(18):5268–72. https://doi.org/10.1158/1078-0432.CCR-05-1554.
117. Gazdar AF. Activating and resistance mutations of EGFR in non-small-cell lung cancer: role in clinical response to EGFR tyrosine kinase inhibitors. Oncogene. 2009;28(Suppl 1):S24–31. https://doi.org/10.1038/onc.2009.198.
118. Ono M, Kuwano M. Molecular mechanisms of epidermal growth factor receptor (EGFR) activation and response to gefitinib and other EGFR-targeting drugs. Clin Cancer Res. 2006;12(24):7242–51. https://doi.org/10.1158/1078-0432.CCR-06-0646.
119. Raymond E, Faivre S, Armand JP. Epidermal growth factor receptor tyrosine kinase as a target for anticancer therapy. Drugs. 2000;60(Suppl 1):15–23 . discussion 41-2. https://doi.org/10.2165/00003495-200060001-00002.
120. Guren TK, Thomsen M, Kure EH, Sorbye H, Glimelius B, Pfeiffer P, et al. Cetuximab in treatment of metastatic colorectal cancer: final survival analyses and extended RAS data from the NORDIC-VII study. Br J Cancer. 2017;116(10):1271–8. https://doi.org/10.1038/bjc.2017.93.
121. Specenier P, Vermorken JB. Cetuximab: its unique place in head and neck cancer treatment. Biologics. 2013;7:77–90. https://doi.org/10.2147/BTT.S43628.
122. Hammerman PS, Janne PA, Johnson BE. Resistance to epidermal growth factor receptor tyrosine kinase inhibitors in non-small cell lung cancer. Clin Cancer Res. 2009;15(24):7502–9. https://doi.org/10.1158/1078-0432.CCR-09-0189.
123. Lynch TJ, Bell DW, Sordella R, Gurubhagavatula S, Okimoto RA, Brannigan BW, et al. Activating mutations in the epidermal growth factor receptor underlying responsiveness of non-small-cell lung cancer to gefitinib. N Engl J Med. 2004;350(21):2129–39. https://doi.org/10.1056/NEJMoa040938.
124. Bokemeyer C, Van Cutsem E, Rougier P, Ciardiello F, Heeger S, Schlichting M, et al. Addition of cetuximab to chemotherapy as first-line treatment for KRAS wild-type metastatic colorectal cancer: pooled analysis of the CRYSTAL and OPUS randomised clinical trials. Eur J Cancer. 2012;48(10):1466–75. https://doi.org/10.1016/j.ejca.2012.02.057.
125. Bell DW, Gore I, Okimoto RA, Godin-Heymann N, Sordella R, Mulloy R, et al. Inherited susceptibility to lung cancer may be associated with the T790M drug resistance mutation in EGFR. Nat Genet. 2005;37(12):1315–6. https://doi.org/10.1038/ng1671.
126. Jones HE, Goddard L, Gee JM, Hiscox S, Rubini M, Barrow D, et al. Insulin-like growth factor-I receptor signalling and acquired resistance to gefitinib (ZD1839; Iressa) in human breast and prostate cancer cells. Endocr Relat Cancer. 2004;11(4):793–814. https://doi.org/10.1677/erc.1.00799.
127. Salesse S, Verfaillie CM. BCR/ABL: from molecular mechanisms of leukemia induction to treatment of chronic myelogenous leukemia. Oncogene. 2002;21(56):8547–59. https://doi.org/10.1038/sj.onc.1206082.
128. Patel AB, O'Hare T, Deininger MW. Mechanisms of resistance to ABL kinase inhibition in chronic myeloid leukemia and the development of next generation ABL kinase inhibi-

tors. Hematol Oncol Clin North Am. 2017;31(4):589–612. https://doi.org/10.1016/j. hoc.2017.04.007.

129. Itonaga H, Tsushima H, Imanishi D, Hata T, Doi Y, Mori S, et al. Molecular analysis of the BCR-ABL1 kinase domain in chronic-phase chronic myelogenous leukemia treated with tyrosine kinase inhibitors in practice: study by the Nagasaki CML Study Group. Leuk Res. 2014;38(1):76–83. https://doi.org/10.1016/j.leukres.2013.10.022.

130. Bewry NN, Nair RR, Emmons MF, Boulware D, Pinilla-Ibarz J, Hazlehurst LA. Stat3 contributes to resistance toward BCR-ABL inhibitors in a bone marrow microenvironment model of drug resistance. Mol Cancer Ther. 2008;7(10):3169–75. https://doi.org/10.1158/1535-7163. MCT-08-0314.

131. Burchert A, Wang Y, Cai D, von Bubnoff N, Paschka P, Muller-Brusselbach S, et al. Compensatory PI3-kinase/Akt/mTor activation regulates imatinib resistance development. Leukemia. 2005;19(10):1774–82. https://doi.org/10.1038/sj.leu.2403898.

132. Barnes DJ, Palaiologou D, Panousopoulou E, Schultheis B, Yong AS, Wong A, et al. Bcr-Abl expression levels determine the rate of development of resistance to imatinib mesylate in chronic myeloid leukemia. Cancer Res. 2005;65(19):8912–9. https://doi.org/10.1158/0008-5472.CAN-05-0076.

133. Graham SM, Jorgensen HG, Allan E, Pearson C, Alcorn MJ, Richmond L, et al. Primitive, quiescent, Philadelphia-positive stem cells from patients with chronic myeloid leukemia are insensitive to STI571 in vitro. Blood. 2002;99(1):319–25.

134. White DL, Dang P, Engler J, Frede A, Zrim S, Osborn M, et al. Functional activity of the OCT-1 protein is predictive of long-term outcome in patients with chronic-phase chronic myeloid leukemia treated with imatinib. J Clin Oncol. 2010;28(16):2761–7. https://doi.org/10.1200/JCO.2009.26.5819.

135. White DL, Saunders VA, Dang P, Engler J, Hughes TP. OCT-1 activity measurement provides a superior imatinib response predictor than screening for single-nucleotide polymorphisms of OCT-1. Leukemia. 2010;24(11):1962–5. https://doi.org/10.1038/leu.2010.188.

136. Haxho F, Allison S, Alghamdi F, Brodhagen L, Kuta VE, Abdulkhalek S, et al. Oseltamivir phosphate monotherapy ablates tumor neovascularization, growth, and metastasis in mouse model of human triple-negative breast adenocarcinoma. Breast Cancer. 2014;6:191–203. https://doi.org/10.2147/BCTT.S74663.

137. O'Shea LK, Abdulkhalek S, Allison S, Neufeld RJ, Szewczuk MR. Therapeutic targeting of Neu1 sialidase with oseltamivir phosphate (Tamiflu(R)) disables cancer cell survival in human pancreatic cancer with acquired chemoresistance. OncoTargets and therapy. 2014;7:117–34. https://doi.org/10.2147/OTT.S55344.

138. Abdulkhalek S, Geen OD, Brodhagen L, Haxho F, Alghamdi F, Allison S, et al. Transcriptional factor snail controls tumor neovascularization, growth and metastasis in mouse model of human ovarian carcinoma. Clin Transl Med. 2014;3(1):28. https://doi.org/10.1186/s40169-014-0028-z.

139. Wood K, Szewczuk MR, Rousseau D, Neufeld RJ. Oseltamivir phosphate released from injectable Pickering emulsions over an extended term disables human pancreatic cancer cell survival. Oncotarget. 2018;9(16):12754–68. https://doi.org/10.18632/oncotarget.24339.

140. Hrynyk M, Ellis JP, Haxho F, Allison S, Steele JA, Abdulkhalek S, et al. Therapeutic designed poly (lactic-co-glycolic acid) cylindrical oseltamivir phosphate-loaded implants impede tumor neovascularization, growth and metastasis in mouse model of human pancreatic carcinoma. Drug Des Devel Ther. 2015;9:4573–86. https://doi.org/10.2147/DDDT.S90170.

141. Allison Logan S, Brissenden AJ, Szewczuk MR, Neufeld RJ. Combinatorial and sequential delivery of gemcitabine and oseltamivir phosphate from implantable poly(d,l-lactic-co-glycolic acid) cylinders disables human pancreatic cancer cell survival. Drug Des Devel Ther. 2017;11:2239–50. https://doi.org/10.2147/DDDT.S137934.

142. Haq S, Samuel V, Haxho F, Akasov R, Leko M, Burov SV, et al. Sialylation facilitates self-assembly of 3D multicellular prostaspheres by using cyclo-RGDfK(TPP) peptide. OncoTargets and therapy. 2017;10:2427–47. https://doi.org/10.2147/OTT.S133563.

143. Akasov R, Haq S, Haxho F, Samuel V, Burov SV, Markvicheva E, et al. Sialylation transmog-rifies human breast and pancreatic cancer cells into 3D multicellular tumor spheroids using cyclic RGD-peptide induced self-assembly. Oncotarget. 2016;7(40):66119–34. https://doi.org/10.18632/oncotarget.11868.

144. Sambi M, Haq S, Samuel V, Qorri B, Haxho F, Hill K, et al. Alternative therapies for meta-static breast cancer: multimodal approach targeting tumor cell heterogeneity. Breast Cancer. 2017;9:85–93. https://doi.org/10.2147/BCTT.S130838.

145. Adams JM, Cory S. Bcl-2-regulated apoptosis: mechanism and therapeutic potential. Curr Opin Immunol. 2007;19(5):488–96. https://doi.org/10.1016/j.coi.2007.05.004.

146. Hardwick JM, Soane L. Multiple functions of BCL-2 family proteins. Cold Spring Harb Perspect Biol. 2013;5(2). https://doi.org/10.1101/cshperspect.a008722.

147. Reed JC. Bcl-2: prevention of apoptosis as a mechanism of drug resistance. Hematol Oncol Clin North Am. 1995;9(2):451–73.

148. Reed JC, Miyashita T, Takayama S, Wang HG, Sato T, Krajewski S, et al. BCL-2 family proteins: regulators of cell death involved in the pathogenesis of cancer and resistance to therapy. J Cell Biochem. 1996;60(1):23–32. https://doi.org/10.1002/(SICI)1097-4644(19960101)60:1%3C23::AID-JCB5%3E3.0.CO;2-5.

149. Konopleva M, Contractor R, Tsao T, Samudio I, Ruvolo PP, Kitada S, et al. Mechanisms of apoptosis sensitivity and resistance to the BH3 mimetic ABT-737 in acute myeloid leukemia. Cancer Cell. 2006;10(5):375–88. https://doi.org/10.1016/j.ccr.2006.10.006.

150. Hervouet E, Cheray M, Vallette FM, Cartron PF. DNA methylation and apoptosis resistance in cancer cells. Cell. 2013;2(3):545–73. https://doi.org/10.3390/cells2030545.

151. Fahrenkrog B. Histone modifications as regulators of life and death in Saccharomyces cere-visiae. Microb Cell. 2015;3(1):1–13. https://doi.org/10.15698/mic2016.01.472.

Chapter 2
Targeting the Tumor Microenvironment to Overcome Resistance to Therapy

Bessi Qorri and Myron R. Szewczuk

Abstract Recent advancements in cancer research have led to a deeper understanding of tumor biology and uncovered the crucial role of the tumor microenvironment (TME) in promoting multistage tumorigenesis. As such, it is widely accepted that the tumor microenvironment is plastic and can shape a tumor's response to therapy and subsequently contribute to the development of resistance. Consequently, therapeutic options for cancer are now transitioning from traditional cancer cell-centric approaches to holistic approaches that incorporate the tumor microenvironment and its complex interactions. However, in order to optimize such therapies and mitigate the challenge of acquired resistance, it is imperative that we understand the complexities of the tumor microenvironment. Doing so will shed light on the interactions between the extracellular matrix, cytokines, growth factors, integrins, proteases, cancer-associated fibroblasts, myeloid cells, tumor-infiltrating lymphocytes, aberrant neovasculature, and exosomal transporters, all of which have been implicated in contributing to the development of resistance to therapy. Clinical success requires cancer therapies that are capable of circumventing multistage tumorigenesis, including aberrant growth factor receptor activation, tumor neovascularization, chemoresistance, immune-mediated tumorigenesis, and the development of metastatic disease. We describe the role of mammalian neuraminidase-1 in complex with matrix metalloproteinase-9 and G protein-coupled receptors tethered to receptor tyrosine kinases and Toll-like receptors in multistage tumorigenesis upending cancer resistance. Here, we highlight an innovative and promising therapy that simultaneously targets many of the components within the TME to overcome acquired resistance.

B. Qorri · M. R. Szewczuk (✉)
Department of Biomedical and Molecular Sciences, Queen's University,
Kingston, ON, Canada
e-mail: bessi.qorri@queensu.ca; szewczuk@queensu.ca

© Springer Nature Switzerland AG 2019
M. R. Szewczuk et al. (eds.), *Current Applications for Overcoming Resistance to Targeted Therapies*, Resistance to Targeted Anti-Cancer Therapeutics 20, https://doi.org/10.1007/978-3-030-21477-7_2

Keywords Acquired resistance · Extracellular matrix · Angiogenesis · Inflammation · Hypoxia · Tumor heterogeneity · Multistage tumorigenesis · Multimodal therapy

Abbreviations

ADAM	A disintegrin and metalloprotease
ADME	Absorption, distribution, metabolism, elimination
AKT	Protein kinase B
AT2R	Angiotensin II receptor type I
BR2	Bradykinin receptor
B_{reg}	Regulatory B-cell
CAF	Cancer-associated fibroblast
CTL	Cytotoxic CD8+ T-cell
EBP	Elastin-binding protein
ECM	Extracellular matrix
EGF	Epidermal growth factor
EGFR	Epidermal growth factor receptor
EMT	Epithelial-to-mesenchymal transition
ERK	Extracellular signal-related kinase
FAK	Focal adhesion kinase
FGF	Fibroblast growth factor
GPCR	G protein-coupled receptor
HA	Hyaluronan
HGF	Hepatocyte growth factor
HIF-1	Hypoxia-inducible factor 1
HIF-2	Hypoxia-inducible factor 2
IFN-γ	Interferon-γ
IGF-1	Insulin growth factor-1
IL	Interleukin
IR	Insulin receptor
IRβ	Insulin receptor β
JAK	Janus kinase
LPA	Lysophosphatidic acid
LPS	Endotoxin lipopolysaccharide
MAPK	Mitogen-activated protein kinase
MDSC	Myeloid-derived suppressor cell
MHC	Major histocompatibility complex
miRNA	MicroRNA
MMP	Matrix metalloprotease
MMPi	Matrix metalloprotease inhibitor
mRNA	Messenger RNA
mTORC1	Mammalian target of rapamycin complex 1

NMBR	Neuromedin B GPCR
NRP	Neuropilin
OP	Oseltamivir phosphate
PDAC	Pancreatic ductal adenocarcinoma
PDGF-1	Platelet-derived growth factor-1
PG	Proteoglycan
PI3K	Phosphoinositide 3-kinase
pIRS1	phosphorylating insulin receptor substrate-1
PPCA	Protective protein cathepsin A
RGD	Arginine-glycine-aspartic acid
RONS	Reactive oxygen and nitrogen species
RTK	Receptor tyrosine kinase
SRK	Src family kinase
STAT	Signal transducer and activator of transcription
TAM	Tumour-associated macrophage
TAN	Tumour-associated neutrophil
TGF-β	Tumour growth factor β
T_H1	CD4+ T helper 1
TIL	Tumour-infiltrating lymphocyte
TKI	Tyrosine kinase inhibitor
TLR	Toll-like receptor
TME	Tumour microenvironment
TNBC	Triple negative breast cancer
TNF-α	Tumour necrosis factor α
T_{reg}	Regulatory T-cell
uPA	Urokinase-type plasminogen activator
VEGF	Vascular endothelial growth factor
VEGFR	Vascular endothelial growth factor receptor

2.1   Introduction

The development of resistance to traditional cytotoxic chemotherapeutic agents and targeted therapy is a significant challenge in the advancement of cancer research [1]. More recently, the tumour microenvironment (TME) has emerged as an essential contributor and moderator of the development of resistance to cancer therapy as it plays a crucial role in all aspects of tumorigenesis: initiation, progression, and metastasis [2, 3]. Correspondingly, cancer therapy needs to move towards a more holistic approach as opposed to traditional cancer cell-centric methods. This is primarily because any of the cell lineages or structural components within the heterogeneous TME stroma to contribute to TME-mediated resistance [1, 4, 5]. Although we have an increased understanding of tumor-stroma interactions and a greater appreciation for their importance in tumorigenesis, significant gaps in our knowledge remain.

The advent of genomic sequencing has resulted in countless reports of distinct genomic profiles associated with tumorigenesis in specific cancer cell types [6–9]. In contrast, the aberrant TME and its many constituents is a consistent feature in several cancer types and present as a novel, broadly applicable therapeutic targets [10, 11]. Despite significant advancements in therapeutic options for cancer, the dynamic TME continues to limit treatment efficacy by modulating drug pharmacokinetics (absorption, distribution, metabolism, elimination; ADME), which can ultimately limit the amount of therapeutic agent that reaches the tumour [1, 12]. In this chapter, we provide an overview of some of the critical components of the TME that contribute to the advent of drug resistance. We then describe a novel signaling platform that is implicated in multistage tumorigenesis and contributes to the acquisition of TME-mediated resistance. Here, we focus on simultaneously targeting the critical compensatory pathways that are characteristic of cancer in a multimodal approach that modulates the TME, to mitigate resistance to targeted therapy.

2.2 Key Components of the Tumor Microenvironment That Contribute to the Acquisition of Resistance

Tumour heterogeneity is central to the development of resistance to therapy. The cancer stem cell and clonal evolution models, which are not mutually exclusive, offer potential explanations for the development of genotypic, phenotypic, and morphological heterogeneity [13–16]. It is now well established that the heterogeneous malignant cell population does not act alone to initiate tumorigenesis but rather interacts in concert with the extracellular matrix (ECM) and stromal cells of the TME to facilitate a chronic inflammatory, immunosuppressive, and pro-angiogenic intra-tumoral environment [17, 18]. Contact-dependent (cell-cell or cell-ECM) and contact-independent (via non-cellular ECM components) interactions within the TME further intensify pro-tumorigenic activity leading to the development of resistance [19, 20]. Moreover, several TME components have been reported to have rather paradoxical roles in tumorigenesis, adding another layer of complexity in the already convoluted process of TME-mediated acquisition of resistance [17, 21].

Nonetheless, targeting the TME holds much promise in reducing the rate of therapy failure. This is because therapies ultimately exert a selective pressure that modulates TME plasticity and evolution, and consequently the response to therapy. The surviving cells are therefore more resistant to the therapeutic effects and stop responding. Figure 2.1 provides an overview of the crucial components of the tumour microenvironment that contribute to the development of resistance. The intricate interactions taking place that promote an immunosuppressive and pro-tumorigenic environment highlight the need for a more inclusive approach when targeting cancer in the clinic. The remainder of this section will focus on the key TME components that are central to the development of resistance to cancer therapies, particularly targeted therapy.

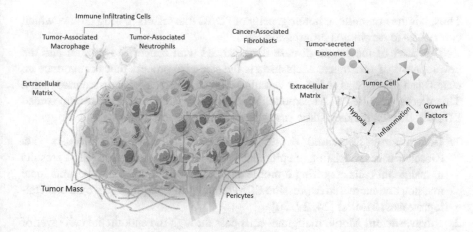

Fig. 2.1 Components of the tumor microenvironment contributing to the acquisition of resistance to therapy. The tumor microenvironment (TME) consists of cellular and non-cellular components that work together to contribute to multistage tumorigenesis and facilitate the development of resistance to therapy. As part of the non-cellular component, the extracellular matrix (ECM) is the dynamic scaffolding comprised of several glycoproteins and proteoglycans that maintains the structural integrity of the tumor mass. The ECM provides a means for several growth factors and cytokines, that are pleiotropic in nature, to initiate autocrine and paracrine signals. The malignant cells result in local stromal cells altering their phenotype to become cancer-associate cells, primarily through the release of tumor-derived exosomes, acting as the primary transporters between tumor and stromal cells. As a result, the stromal cells including cancer-associated fibroblasts (CAFs), tumor infiltrating lymphocytes (TILs) such as tumor associated macrophages (TAMs) and tumor associated neutrophils (TANs) and myeloid cells, which work with the non-cellular TME components to generate a tumorigenic and immunosuppressive environment. *TME* tumor microenvironment; *ECM* extracellular matrix; *CAF* cancer-associated fibroblast; *TIL* tumor infiltrating lymphocyte; *TAM* tumor associated macrophage; *TAN* tumor associated neutrophil

2.2.1 Extracellular Matrix Regulation of Invasion and Metastasis

The extracellular matrix is the dynamic network of non-cellular components that provides the structural scaffolding for all tissues of the body. The process of ECM remodeling, which consists of the continuous degradation, modification, and deposition of ECM components, is critical for several processes in human development, including embryogenesis and wound healing. However, perturbations in the homeostatic process of ECM remodelling is associated with several pathologic conditions [22, 23]. In the context of cancer, the ECM provides the biochemical and biomechanical milieu for malignant cells to exist and forms a robust semi-permeable matrix that prevents drug penetration into the tumor, contributing to the development of resistance [24, 25]. This is particularly evident in pancreatic ductal adenocarcinoma (PDAC), in which the extremely dense ECM acts as a physical barrier that prevents therapeutic molecules from reaching their tumour target site [26].

Thus, it is the non-cellular heterogeneity of PDAC that results in drug failure, which contributes to carcinoma progression.

The onset of metastatic disease is associated with cancer progression and the development of resistance. Metastasis is the stepwise process that occurs once an established tumour has sufficient vascularization and increased invasive propensity. This process requires ECM remodelling for tumour growth and metastatic spread [27, 28]. Briefly, the metastatic cascade involves three important steps:

1. **Detachment:** Decreased expression of cell-cell adhesion molecules (i.e. E-cadherin) and initiation of epithelial-to-mesenchymal transition (EMT) results in malignant cells acquiring a motile and invasive phenotype that permits local invasion and increased expression ECM remodelling enzymes (i.e. matrix metalloproteases; MMPs) [24, 29, 30].
2. **Intravasation:** Motile malignant cells pass through the endothelial cell layer of the aberrant tumor vasculature and enter the bloodstream [31, 32].
3. **Extravasation:** Malignant cells that survive in the bloodstream exit at a secondary site and establish a pre-metastatic niche that supports and promotes cancer cell growth and the formation of distant metastases [33, 34].

The dynamic process of ECM remodelling and increased protein deposition observed in tumorigenesis is largely comparable to ECM remodeling processes characteristic of wound healing. However, tumours are frequently referred to as "wounds that fail to heal," and are structurally stiffer than the surrounding healthy tissue [35, 36]. The stiff ECM and resulting lack of ECM plasticity are due to the increased deposition of fibronectin, collagens and other matrix proteins, which promote tumour growth and metastasis by interfering with cell-cell adhesion, cell polarity and amplification of growth factor signalling [37–40]. The major ECM macromolecules can be broadly classified into collagens, elastin and myofibrillar proteins, proteoglycans (PGs) and hyaluronan (HA), and non-collagenous matrix glycoproteins.

Collagen is the major source of structural integrity within the ECM. Generally, collagen associates with elastin to provide recoil ability for tissues with repeated stretches. Additionally, fibronectin (FN), particularly the arginine-glycine-aspartic acid (RGD) motif, plays a crucial role in the ECM, facilitating cell attachment and function [37]. However, the role of these ECM constituents is rather pleiotropic, exerting additional effects on surrounding cell behaviour, such as promoting migration and metastasis. For example, increased levels of type I collagen promote a mesenchymal phenotype characteristic of EMT due to disrupted E-cadherin/β--catenin signalling [41]. However, the detailed and specific roles of these macromolecules in the tumorigenic ECM are beyond the scope of this chapter but have been described in detail elsewhere [37, 42, 43].

Hanahan and Weinberg reported that the deregulated ECM modulates the classical hallmarks of cancer such as evasion of growth suppressors, evasion of apoptosis, replicative immortality, sustained angiogenesis, tissue invasion and metastasis, and self-sufficient growth [44]. The cancerous ECM also modulates the avoidance of immune destruction and deregulation of cellular energetics, the two emerging hallmarks of cancer [44, 45]. In general, the ECM provides binding sites for growth factors, controls adhesion and movement of cells, maintains structural integrity and anchorage, controls release and presentation to target cells, and transmits signals to activate critical intracellular signalling pathways [46, 47]. The binding of ECM molecules to cell surface receptors activates the mitogen-activated protein kinase (MAPK)/extracellular signal-related kinase (ERK) pathway and the phosphoinositide 3-kinase (PI3K) pathway. These pathways enhance migration via tumour growth factor β (TGF-β) signalling and through focal adhesion kinase (FAK) signalling, which is also implicated in angiogenesis [45, 48].

2.2.2 Soluble Factors in the Tumor Microenvironment Modulate Tumor-Stromal Crosstalk

Cytokines, integrins and proteases are small, secreted soluble molecules in the TME that enhance paracrine signalling between malignant cells and tumour-associated cells [49, 50]. These soluble molecules pose a significant challenge in terms of modulating the TME as they have been found to have pleiotropic and paradoxical effects [51]. Detailed effects of these soluble pleiotropic factors are described elsewhere [52, 53].

Cytokines Malignant cells undergoing EMT are associated with increased secretion of cytokines, which are considered critical mediators of the inflammatory and immune responses [54, 55]. The subsequent augmented tumour-stromal crosstalk further exacerbates cytokine, integrin, and protease production, facilitating and promoting tumour growth and angiogenesis in a positive cancer feedback loop [56, 57]. Pleiotropic cytokines in the TME result in paradoxical outcomes, with the pro- or anti-tumoral response of cytokines depending on factors including the local cytokine concentration, tumour expression site, and stage of carcinogenesis [58]. For example, tumour necrosis factor α (TNF-α) has a significantly pro-tumorigenic effect during cancer initiation and the early stages of carcinogenesis rather than during cancer progression. Furthermore, TGF-β initially acts as a tumour suppressor; however, later on during cancer progression, TGF-β induces EMT and promotes invasion and metastasis, exerting a pro-tumorigenic effect [59]. Many other cytokines comprising the interleukin (IL) family, such as IL-6 also play an important role in tumorigenesis. IL-6 activates the Janus kinase (JAK)/signal transducers and activators of transcription (STAT) signalling pathway, an essential pathway for cell proliferation and tumour growth. As a result, elevated circulating IL-6 levels are associated with a poor cancer patient prognosis [58].

The tumour microenvironment is also rich in polypeptide growth factors that mediate cell-cell communication within distinct cellular populations [49]. The significant growth factors present in the TME include the epidermal growth factor (EGF), vascular endothelial growth factor (VEGF), hepatocyte growth factor

(HGF), fibroblast growth factor (FGF), platelet-derived growth factor-1 (PDGF-1), and insulin growth factor-1 (IGF-1) [49, 52]. Upregulation of these growth factors and their respective receptor tyrosine kinases (RTKs) is characteristic of most human malignancies. Their sustained signalling is associated with a broad spectrum of tumorigenic activity, including stem cell differentiation, migration and invasion, mediation of stromal-epithelial crosstalk, and angiogenesis [52]. To further complicate growth factor signaling in tumorigenesis, several of these growth factors share similar downstream signalling pathways, including the PI3K/AKT and the MAPK pathways [60]. Thus, the cross-activation of growth factor signalling pathways is a significant challenge in targeted therapy due to shared downstream signalling cascades [60].

Similarly, chemokines, cytokines that induce direct chemotaxis via G protein-coupled receptor (GPCR) signalling, have been implicated in malignant cell growth, angiogenesis, metastasis and anti-tumour immune responses [61]. Raman and colleagues have provided a comprehensive review of chemokines that are involved in tumour growth [62]. However, CXCL8 is one of the most extensively studied chemokines and exhibits proangiogenic activity by upregulating MMP-2 and -9 secretion in tumour endothelial cells [63–65]. The resulting degradation of the surrounding ECM permits endothelial cell migration crucial for angiogenesis and metastasis as discussed in Sect. 2.2.1. A study investigating cytokine and chemokine levels in response to BRAF inhibitor therapy for BRAF-mutant melanoma patients reinforced the idea that cytokines and chemokines exert their effects locally in a paracrine or autocrine fashion within the TME rather than systemically [66]. Here, there were no reported changes in cytokine and chemokine levels following BRAF therapy.

Integrins Both normal and malignant cells express integrins, multifunctional adhesion receptors that recognize the short arginine-glycine-aspartic acid (RGD) amino acid sequence of many ECM proteins such as fibronectin [67]. However, the role of integrins extends beyond cell adhesion, as these receptors act as conduits that mediate bidirectional signal transmission between the ECM and cells and vice versa. Integrin-mediated signalling involves FAK and Src family kinase (SRK) signalling, which play critical roles in tissue invasion and cell migration [68]. This bidirectional integrin signalling which directly connects extracellular inputs with intracellular outputs makes integrins favourable targets for cancer therapy. Despite favourable preclinical outcomes with targeting integrin function, these results were not translated to clinical trials [69]. This is likely due to the complexity of integrin function and crosstalk with growth factors in the TME. For example, integrin signalling incorporates interactions with growth factors and their receptors, through either direct activation or by sharing similar downstream signalling axes such as the PI3K/AKT and MAPK pathways [70, 71]. Consequently, integrin activity can modulate how cells respond to growth factors, adding another layer of complexity to the TME and tumor progression.

Proteases There are several proteases within the TME, including cathepsin B, urokinase-type plasminogen activator (uPA), matrix metalloproteases (MMPs), and a disintegrin and metalloproteases (ADAMs) [72]. However, MMPs are the predominant class of proteases and are capable of processing almost all of the ECM components and soluble factors within the TME [50, 73]. Not surprisingly, it has been reported that MMPs play a crucial role in many aspects of tumorigenesis. Despite the identification of 23 mammalian MMPs, MMP-9 has been extensively studied with respect to the ECM. MMP-9 has been reported to play a significant role in ECM degradation and vessel formation, acting as an integral player in ECM remodelling. We have previously reported on the widespread role of MMP-9 in ECM remodelling, including interactions with integrins, to modulate the ECM in healthy and pathologic conditions by regulating the activity of the EGF receptor (EGFR), insulin receptor (IR), and several Toll-like receptors (TLRs), and ultimately contributing to several tumorigenic processes including angiogenesis and metastasis [74]. In the past, there have been several clinical trials investigating the efficacy of MMP inhibitors (MMPis). However, these clinical studies demonstrated no compelling efficacy of MMPis and reported significant toxicities in normal tissues [39]. These disappointing results are likely due to both the wide range of MMP function, which can exert both pro- and anti-tumorigenic effects, as well as the non-specific targeting of MMP inhibitors, resulting in widespread adverse effects.

2.2.3   Inflammation and Immunity Modulate the Tumorigenic Niche

Inflammation has been linked to cancer as early as 1864 when Virchow observed inflammatory cell infiltration in the tumour stroma [75]. Although the inflammatory responses of the innate and adaptive immune systems generally function to prevent tissue damage, excess inflammation can be detrimental to the host. This paradoxical role of inflammation is particularly evident in tumorigenesis, where acute inflammation exerts an immunoprotective role that limits cancer progression, while chronic inflammation promotes tumour growth and invasion [55].

Immune cells in the TME that facilitate the immune response to cancer include cancer-associated fibroblasts (CAFs), tumor-associated macrophages (TAMs), tumor-associated neutrophils (TANs), myeloid-derived suppressor cells (MDSCs) and tumor-infiltrating lymphocytes (TILs). Collectively, these cells secrete cytokines and growth factors that promote growth and metastasis while maintaining an overall immunosuppressive environment. Briefly, in response to tissue damage, immune cells release proinflammatory TNF-α, IL-1β, IL-6, and IL-8 cytokines, which induce reactive oxygen and nitrogen species (RONS). The resulting DNA damage then facilitates tumour initiation if inflammation persists. These proinflammatory cytokines also disrupt the epithelial barrier and recruit additional inflammatory cell infiltration, acting in a positive feedback loop to promote tumour growth, invasion, and angiogenesis through the stimulation of additional cytokines and growth factors. Anti-inflammatory cytokines such as IL-10 and TGF-β also contribute to malignant progression by enhancing tumour immune evasion [58]. The details of innate and adaptive immune cells are covered in detail elsewhere [76, 77]; however, we have provided a succinct overview to demonstrate the complex immune responses that exacerbate inflammation and tumorigenesis in a feed-forward manner.

Cancer-Associated Fibroblasts Fibroblasts are generally activated in wound healing as part of the normal inflammatory immune response and return to their quiescent state [78]. In the context of cancer, growth factors and other soluble molecules within the TME transform fibroblasts into CAFs through the process of EMT. This results in CAFs being morphologically and metabolically different from fibroblasts. Consequently, the constitutively active CAFs exert a wide variety of pro-tumorigenic effects due to enhanced ECM production and unique cytokine secretion [79]. Within the TME, CAFs synthesize several of the crucial ECM components and comprise a significant component of the cancer stroma, contributing to the development of a biophysical barrier for drug delivery as a result of increased ECM deposition [80].

Paget's "seed and soil" theory of cancer progression and metastasis states that tumour progression and spread is dependent on the interaction and cooperation between the cancer cells (seed) and the microenvironment (soil) [81]. CAFs directly modify the ECM architecture by depositing ECM proteins and indirectly by stimulating growth factors such as VEGF, PDGF, and HGF to induce angiogenesis and promote inflammation. Furthermore, CAFs are characterized by an increased expression of MMPs, which further contribute to the process of ECM remodeling [81]. Thus, CAFs play an essential role in the development of a metastatic niche (soil) by modulating the process of ECM remodelling to promote malignant progression and spread.

Myeloid Cells Myeloid cells comprise part of the stromal cells of the TME and differentiate into tumor-associated macrophage (TAMs), tumor-associated neutrophils (TANs), and myeloid-derived suppressor cells (MDSCs), each which individually and collectively contribute to the development of resistance to therapy. These cells can be polarized towards being tumorigenic or anti-tumorigenic and are characterized by changes in metabolic processes and cytokine production, altering cell phenotype and their response to the environment [82]. Collectively, myeloid cells can exert profound antitumor functions directly or indirectly by modulating cytotoxic CD8+ T-cell activation.

Within the TME, TAMs are primarily polarized to M2 phenotypes, which have greater tumorigenic activity compared to M1 TAMs [76]. These M2 TAMs contribute to the development of drug resistance by inducing EMT, ECM remodelling and angiogenesis via the secretion of specific cytokines, MMPs and growth factors [83]. TAMs secrete high levels of angiogenic VEGF and MMP-9 and are thought to be responsible, in part, for the tumour angiogenic switch. Moreover, TAMs are capable of adapting to hypoxia and subsequently accumulate in hypoxic regions, which further enhances and promotes proangiogenic events. As a result, TAM accumulation in the TME is associated with a poor prognosis. Perhaps not surprisingly, TANs are also polarized to tumour progressive and immunosuppressive (N2) types within the TME. These cells contribute to the development of resistance by secreting MMP-2 and HGF, which promote ECM remodelling and subsequent tumour invasion and metastasis, as well as MMP-9 and VEGF, which promote angiogenesis [83]. Finally, MDSCs, a group of immunosuppressive cells with variable phenotypes, can differentiate into TAMs or promote the M2 polarization of TAMs. Additionally, MDSCs promote the development of immunosuppressive regulatory T-cells (T_{regs}) [21, 76]. Thus, myeloid cells within the TME promote a tumorigenic environment due to their shared and overlapping protumorigenic functions.

Tumor Infiltrating Lymphocytes Within the TME, lymphocytes have been reported to have several different roles. For example, cytotoxic CD8+ T-cells (CTLs), also referred to as the "tumor killing" cells, exert their effects following recognition of major histocompatibility complex (MHC) class I antigens on the surface of malignant cells [84]. CTL activity is supported by CD4+ T helper 1 (T_H1)-cells which produce IL-2 and interferon-γ (IFN-γ). Collectively, these cells and cytokines are correlated with better cancer prognoses [83]. As a result, the efficacy of their antitumor effects is dependent upon their ability to become activated following recognition of tumour antigens. However, myeloid cells and cytokines within the TME suppress their antitumor effects [85]. Additionally, T_{regs}, which are characterized by FOXP3 and CD25 expression, exert a potent immunosuppressive effect via IL-10 and TGF-β secretion. Consequently, elevated T_{reg} levels are associated with an adverse prognosis [83]. Interestingly, B-cells are reported to be generally located at the invasive margin of tumours. The infiltration of B-cells in the TME has been associated with conflicting prognoses. However, the presence of the immunosuppressive population of IL-10 producing B-cells (B_{regs}) has been reported to increase tumor burden and inhibit tumor-specific immune responses [77].

2.2.4   The Angiogenic Switch in Tumorigenesis

Aberrant vasculature is considered one of the hallmarks of cancer. Irregular, leaky vascular endothelial membranes in combination with poor lymphatic drainage result in a complex tumor topography with regions of variable interstitial pressure and nutrient and oxygen gradients [79]. Hypoxic regions and nutrient deficient regions exert additional selective pressures and further exacerbate tumour heterogeneity and contributing to the advent of resistance to therapy, influencing clinical outcome. Thus far, it is evident that the TME is a complex signalling network involving interactions between cellular and non-cellular components to facilitate tumorigenesis. As discussed in Sect. 2.2.3, the immune response within the TME results in the production of several proangiogenic factors, suggesting that the processes of inflammation and angiogenesis operate concurrently to contribute to tumorigenesis.

VEGF is the predominant angiogenic factor in the TME and stimulates angiogenesis and neovascularization by binding to the VEGF receptor (VEGFR) expressed on tumour cells [83, 86, 87]. Neuropilins (NRPs) are also implicated in VEGF signaling and angiogenesis as they regulate the trafficking and function of RTKs and integrins [87]. Pleiotropic IL-6 has been associated with aberrant tumour vascularization as it disrupts the equilibrium between positive and negative angiogenic regulatory molecules, triggering the tumor angiogenic switch [88]. The angiogenic switch occurs when angiogenesis is activated by factors that induce chemotaxis of endothelial cells to direct homing to the tumour [89]. Although we have seen some success following targeted antiangiogenic therapies such as bevacizumab, the subsequent hypoxia and hypoxia-related metabolic symbiosis, invasion and metastasis and vascular mimicry, leads to the development of resistance [90, 91]. This outcome is likely due to hypoxia promoting the activation of hypoxia-inducible factor 1 (HIF-1) and hypoxia-inducible factor 2 (HIF-2), which induce the expression of pro-tumoral genes in TAMs [92]. This is another example of a positive feedback loop in cancer that exacerbates tumorigenesis, reinforcing the idea that inflammation and angiogenesis are closely linked in tumorigenesis, with the same molecular events triggering both processes [93].

2.2.5 Exosomes Are the Transporters of the Tumor Microenvironment

Exosomes are small extracellular membrane-bound vesicles that contain genetic material including messenger RNA (mRNA) and microRNA (miRNA), proteins and lipids [94]. Recently, exosomes have emerged as an integral component of TME-mediated resistance to therapy as they are implicated in all stages of tumorigenesis [94]. Thus far, it is evident that the TME modulates its effects by cell-cell interactions. As a result, exosomes are an important paracrine signalling mechanism that facilitates this cell-cell communication. Broadly, exosomes act as signalling complexes to stimulate target cells, transmit receptors between cells, transport functional proteins to receptor cells and deliver genetic information to cells. These vesicles are secreted from cells via endocytic pathways and have internalization signal receptors on their surface membrane that are recognized by recipient cells to initiate endocytosis or phagocytosis of the exosome [95]. Once inside their target cells, exosomes can exert their effects.

In Sect. 2.2.1, we highlighted the importance of cancer-associated fibroblasts in the tumour microenvironment. Recently, CAF-derived exosomes have been reported to be significant contributors to resistance [95]. Exosomes from cancer cells induce phenotypic and functional changes that promote the differentiation of fibroblasts into CAFs [95]. CAFs, in turn, produce more exosomes than normal fibroblasts. These CAF-derived exosomes have been reported to contribute to the reprogramming of TME constituents [96]. Conveniently, cancer cells produce more exosomes under hypoxic conditions than normoxic conditions permitting cell-cell communication typical of tumor microenvironment conditions [94]. Additionally, exosomes from these malignant cells in hypoxic conditions have been found to contain more miRNA than exosomes from healthy cells. Alarmingly, these cancer-derived exosomes can transfer metastatic potential and facilitate tumour growth and metastasis [97]. Li and Nabet have eloquently described the role of exosomes in the TME-mediated resistance to therapy [98].

2.3   Targeting the Tumor Microenvironment to Overcome Resistance to Therapy

Advancements in our understanding of cancer have resulted in the development of several therapies. In particular, targeted therapies represent a breakthrough in cancer research and have demonstrated major clinical success in the treatment of many types of cancer by targeting key tumorigenic components. However, relapse as a result of the development of resistance is common and continues to pose a significant challenge to researchers and clinicians. In the context of acquired resistance to targeted therapy, there are three generally established mechanisms through which resistance develops:

1. Alteration of the target protein,
2. Reactivation of downstream signalling, and
3. Activation of compensatory pathways [99].

Our expanded understanding of the complex process of tumorigenesis has highlighted that in addition to conventional mechanisms of resistance to targeted therapy, there also exist tumour cell-extrinsic mechanisms of resistance. The first half of this chapter, Sect. 2.2, set out to describe the crucial role of the many TME constituents in tumorigenesis, as well as how they interact and collectively contribute to the development of resistance. The specific details of the many subtypes of each of the TME components were not discussed in detail as they have been thoroughly reviewed elsewhere and are beyond the scope of this chapter. Instead, we shed light on the pleiotropic nature of the vast number of TME components. Despite some clinical success, targeted therapies, just like any other therapy, exert selective pressure on the tumour microenvironment, shaping the remaining cells by driving clonal selection and drug resistance [99]. Consequently, single-agent targeted therapy is not enough for the effective treatment of cancer. Thus, it is imperative that we transition from a malignant cell-centric approach to also incorporate the interactions within the tumour microenvironment.

In attempts to mitigate the development of resistance to targeted therapy as a result of clonal selection that is characteristic of single-agent targeted therapies, combination therapy has emerged as a favourable option. Generally, combination or polytherapy is designed to target:

1. Several components of the same downstream signalling pathways, or
2. Multiple compensatory signalling pathways simultaneously [99].

However, an alternative, yet challenging approach is the identification of novel therapeutic targets that modulate the tumour microenvironment and TME-mediated resistance.

2.3.1 Discovering a Novel Role of Neuraminidase-1 Activity in Multistage Tumorigenesis

Our group has reported on a signalling platform that consists of crosstalk between mammalian lysosomal neuraminidase-1 (Neu-1), MMP-9 and GPCRs, all of which are essential for regulating the downstream activity of several receptor tyrosine kinases (RTKs) following binding of their ligand (Fig. 2.2) [100]. As outlined above, the upregulated activity of RTKs has been implicated in the establishment of the TME and multistage tumorigenesis; therefore, modulating their overactivity presents as an important therapeutic avenue to explore. The initial report of a direct link between receptor glycosylation and activation of RTK signalling was with the neurotrophic TrkA receptor [101]. Woronowicz et al. reported that ligand (nerve growth factor; NGF) binding to its RTK (TrkA receptor) induces membrane siali-dase activity that specifically targets and desialylates α-2,3 sialyl linked β-galactosyl sugar residues on the TrkA receptor [101].

Additional work uncovered the mechanism by which NGF-mediated TrkA receptor desialylation occurs [102]. Central to this signalling is the existence of a tripartite alliance between Neu-1, GPCR-signaling $G\alpha_i$ subunit proteins and MMP-9 on the cell surface of TrkA receptor expressing cells [102]. The pathway, as depicted in Fig. 2.2, suggests that NGF binding to the TrkA receptor induces an allosteric conformational change which potentiates GPCR-signaling via $G\alpha_i$ to activate MMP-9 which in turn induces Neu-1 activity [100]. It was also found that elastin-binding protein (EBP) exists as part of the multi-enzymatic complex that contains Neu-1 and protective protein cathepsin A (PPCA). Thus, MMP-9 and its elastin-degrading activity are necessary to remove EBP from the complex so that Neu-1 is activated and can desialylate terminal α-2,3 sialyl residues. Under normal, unstimu-lated conditions, the α-2,3 sialyl residues provide steric hindrance that prevents receptor association and activation. However, due to Neu-1 activity, the α-2,3 sialic acid-mediated steric hindrance is relieved, permitting receptor association and acti-vation [102].

Interestingly, Amith et al. demonstrated that Neu-1 also forms a complex with mammalian Toll-like receptors (TLRs)-2, −3, and − 4 on the surface of macro-

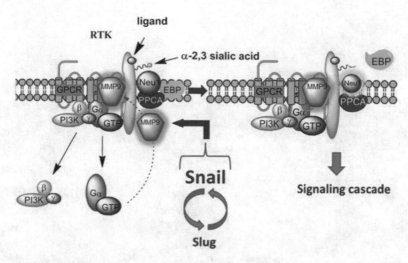

Fig. 2.2 Neuraminidase-1 (Neu-1) and matrix metalloprotease-9 (MMP-9) crosstalk in alliance with G protein-coupled receptors (GPCRs) regulates receptor tyrosine kinase (RTK) signalling. Ligand binding to its respective RTK results in an allosteric conformational change that initiates GPCR subunit $G\alpha_i$ signalling to activate MMP-9. The elastin-degrading activity of MMP-9 removes elastin binding protein (EBP) from the multi-enzymatic complex consisting of EBP, Neu-1 and protective protein cathepsin A (PPCA). Activated Neu-1 hydrolyzes α-2,3 sialyl linked β-galactosyl sugar residue on the receptor, relieving steric hindrance and facilitating receptor dimerization and subsequent activation. Note: In the context of epidermal growth factor receptor (EGFR) activation via epidermal growth factor (EGF) binding, transcription factor Snail has been shown to upregulate MMP-9 transcription, indirectly promoting RTK glycosylation modification via Neu-1-MMP-9 crosstalk that is necessary for EGFR signalling. *Neu-1* neuraminidase-1; *MMP-9* matrix metalloprotease-9; *GPCR* G protein-coupled receptor; *RTK* receptor tyrosine kinase; *PI3K* phosphatidylinositol 3-kinase; *GTP* guanine triphosphate; *EBP* elastin-binding protein; *PPCA* protective protein cathepsin A. Taken in part from © 2013 Abdulkhalek et al. [100]. Publisher and licensee Dove Medical Press Ltd. This is an Open Access article which permits unrestricted noncommercial use, provided the original work is properly cited, and © 2014 Abdulkhalek et al. [111]. Licensee Springer. This is an Open Access article distributed under the terms of the Creative Commons Attribution License (http://creativecommons.org/licenses/by/4.0), which permits unrestricted use, distribution, and reproduction in any medium, provided the original work is properly credited

phages (Fig. 2.3). Similar to the TrkA receptor findings, Neu-1 activity was found to be dependent on ligand-induced TLR activation, which in turn is essential for TLR activation and downstream signalling [103, 104]. Not surprisingly, TLR signalling has been reported to potentiate GPCR signalling via $G\alpha_i$ subunit proteins [105]. Here, endotoxin lipopolysaccharide (LPS) binding to TLR4 was found to potentiate $G\alpha_i$ subunit signalling and subsequent MMP-9 activation to induce Neu-1 activity.

Remarkably, this same Neu-1 and MMP-9 crosstalk is essential for the activation of EGFR and the insulin receptor (IR) following EGF and insulin binding, respectively [106–108]. In Sect. 2.2.1, we highlighted the elevated growth factor and growth factor receptor expression levels associated with many malignancies that

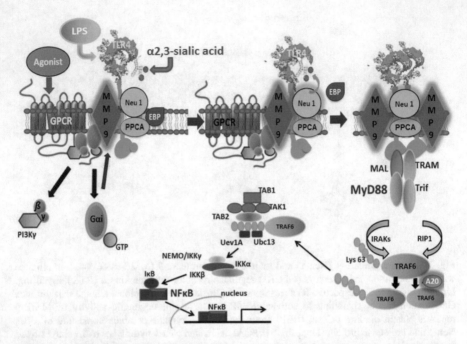

Fig. 2.3 Agonist-bound GPCRs tethered to TLR-4 and MMP-9 induce Neu-1 sialidase activity in macrophages. Endotoxin polysaccharide (LPS) binding to TLR-4 induces the activity of GPCR tethered to TLR-4 and MMP-9. Additionally, GPCR agonists involve the activation of GPCR-signaling via $G\alpha_i$ to induce MMP-9, which removes elastin-binding protein (EBP) to activate Neu-1 in complex with protective protein cathepsin A (PPCA). Activated Neu-1 hydrolyzes α-2,3 sialic acid residues at the ectodomain of the TLR-4 receptor to facilitate receptor association, MyD88 recruitment, and subsequent downstream NF-κB activation. Thus, agonist-bound GPCRs can preferentially activate TLR signaling in the absence of TLR agonists. *TLR-4* toll-like receptor 4; *GPCR* G protein-coupled receptor; *Neu-1* neuraminidase-1; *PPCA* protective protein cathepsin A; *GTP* guanine triphosphate; *EBP* elastin-binding protein; *MyD88* myeloid differentiation primary response gene 88; *LPS* endotoxic polysaccharide. Taken from © 2013 Abdulkhalek et al. [100]. Publisher and licensee Dove Medical Press Ltd. This is an Open Access article which permits unrestricted noncommercial use, provided the original work is properly cited

contribute to several tumorigenic processes [52]. Specifically, elevated EGFR is characteristic of several cancer types, including pancreatic and ovarian cancer. These EGFR-overexpressing malignant cells are also associated with reduced levels of cell adhesion molecule E-cadherin as a result of EMT [109]. It was previously reported that EGFR activation promotes PI3K-dependent induction of MMP-9 to facilitate cell invasion. In particular, overexpression of MMP-9 has been shown to result in the loss of E-cadherin and junctional integrity as well as the promotion of a migratory and invasive phenotype in ovarian cancer [110]. Additionally, transcription factor Snail, a repressor of E-cadherin, is associated with the expression of MMP-9. Abdulkhalek et al., discovered a Snail-MMP-9 signalling axis, whereby Snail plays a role in the transcriptional upregulation of MMP-9, ultimately amplifying MMP-9-Neu-1 crosstalk in regulating EGFR activation Fig. 2.2 [111]. In this study, silencing Snail in A2780 ovarian tumor cells completely abrogated tumor vascularization, tumor growth and spread to the lungs in an immunocompromised mouse model [111].

The discovery of this novel signaling paradigm that regulates receptor activation that is conserved across several receptors critical in tumorigenesis suggests that receptor glycosylation is an avenue that warrants additional investigation. Concerning the role of Neu-1 activity in regulating broad receptor activation following ligand binding, this enzyme presents as a unique target that modulates several TME components that contribute to metastatic disease and the advent of resistance to therapy. Theoretically, by inhibiting Neu-1 activity, EGFR, IR, TrkA, and TLR signaling, which is implicated in promoting migration and invasion, chemotherapy resistance and neovascularization, can be prevented, despite the presence of elevated levels of their growth factors, which would typically promote constitutive receptor signaling.

2.3.2 Role of GPCR Transactivation in Neuraminidase-1 Activity

The discovery of Neu-1-MMP-9 crosstalk in alliance with GPCRs, a signaling platform that is strikingly similar across several RTKs, was discussed in detail in Sect. 2.2.2. GPCRs are the largest family of cell-surface signal-transduction molecules in mammalian cells. It is well understood that agonist-bound GPCRs activate MMP-9 and are thought to subsequently induce Neu-1 activity. Abdulkhalek et al. have reviewed the role of this novel GPCR-signaling platform and the implications that it has on several human disease states [100]. This crosstalk is particularly interesting because not only is GPCR signalling critical for growth factor RTK activation including TrkA, EGFR, and IR, but RTKs can also be transactivated by GPCR agonists as shown in (Figs. 2.3 and 2.4) [100].

Abdulkhalek et al. reported on GPCR agonists inducing Neu-1 activity in macrophages by transactivating TLR receptors independently of TLR ligands (Fig. 2.3) [112]. Here, our understanding of the importance of Neu-1-MMP-9 crosstalk for TLR signaling was further extended. It was reported that GPCR agonists bombesin, bradykinin, lysophosphatidic acid (LPA), cholesterol, angiotensin-1 and -2 induce Neu-1 activity. This concept was further expanded to GPCR agonists transactivating insulin receptor signalling. Haxho et al. reported on this same signalling platform consisting of neuromedin B GPCR (NMBR)-Neu-1-MMP-9 crosstalk tethered to insulin receptor β (IRβ) subunits [113]. Similarly, bradykinin (BR$_2$) and angiotensin II receptor type I (AT$_2$R) were found to exist in a multimeric receptor complex with NMBR, IRβ and Neu-1 (Fig. 2.4). In this report, bradykinin and angiotensin II binding to their respective GPCRs resulted in the potentiation of Neu-1-MMP-9 crosstalk that is essential for IRβ activation, namely phosphorylating insulin receptor substrate-1 (pIRS1) and initiating insulin signalling in the absence of insulin. This finding of GPCR bias agonism or "functional selectivity" has significant implications

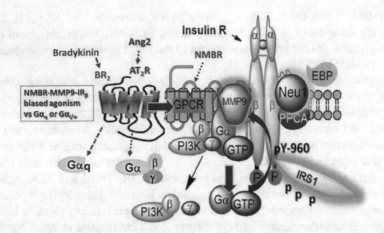

Fig. 2.4 Mechanism of GPCR bias agonism towards insulin receptor activation. The bradykinin (BR₂) and angiotensin II receptor type I (AT₂R) exist in a multimeric receptor complex with the neuromedin B GPCR (NMBR), IRβ and Neu-1. Bradykinin and angiotensin II binding to their respective GPCRs results in the preferential activation of IR signalling by forming a complex with NMBR. The biased GPCR-signaling platform potentiates Neu-1 and MMP-9 crosstalk on the cell surface that is essential for IRβ tyrosine kinases, leading to phosphorylation and subsequent activation of insulin receptor substrate 1 (IRS1), initiating the phosphoinositide 3-kinase-protein kinase B (PI3K-AKT) pathway and others in the absence of insulin. *Neu-1* neuraminidase 1; *GPCR* G protein-coupled receptor, *BR₂* bradykinin receptor; *AT₂R* angiotensin II receptor type 1; *NMBR* neuromedin B G protein-coupled receptor; *MMP-9* matrix metalloprotease-9; *IRS1* insulin receptor substrate 1 (IRS1), *PI3K-AKT* phosphoinositide 3-kinase-protein kinase B; *GTP* guanine triphosphate. Taken in part from © 2014 Alghamdi et al. [107] and © 2017 Haxho et al. [113]. Published by Elsevier Inc. This is an open access article under the CC BY-NC-ND license (http://creativecommons.org/licenses/by-nc-nd/3.0/). This is an Open Access article which permits unrestricted non-commercial use

in many health and disease states. The application of biased GPCR agonism with the insulin receptor and its implication on the development of metabolic syndrome has been extensively reviewed by Liauchonak et al. [114]. Specifically, GPCR-IR crosstalk was reported to be implicated in pancreatic cancer [115, 116]. This GPCR-IR crosstalk revealed IR-dependent potentiation of mitogenic agonist neurotensin and its relation to the mammalian target of rapamycin complex 1 (mTORC1) pathway [117]. Subsequently, activation of the PI3K-AKT pathway contributes to tumorigenic pathways implicated in pancreatic cancer development [118].

2.3.3 Targeting Neuraminidase-1 Activity as the Achilles Heel of the Tumor Microenvironment

Despite many targeted therapies for growth factors and their receptors, the development of resistance to tyrosine kinase inhibitors (TKIs) remains a significant challenge in cancer therapy [119]. Fortunately, we have uncovered the crucial role

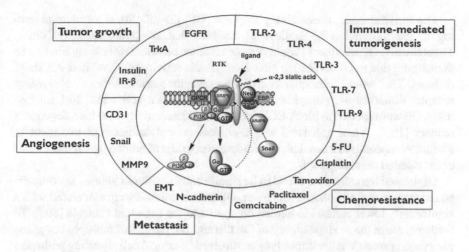

Fig. 2.5 Novel signalling platform implicated in multistage tumorigenesis. Neuraminidase-1 (Neu-1) exists in a tripartite complex with matrix metalloprotease-9 (MMP-9) and G protein-coupled receptors (GPCRs) and regulates the activity of receptor tyrosine kinases (RTKs) and intracellular Toll-like receptors (TLRs) in malignant cells. This signaling platform regulates multistage tumorigenesis, including tumor growth, invasive and metastatic propensity, angiogenesis, immune-mediated tumorigenesis and chemoresistance. *Neu-1* neuraminidase-1; *MMP-9* matrix metalloprotease-9; *GPCR* G protein-coupled receptor; *RTK* receptor tyrosine kinase; *TLR* Toll-like receptor; *EGFR* epidermal growth factor receptor; *EMT* epithelial-to-mesenchymal transition; *EBP* elastin binding protein; *PPCA* protective protein cathepsin A. Taken from © 2016 Haxho et al. [120]. This is an open-access article distributed under the terms of the Creative Commons Attribution License, which permits unrestricted use, distribution, and reproduction in any medium, provided the original author and source are credited

of Neu-1 in sialidase-mediated regulation of tumorigenesis, surpassing the role of Neu-1 previously expected. Haxho et al. reviewed the signalling of Neu-1 mediated desialylation and its implications, particularly in tumorigenesis (Fig. 2.5) [120]. In Sect. 2.2.1, we highlighted the crucial and rather pleiotropic role of growth factor-mediated signalling in several aspects of tumorigenesis, including invasion, migration, and angiogenesis. Many malignancies are characterized by the overexpression of growth factor receptors as well as elevated levels of growth factors within the tumour microenvironment [52]. Moreover, growth factor binding to their respective receptors share several downstream signalling pathways, resulting in the added challenge of receptor cross-activation [60].

Collectively, these results suggest that Neu-1 activity is crucial for the activation of several receptors that play critical roles in tumorigenesis. Therefore, neuraminidase-1 presents as a promising target for the broad targeting of several key tumorigenic signalling pathways. Even more favourable is that as a result of similar downstream cascades of these essential receptors, targeting neuraminidase-1 activity can subsequently prevent their cross-activation. Thus, it appears as though Neuraminidase-1 activity is the 'Achilles Heel' of tumour microenvironment-mediated resistance, targeting Neu-1 can have significant anticancer effects.

The antiviral agent, oseltamivir phosphate (OP) (Tamiflu®), is a structural analog of the terminal α-2,3 sialic acid residues that are hydrolyzed by Neu-1. Theoretically, OP treatment should disable receptor activation following binding to their ligand due to OP inhibiting Neu-1 enzymatic activity of cleaving α-2,3 sialyl residues. This would subsequently maintain receptor steric hindrance, preventing receptor dimerization, phosphorylation and downstream activation. Not surprisingly, OP was reported to block EGF-induced sialidase activity in a dose-dependent manner [106]. When translated to pre-clinical animal studies, OP treatment in immunocompromised mice with heterotopic xenografts of human pancreatic cancer cells impeded tumour growth.

OP-treated tumours were found to be significantly smaller in volume in comparison to their untreated cohorts. Moreover, OP treated animals were associated with a significantly lower metastatic burden compared to the untreated controls [106]. To further confirm the *in vivo* efficacy of OP therapy, the profiles of multiple key phosphorylated proteins in the tumor lysates involved in critical cell signaling pathways were investigated [106]. Not surprisingly, individual tumors taken from the OP treated cohorts expressed significantly less phosphorylation (i.e. activated form) of EGFR-Tyr1173, Akt-Thr308 and PDGFRα-Tyr754, proteins that are important for the establishment of the TME.

Due to the significant effects of OP on tumor growth and metastatic burden, OP efficacy was also tested in human pancreatic cancer PANC-1 cells with acquired resistance to cisplatin and gemcitabine [121]. OP treatment demonstrated a chemosensitizing effect for both resistant cell lines. Collectively, these results suggest that OP-targeting Neu-1 activity can effectively shut down downstream signalling pathways that are implicated in metastasis and the development of chemotherapy resistance.

EMT is generally characterized by a loss of E-cadherin expression and an upregulation of N-cadherin, permitting a more motile and aggressive phenotype that is characteristic of invasive mesenchymal cells, allowing for the initiation of the metastatic cascade [24, 29, 30]. To confirm if OP decreased tumour burden by interfering with EMT, immunohistochemical analysis of paraffin-embedded tumours of heterotopic xenografts of PANC-1 cells in immunodeficient mice was performed for standard EMT markers E-cadherin and N-cadherin [121]. Expression of both cadherins was investigated in PANC1 cells and their resistant variants. Treatment with OP resulted in significantly increased expression of E-cadherin and decreased N-cadherin expressions in all cell lines.

To confirm that OP monotherapy was translatable in other cancers, its anticancer effects were further investigated in a mouse model of human triple-negative breast adenocarcinoma [122]. In these studies, not only was OP monotherapy similarly able to dose-dependently decrease tumour vascularization, growth, and invasiveness in heterotopic xenografts of triple negative breast cancer (TNBC) MDA-MB-231 cells in an immunocompromised mouse model [122]. As shown in Fig. 2.6, OP treatment was also associated with higher levels of E-cadherin with a concomitant reduction in N-cadherin levels, unlike their untreated cohorts, confirming the results observed in pancreatic cancer mouse models [122].

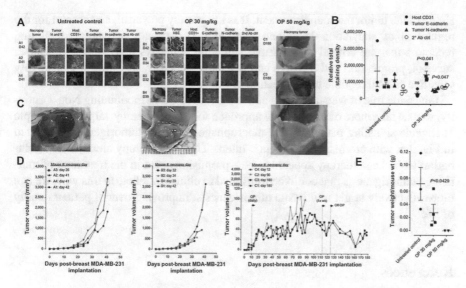

Fig. 2.6 OP monotherapy ablates tumour vascularization, growth and invasiveness in heterotopic xenografts of TNBC MDA-MB-231 in cells in a mouse model. Taken from © 2014 Haxho et al. [122]. This work is published by Dove Medical Press Limited and licensed under Creative Commons Attribution—Non-Commercial License. The full terms of the License are available at http://creativecommons.org/licenses/by-nc/3.0/. Non-commercial uses of the work are permitted without any further permission from Dove Medical Press Limited, provided the work is properly attributed

2.4 Conclusions

Taken together, the studies summarized in this chapter clearly indicate a critical role for the tumor microenvironment as a significant contributor to the development of cancer resistance. A closer look at the TME reveals that there is continuous cross-talk between tumor cells, stromal cells and non-cellular components that collectively promote multistage tumorigenesis and shape tumor response to therapy. Research progress to date provides a better understanding of the rational design of combinational therapies targeting both the tumor and the more genetically stable tumor microenvironment components. In light of this information, we present the application of a novel signaling platform that contributes to several processes related to the establishment of the TME and represents a promising therapeutic target.

The Snail–MMP-9 signaling axis involvement in tumor neovascularization suggests that the modification of glycosylation on growth factor receptors involves the activation of Neu-1. It follows that the molecular-targeting with OP treatment of Neu-1 tethered to these receptors would be critically dose-dependent. Given the ability of OP to increase E-cadherin expression and decrease N-cadherin expression in malignant cells, tumors treated with OP may become more adherent to the surrounding tissue and fail to metastasize. Collectively, these data demonstrate that OP effectively targets Neu-1 activity. In this way, Neu-1 activity represents the "Achilles

Heel" of the tumor microenvironment. It is immensely powerful, and crucial for the regulation of sialylation-dependent regulation of receptor activation, including receptors that are critical for multiple signaling pathways detrimental for cancer survival, progression and invasive and resistant propensity. As well, it is also very sensitive and susceptible to OP treatment.

Given the role of Neu-1 activity and the effect of OP in modulating Neu-1 activity, we can take more of a horizontal approach for cancer therapy, targeting multiple oncogenic signaling pathways and macrophage-mediated tumorigenesis, depicted in Fig. 2.5, with promising therapeutic intent. Thus, OP therapy alone or in combination with chemotherapy appears to be a promising agent in the treatment of multistage tumorigenesis that could be translated to clinical studies. In this way, we can more effectively target multistage tumorigenesis, improving overall patient quality of life.

References

1. Holohan C, Van Schaeybroeck S, Longley DB, Johnston PG. Cancer drug resistance: an evolving paradigm. Nat Rev Cancer. 2013;13(10):714.
2. Wang M, Zhao J, Zhang L, Wei F, Lian Y, Wu Y, et al. Role of tumor microenvironment in tumorigenesis. J Cancer. 2017;8(5):761.
3. Hui L, Chen Y. Tumor microenvironment: sanctuary of the devil. Cancer Lett. 2015;368(1): 7–13. https://doi.org/10.1016/j.canlet.2015.07.039.
4. Chen F, Zhuang X, Lin L, Yu P, Wang Y, Shi Y, et al. New horizons in tumor microenvironment biology: challenges and opportunities. BMC Med. 2015;13(1):45.
5. Sun Y. Translational horizons in the tumor microenvironment: harnessing breakthroughs and targeting cures. J Med Res Rev. 2015;35(2):408–36.
6. Chen Y-C, Gotea V, Margolin G, Elnitski L. Significant associations between driver gene mutations and DNA methylation alterations across many cancer types. PLoS Comput Biol. 2017;13(11):e1005840. https://doi.org/10.1371/journal.pcbi.1005840.
7. Wheeler DA, Wang L. From human genome to cancer genome: the first decade. Genome Res. 2013;23(7):1054–62. https://doi.org/10.1101/gr.157602.113.
8. Lu L, Bi J, Bao L. Genetic profiling of cancer with circulating tumor DNA analysis. J Genet Genomics. 2018;45(2):79–85. https://doi.org/10.1016/j.jgg.2017.11.006.
9. Bartsch H, Dally H, Popanda O, Risch A, Schmezer P. Genetic risk profiles for cancer susceptibility and therapy response. Recent Results Cancer Res. 2007;174:19–36.
10. Mbeunkui F, Johann DJ Jr. Cancer and the tumor microenvironment: a review of an essential relationship. Cancer Chemother Pharmacol. 2009;63(4):571–82. https://doi.org/10.1007/s00280-008-0881-9.
11. Joyce JA. Therapeutic targeting of the tumor microenvironment. Cancer Cell. 2005;7(6): 513–20.
12. Son B, Lee S, Youn H, Kim E, Kim W, Youn B. The role of tumor microenvironment in therapeutic resistance. Oncotarget. 2017;8(3):3933.
13. Lovly CM, Salama AK, Salgia R. Tumor heterogeneity and therapeutic resistance. Am Soc Clin Oncol Educ Book. 2016;36:e585–e93.
14. Prasetyanti PR, Medema JP. Intra-tumor heterogeneity from a cancer stem cell perspective. Mol Cancer. 2017;16(1):41.
15. Shlush LI, Hershkovitz D. Clonal evolution models of tumor heterogeneity. Am Soc Clin Oncol Educ Book. 2015;35:e662–5.

16. McGranahan N, Swanton C. Clonal heterogeneity and tumor evolution: past, present, and the future. Cell. 2017;168(4):613–28.
17. Fang H, DeClerck YA. Targeting the tumor microenvironment: from understanding pathways to effective clinical trials. Cancer Res. 2013;73(16):4965–77.
18. Pitt J, Marabelle A, Eggermont A, Soria J-C, Kroemer G, Zitvogel L. Targeting the tumor microenvironment: removing obstruction to anticancer immune responses and immunotherapy. Ann Oncol. 2016;27(8):1482–92.
19. Ungefroren H, Sebens S, Seidl D, Lehnert H, Hass R. Interaction of tumor cells with the microenvironment. Cell Commun Signal. 2011;9(1):18.
20. Morin PJ. Drug resistance and the microenvironment: nature and nurture. Drug Resist Updat. 2003;6(4):169–72.
21. Son B, Lee S, Youn H, Kim E, Kim W, Youn B. The role of tumor microenvironment in therapeutic resistance. Oncotarget. 2016;8(3):3933–45. https://doi.org/10.18632/oncotarget. 13907.
22. Bonnans C, Chou J, Werb Z. Remodelling the extracellular matrix in development and disease. Nat Rev Mol Cell Biol. 2014;15(12):786. https://doi.org/10.1038/nrm3904.
23. Karsdal MA, Nielsen MJ, Sand JM, Henriksen K, Genovese F, Bay-Jensen A-C, et al. Extracellular matrix remodeling: the common denominator in connective tissue diseases possibilities for evaluation and current understanding of the matrix as more than a passive architecture, but a key player in tissue failure. Assay Drug Dev Technol. 2013;11(2):70–92.
24. Samuel MS, Poltavets V, Pitson SM, Kochetkova M. The role of the extracellular matrix and its molecular and cellular regulators in cancer cell plasticity. Front Oncol. 2018;8:431.
25. Minchinton AI, Tannock IF. Drug penetration in solid tumours. Nat Rev Cancer. 2006;6(8):583.
26. Weniger M, Honselmann K, Liss A. The extracellular matrix and pancreatic cancer: a complex relationship. Cancers. 2018;10(9):316.
27. Walker C, Mojares E, del Río Hernández A. Role of extracellular matrix in development and cancer progression. Int J Mol Sci. 2018;19(10):3028.
28. Talmadge JE, Fidler IJ. AACR centennial series: the biology of cancer metastasis: historical perspective. Cancer Res. 2010;70(14):5649–69. https://doi.org/10.1158/0008-5472.
29. Guan X. Cancer metastases: challenges and opportunities. Acta Pharm Sin B. 2015;5(5): 402–18.
30. Buchheit CL, Weigel KJ, Schafer ZT. Cancer cell survival during detachment from the ECM: multiple barriers to tumour progression. Nat Rev Cancer. 2014;14(9):632.
31. Quail DF, Joyce JA. Microenvironmental regulation of tumor progression and metastasis. Nat Med. 2013;19(11):1423.
32. Chiang SP, Cabrera RM, Segall JE. Tumor cell intravasation. Am J Phys Cell Phys. 2016;311(1):C1–C14.
33. Fidler IJ. The pathogenesis of cancer metastasis: the 'seed and soil' hypothesis revisited. Nat Rev Cancer. 2003;3(6):453.
34. Arvelo F, Sojo F, Cotte C. Tumour progression and metastasis. Ecancermedicalscience. 2016;10:617.
35. Schafer M, Werner S. Cancer as an overhealing wound: an old hypothesis revisited. Nat Rev Mol Cell Biol. 2008;9(8):628–38. https://doi.org/10.1038/nrm2455.
36. Butcher DT, Alliston T, Weaver VM. A tense situation: forcing tumour progression. Nat Rev Cancer. 2009;9(2):108–22. https://doi.org/10.1038/nrc2544.
37. Frantz C, Stewart KM, Weaver VM. The extracellular matrix at a glance. J Cell Sci. 2010;123(24):4195.
38. Xiong G-F, Xu R. Function of cancer cell-derived extracellular matrix in tumor progression. Cancer Metastasis Treat. 2016;2(9):357.
39. Cox TR, Erler JT. Remodeling and homeostasis of the extracellular matrix: implications for fibrotic diseases and cancer. Front Oncol. 2011;4(2):165–78.
40. Murphy-Ullrich JE, Sage EH. Revisiting the matricellular concept. Matrix Biol. 2014;37:1–14.

41. Jang M, Koh I, Lee JE, Lim JY, Cheong J-H, Kim P. Increased extracellular matrix density disrupts E-cadherin/β-catenin complex in gastric cancer cells. Biomater Sci. 2018;6(10):2704–13. https://doi.org/10.1039/C8BM00843D.
42. Järveläinen H, Sainio A, Koulu M, Wight TN, Penttinen R. Extracellular matrix molecules: potential targets in pharmacotherapy. Pharmacol Rev. 2009;61(2):198–223. https://doi.org/10.1124/pr.109.001289.
43. Sainio A, Järveläinen H. Extracellular matrix macromolecules: potential tools and targets in cancer gene therapy. Mol Cell Ther. 2014;2:14. https://doi.org/10.1186/2052-8426-2-14.
44. Hanahan D, Weinberg RA. Hallmarks of cancer: the next generation. Cell. 2011;144(5):646–74. https://doi.org/10.1016/j.cell.2011.02.013.
45. Pickup MW, Mouw JK, Weaver VM. The extracellular matrix modulates the hallmarks of cancer. EMBO Rep. 2014;15(12):1243–53.
46. Filipe EC, Chitty JL, Cox TR. Charting the unexplored extracellular matrix in cancer. Int J Exp Pathol. 2018;99(2):58–76.
47. Malandrino A, Mak M, Kamm RD, Moeendarbary E. Complex mechanics of the heterogeneous extracellular matrix in cancer. Extreme Mech Lett. 2018;21:25–34.
48. Lu P, Weaver VM, Werb Z. The extracellular matrix: a dynamic niche in cancer progression. J Cell Biol. 2012;196(4):395.
49. Jones VS, Huang R-Y, Chen L-P, Chen Z-S, Fu L, Huang R-P. Cytokines in cancer drug resistance: cues to new therapeutic strategies. Biochim Biophys Acta Rev Cancer. 2016;1865(2):255–65.
50. Guo S, Deng CX. Effect of stromal cells in tumor microenvironment on metastasis initiation. Int J Biol Sci. 2018;14(14):2083–93. https://doi.org/10.7150/ijbs.25720.
51. Dranoff G. Cytokines in cancer pathogenesis and cancer therapy. Nat Rev Cancer. 2004;4:11. https://doi.org/10.1038/nrc1252.
52. Zhang X, Nie D, Chakrabarty S. Growth factors in tumor microenvironment. Front Biosci. 2010;15:151–65.
53. Jones VS, Huang RY, Chen LP, Chen ZS, Fu L, Huang RP. Cytokines in cancer drug resistance: cues to new therapeutic strategies. Biochim Biophys Acta. 2016;1865(2):255–65. https://doi.org/10.1016/j.bbcan.2016.03.005.
54. Ho EA, Piquette-Miller M. Regulation of multidrug resistance by pro-inflammatory cytokines. Curr Cancer Drug Targets. 2006;6(4):295–311.
55. Malek TR. The biology of interleukin-2. Annu Rev Immunol. 2008;26:453–79.
56. Turner MD, Nedjai B, Hurst T, Pennington DJ. Cytokines and chemokines: at the crossroads of cell signalling and inflammatory disease. Biochim Biophys Acta Mol Cell Res. 2014;1843(11):2563–82.
57. Palena C, Hamilton DH, Fernando RI. Influence of IL-8 on the epithelial–mesenchymal transition and the tumor microenvironment. Future Oncol. 2012;8(6):713–22.
58. Landskron G, De la Fuente M, Thuwajit P, Thuwajit C, Hermoso MA. Chronic inflammation and cytokines in the tumor microenvironment. J Immunol Res. 2014;2014:19. https://doi.org/10.1155/2014/149185.
59. Szlosarek P, Charles KA, Balkwill FR. Tumour necrosis factor-alpha as a tumour promoter. Eur J Cancer. 2006;42:745–50. https://doi.org/10.1016/j.ejca.2006.01.012.
60. Corso S, Giordano S. Cell-autonomous and non-cell-autonomous mechanisms of HGF/MET-driven resistance to targeted therapies: from basic research to a clinical perspective. Cancer Discov. 2013;3(9):978–92. https://doi.org/10.1158/2159-8290.
61. Schneider GP, Salcedo R, Welniak LA, Howard OZ, Murphy WJ. The diverse role of chemokines in tumor progression: prospects for intervention. Int J Mol Med. 2001;8(3):235–44.
62. Raman D, Baugher PJ, Thu YM, Richmond A. Role of chemokines in tumor growth. Cancer Lett. 2007;256(2):137–65. https://doi.org/10.1016/j.canlet.2007.05.013.
63. Li A, Varney ML, Valasek J, Godfrey M, Dave BJ, Singh RK. Autocrine role of interleukin-8 in induction of endothelial cell proliferation, survival, migration and MMP-2 production and angiogenesis. Angiogenesis. 2005;8(1):63–71.

64. McCawley LJ, Matrisian LM. Matrix metalloproteinases: multifunctional contributors to tumor progression. Mol Med Today. 2000;6(4):149–56.
65. Singh S, Sadanandam A, Singh RK. Chemokines in tumor angiogenesis and metastasis. Cancer Metastasis Rev. 2007;26(3–4):453–67.
66. Wilmott JS, Haydu LE, Menzies AM, Lum T, Hyman J, Thompson JF, et al. Dynamics of chemokine, cytokine, and growth factor serum levels in BRAF-mutant melanoma patients during BRAF inhibitor treatment. J Immunol. 2014;192(5):2505. https://doi.org/10.4049/jimmunol.1302616.
67. Raab-Westphal S, Marshall JF, Goodman SL. Integrins as therapeutic targets: successes and cancers. Cancers. 2017;9(9):110. https://doi.org/10.3390/cancers9090110.
68. Jinka R, Kapoor R, Sistla PG, Raj TA, Pande G. Alterations in cell-extracellular matrix interactions during progression of cancers. Int J Cell Biol. 2012;2012:8. https://doi.org/10.1155/2012/219196.
69. Hamidi H, Pietilä M, Ivaska J. The complexity of integrins in cancer and new scopes for therapeutic targeting. Br J Cancer. 2016;115(9):1017–23. https://doi.org/10.1038/bjc.2016.312.
70. Desgrosellier JS, Cheresh DA. Integrins in cancer: biological implications and therapeutic opportunities. Nat Rev Cancer. 2010;10(1):9–22. https://doi.org/10.1038/nrc2748.
71. Ivaska J, Heino J. Cooperation between integrins and growth factor receptors in signaling and endocytosis. Annu Rev Cell Dev Biol. 2011;27:291–320. https://doi.org/10.1146/annurev-cellbio-092910-154017.
72. Mason SD, Joyce JA. Proteolytic networks in cancer. Trends Cell Biol. 2011;21(4):228–37. https://doi.org/10.1016/j.tcb.2010.12.002.
73. Koblinski JE, Ahram M, Sloane BF. Unraveling the role of proteases in cancer. Clin Chim Acta. 2000;291(2):113–35. https://doi.org/10.1016/S0009-8981(99)00224-7.
74. Qorri B, Kalaydina R-V, Velickovic A, Kaplya Y, Decarlo A, Szewczuk MR. Agonist-biased signaling via matrix metalloproteinase-9 promotes extracellular matrix remodeling. Cell. 2018;7(9):117. https://doi.org/10.3390/cells7090117.
75. Korkaya H, Liu S, Wicha MS. Breast cancer stem cells, cytokine networks, and the tumor microenvironment. J Clin Invest. 2011;121(10):3804–9.
76. Santoni M, Massari F, Amantini C, Nabissi M, Maines F, Burattini L, et al. Emerging role of tumor-associated macrophages as therapeutic targets in patients with metastatic renal cell carcinoma. Cancer Immunol Immunother. 2013;62(12):1757–68.
77. Prenen H, Mazzone MJC, Sciences ML. Tumor-associated macrophages: a short compendium. Cell Mol Life Sci. 2019;76:1447–58.
78. Ishii G, Ochiai A, Neri S. Phenotypic and functional heterogeneity of cancer-associated fibroblast within the tumor microenvironment. Adv Drug Deliv Rev. 2016;99:186–96.
79. Junttila MR, de Sauvage F. Influence of tumour micro-environment heterogeneity on therapeutic response. Nature. 2013;501(7467):346.
80. LeBleu VS, Kalluri R. A peek into cancer-associated fibroblasts: origins, functions and translational impact. Dis Model Mech. 2018;11(4):dmm029447. https://doi.org/10.1242/dmm.029447.
81. Akhtar M, Haider A, Rashid S, Al-Nabet A. Paget's "Seed and Soil" theory of cancer metastasis: an idea whose time has come. Adv Anat Pathol. 2019;26(1):69–74. https://doi.org/10.1097/pap.0000000000000219.
82. Biswas SK, Mantovani A. Macrophage plasticity and interaction with lymphocyte subsets: cancer as a paradigm. Nat Immunol. 2010;11(10):889.
83. Balkwill FR, Capasso M, Hagemann T. The tumor microenvironment at a glance. J Cell Sci. 2012;125(23):5591. https://doi.org/10.1242/jcs.116392.
84. Lorusso G, Rüegg C. The tumor microenvironment and its contribution to tumor evolution toward metastasis. Histochem Cell Biol. 2008;130(6):1091–103.
85. Hanahan D, Coussens LM. Accessories to the crime: functions of cells recruited to the tumor microenvironment. Cancer Cell. 2012;21(3):309–22. https://doi.org/10.1016/j.ccr.2012.02.022.

86. Dankbar B, Padró T, Leo R, Feldmann B, Kropff M, Mesters RM, et al. Vascular endothelial growth factor and interleukin-6 in paracrine tumor-stromal cell interactions in multiple myeloma. Blood. 2000;95(8):2630–6.
87. Goel HL, Mercurio AM. VEGF targets the tumour cell. Nat Rev Cancer. 2013;13(12):871.
88. Nilsson MB, Langley RR, Fidler IJ. Interleukin-6, secreted by human ovarian carcinoma cells, is a potent proangiogenic cytokine. Cancer Res. 2005;65(23):10794–800.
89. Sakurai T, Kudo M. Signaling pathways governing tumor angiogenesis. Oncology. 2011;81(Suppl 1):24–9. https://doi.org/10.1159/000333256.
90. Waldner MJ, Neurath MF. Targeting the VEGF signaling pathway in cancer therapy. Expert Opin Ther Targets. 2012;16(1):5–13.
91. Ma S, Pradeep S, Hu W, Zhang D, Coleman R, Sood A. The role of tumor microenvironment in resistance to anti-angiogenic therapy. F1000Res. 2018;7:326.
92. Guo C, Buranych A, Sarkar D, Fisher PB, Wang XY. The role of tumor-associated macrophages in tumor vascularization. Vasc Cell. 2013;5(1):20. https://doi.org/10.1186/2045-824x-5-20.
93. Ono M. Molecular links between tumor angiogenesis and inflammation: inflammatory stimuli of macrophages and cancer cells as targets for therapeutic strategy. Cancer Sci. 2008;99(8):1501–6.
94. Hu C, Chen M, Jiang R, Guo Y, Wu M, Zhang X. Exosome-related tumor microenvironment. J Cancer. 2018;9(17):3084.
95. Fu H, Yang H, Zhang X, Xu W. The emerging roles of exosomes in tumor-stroma interaction. J Cancer Res Clin Oncol. 2016;142(9):1897–907. https://doi.org/10.1007/s00432-016-2145-0.
96. Kahlert C, Kalluri R. Exosomes in tumor microenvironment influence cancer progression and metastasis. J Mol Med. 2013;91(4):431–7. https://doi.org/10.1007/s00109-013-1020-6.
97. Milane L, Singh A, Mattheolabakis G, Suresh M, Amiji MM. Exosome mediated communication within the tumor microenvironment. J Control Release. 2015;219:278–94. https://doi.org/10.1016/j.jconrel.2015.06.029.
98. Zhang C, Ji Q, Yang Y, Li Q, Wang Z. Exosome: function and role in cancer metastasis and drug resistance. Technol Cancer Res Treat. 2018;17:1533033818763450.
99. Harrison PT, Huang PH. Exploiting vulnerabilities in cancer signalling networks to combat targeted therapy resistance. Essays Biochem. 2018;62(4):583–93.
100. Abdulkhalek S, Hrynyk M, Szewczuk MR. A novel G-protein-coupled receptor-signaling platform and its targeted translation in human disease. Res Rep Biochem. 2013;2013(1):17–30.
101. Woronowicz A, Amith SR, De Vusser K, Laroy W, Contreras R, Basta S, et al. Dependence of neurotrophic factor activation of Trk tyrosine kinase receptors on cellular sialidase. Glycobiology. 2007;17(1):10–24. https://doi.org/10.1093/glycob/cwl049.
102. Jayanth P, Amith SR, Gee K, Szewczuk MR. Neu1 sialidase and matrix metalloproteinase-9 cross-talk is essential for neurotrophin activation of Trk receptors and cellular signaling. Cell Signal. 2010;22(8):1193–205. https://doi.org/10.1016/j.cellsig.2010.03.011.
103. Amith SR, Jayanth P, Franchuk S, Siddiqui S, Seyrantepe V, Gee K, et al. Dependence of pathogen molecule-induced toll-like receptor activation and cell function on Neu1 sialidase. Glycoconj J. 2009;26(9):1197.
104. Amith SR, Jayanth P, Franchuk S, Finlay T, Seyrantepe V, Beyaert R, et al. Neu1 desialylation of sialyl α-2, 3-linked β-galactosyl residues of TOLL-like receptor 4 is essential for receptor activation and cellular signaling. Cell Signal. 2010;22(2):314–24.
105. Abdulkhalek S, Amith SR, Franchuk SL, Jayanth P, Guo M, Finlay T, et al. Neu1 sialidase and matrix metalloproteinase-9 cross-talk is essential for Toll-like receptor activation and cellular signaling. J Biol Chem. 2011;286(42):36532–49. https://doi.org/10.1074/jbc.M111.237578.
106. Gilmour AM, Abdulkhalek S, Cheng TSW, Alghamdi F, Jayanth P, O'Shea LK, et al. A novel epidermal growth factor receptor-signaling platform and its targeted translation in pancreatic cancer. Cell Signal. 2013;25(12):2587–603. https://doi.org/10.1016/j.cellsig.2013.08.008.

107. Alghamdi F, Guo M, Abdulkhalek S, Crawford N, Amith SR, Szewczuk MR. A novel insulin receptor-signaling platform and its link to insulin resistance and type 2 diabetes. Cell Signal. 2014;26(6):1355–68. https://doi.org/10.1016/j.cellsig.2014.02.015.
108. Haxho F, Neufeld R, Szewczuk M. Novel insulin receptor signaling platform. Int J Diabetes Clin Res. 2014;1(005):1–10.
109. Dahl KDC, Symowicz J, Ning Y, Gutierrez E, Fishman DA, Adley BP, et al. Matrix metalloproteinase 9 is a mediator of epidermal growth factor–dependent E-cadherin loss in ovarian carcinoma cells. Cancer Res. 2008;68(12):4606–13.
110. Ellerbroek SM, Halbleib JM, Benavidez M, Warmka JK, Wattenberg EV, Stack MS, et al. Phosphatidylinositol 3-kinase activity in epidermal growth factor-stimulated matrix metalloproteinase-9 production and cell surface association. Cancer Res. 2001;61(5):1855–61.
111. Abdulkhalek S, Geen OD, Brodhagen L, Haxho F, Alghamdi F, Allison S, et al. Transcriptional factor snail controls tumor neovascularization, growth and metastasis in mouse model of human ovarian carcinoma. Clin Transl Med. 2014;3:28. https://doi.org/10.1186/s40169-014-0028-z.
112. Abdulkhalek S, Guo M, Amith SR, Jayanth P, Szewczuk MR. G-protein coupled receptor agonists mediate Neu1 sialidase and matrix metalloproteinase-9 cross-talk to induce transactivation of TOLL-like receptors and cellular signaling. Cell Signal. 2012;24(11):2035–42.
113. Haxho F, Haq S, Szewczuk MR. Biased G protein-coupled receptor agonism mediates Neu1 sialidase and matrix metalloproteinase-9 crosstalk to induce transactivation of insulin receptor signaling. Cell Signal. 2018;43:71–84. https://doi.org/10.1016/j.cellsig.2017.12.006.
114. Liauchonak I, Dawoud F, Riat Y, Qorri B, Sambi M, Jain J, et al. The biased G-protein-coupled receptor agonism bridges the gap between the insulin receptor and the metabolic syndrome. Int J Mol Sci. 2018;19(2):575.
115. Kisfalvi K, Rey O, Young SH, Sinnett-Smith J, Rozengurt E. Insulin potentiates Ca2+ signaling and phosphatidylinositol 4,5-bisphosphate hydrolysis induced by Gq protein-coupled receptor agonists through an mTOR-dependent pathway. Endocrinology. 2007;148(7):3246–57. https://doi.org/10.1210/en.2006-1711.
116. Young SH, Rozengurt E. Crosstalk between insulin receptor and G protein-coupled receptor signaling systems leads to Ca(2)+ oscillations in pancreatic cancer PANC-1 cells. Biochem Biophys Res Commun. 2010;401(1):154–8. https://doi.org/10.1016/j.bbrc.2010.09.036.
117. Yoon MS, Choi CS. The role of amino acid-induced mammalian target of rapamycin complex 1(mTORC1) signaling in insulin resistance. Exp Mol Med. 2016;48(1):e201. https://doi.org/10.1038/emm.2015.93.
118. Hahn-Windgassen A, Nogueira V, Chen CC, Skeen JE, Sonenberg N, Hay N. Akt activates the mammalian target of rapamycin by regulating cellular ATP level and AMPK activity. J Biol Chem. 2005;280(37):32081–9. https://doi.org/10.1074/jbc.M502876200.
119. Wong HH, Lemoine NR. Novel therapies for pancreatic cancer: setbacks and progress. Future Oncol. 2010;6(7):1061–4.
120. Haxho F, Neufeld RJ, Szewczuk MR. Neuraminidase-1: a novel therapeutic target in multistage tumorigenesis. Oncotarget. 2016;7(26):40860–81. https://doi.org/10.18632/oncotarget.8396.
121. O'Shea LK, Abdulkhalek S, Allison S, Neufeld RJ, Szewczuk MR. Therapeutic targeting of Neu1 sialidase with oseltamivir phosphate (Tamiflu®) disables cancer cell survival in human pancreatic cancer with acquired chemoresistance. Onco Targets Ther. 2014;7:117–34.
122. Haxho F, Allison S, Alghamdi F, Brodhagen L, Kuta VEL, Abdulkhalek S, et al. Oseltamivir phosphate monotherapy ablates tumor neovascularization, growth, and metastasis in mouse model of human triple-negative breast adenocarcinoma. Breast Cancer: Targets and Therapy 2014:6 191–203. https://doi.org/10.2147/BCTT.S74663.

Chapter 3
Current Challenges and Applications of Oncolytic Viruses in Overcoming the Development of Resistance to Therapies in Cancer

Jessica Swanner, W. Hans Meisen, Ryan M. McCormack, Cole T. Lewis, Bangxing Hong, and Balveen Kaur

Abstract Oncolytic viruses (OVs) are designed to ablate cancerous cells while sparing non-malignant cells and tissues. In the wake of an active tumor infection, OVs can activate an anti-tumor immune response. Currently, an oncolytic Herpes simplex 1 (HSV-1) derived virus encoding for granulocyte-macrophage colony stimulating factor (GM-CSF) is approved in the US and Europe as a treatment for metastatic melanoma, and an oncolytic adenovirus (oAd) is approved in China for head and neck cancer therapy. Despite the approved use for these indications, this promising biological therapy is currently under-used. However, a multitude of viruses are actively being explored in preclinical animal models and clinically in patients with different malignancies for safety and efficacy. Several ongoing clinical trials evaluate OV utility in combination with other therapies, such as chemotherapeutics and immune checkpoint inhibitors. In this chapter, we highlight some of the barriers faced by OVs and discuss methods used to convert these challenges into opportunities for improvement. Major advancements in this field include engineering OVs to deliver payloads with anti-angiogenic, immune modulatory, or extracellular matrix degrading proteins, as well as in combination with immunotherapies, DNA damaging agents, and stem cells to enhance the therapeutic efficacy of OVs. Despite facing some challenges, there is continued enthusiasm for this innovative and promising biological arsenal in treating cancer.

J. Swanner · R. M. McCormack · C. T. Lewis · B. Hong · B. Kaur (✉)
Department of Neurosurgery, McGovern Medical School, University of Texas Health Science Center at Houston, Houston, TX, USA
e-mail: Jessica.L.Swanner@uth.tmc.edu; Ryan.M.McCormack@uth.tmc.edu; Cole.Lewis@uth.tmc.edu; Bangxing.Hong@uth.tmc.edu; balveen.kaur@uth.tmc.edu

W. H. Meisen
Cell and Gene Therapy Group, Amgen Inc., South San Francisco, CA, USA
e-mail: wmeisen@amgen.com

© Springer Nature Switzerland AG 2019
M. R. Szewczuk et al. (eds.), *Current Applications for Overcoming Resistance to Targeted Therapies*, Resistance to Targeted Anti-Cancer Therapeutics 20, https://doi.org/10.1007/978-3-030-21477-7_3

Keywords Oncolytic viral therapy · Overcoming virotherapy resistance · Biotherapy · Resistance · Anti-angiogenic · Combination therapy · Immunotherapy

Abbreviations

ATP	Adenosine triphosphate
BAI1	Brain angiogenesis inhibitor 1
BiTE	Bispecific T-cell engager
CAR	Chimeric antigen receptor
cGAS	GMP-AMP synthase
CPA	Cyclophosphamide
CV	Coxsackievirus
CXCR4	C-X-C chemokine receptor type 4
DAF	Decay-accelerating factor
DAMP	Damage associated molecular pattern
DDR	DNA damage response
DFS	Disease-free survival
dnFGFR	Dominant-negative FGF receptor
ECM	Extracellular matrix
EGF	Epidermal growth factor
EMT	Epithelial to mesenchymal transition
ER	Endoplasmic reticulum
FGF	Fibroblast growth factor
GADD34	Growth arrest and DNA damage-inducible protein
GM-CSF	Granulocyte-macrophage colony-stimulating factor
HA	Hyaluronan
HDACi	Histone deacetylase inhibitor
HIF	Hypoxia-inducing factor
HMGB1	High Mobility Group Box Protein 1
ICAM-1	Intercellular adhesion molecule 1
IFN	Interferon
IFNR	IFN receptor
IL	Interleukin
IRF	Interferon regulatory factor 3
JAK	Janus family kinase
JAM-1	Junctional adhesion molecule 1
MCP-1	Monocyte chemoattractant protein-1
MDSC	Myeloid-derived suppressor cell
MGMT	O(6)-methylguanine-DNA methyltransferase
MMP	Matrix metalloproteinase
MRB	Maraba Virus
MSC	Mesenchymal stem cell
MV	Measles Virus

NF-κB	Nuclear factor kappa-light-chain-enhancer of activated B-cells
NK	Natural killer
NSC	Neural Stem Cell
NSCLC	Non-small cell lung cancer
oAd	Oncolytic adenoviruses
OS	Overall survival
OV	Oncolytic virus
PARP	Poly ADP ribose polymerase
PBMC	Peripheral blood mononuclear cell
PDAC	Pancreatic ductal adenocarcinoma
PDGF	Platelet-derived growth factor
PKR	Protein kinase R
PV	Poliovirus
ReoT3D	Reovirus type 3 Dearing
shRNA	Short hairpin RNA
Smac	Supramolecular activation complex
STAT	Signal transducer and activator of transcription
STING	Stimulator of interferon genes
TAM	Tumor associated macrophage
TBK1	TANK-binding kinase 1
TIMP	Tissue inhibitor of Matrix metalloproteinases
TMZ	Temozolomide
TNF-α	Tumor necrosis factor alpha
VEGF	Vascular endothelial factor
Vstat120	Vasculostatin
VSV	Vesicular stomatitis virus
VV	Vaccinia virus

3.1 Introduction

Oncolytic virus (OV) therapy is a promising biological treatment that exploits the deregulation of neoplastic cell signaling, including resistance to apoptosis, uncontrolled cellular proliferation, and defective immune signaling, to preferentially replicate in, spread, and destroy tumor cells (Fig. 3.1). Since most OVs are not target-specific, they can be utilized in a variety of cancer types. Additionally, OVs can initiate anti-tumor immune responses, extending their effects beyond the site of virus inoculation.

The world's first approved oncolytic virus was Oncorine, an attenuated adenovirus approved in China that was marketed for head and neck cancer patients [1]. At the time of writing this chapter, Imlygic, an engineered Herpes simplex virus 1 (HSV-1) derived virus, was the only approved oncolytic virus in Europe and the United States [2]. While these advances are promising, the utility of this approach for other malignancies continues to be explored in both preclinical animal models and in the clinic.

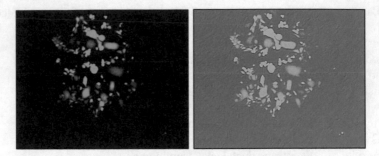

Fig. 3.1 Viral spread and plaque formation. Oncolytic viruses can infect and replicate in tumor cells. Upon viral burst, the tumor cells are lysed, releasing viral particles to surrounding tumor cells, resulting in secondary infections, viral spread, and plaque formation. Here, there is a Vero cell plaque with an oncolytic HSV-1 derived virus encoded for GFP. GFP positive infected cells outline a clear plaque in the monolayer of Vero cells seen in the bright field

In this chapter, we will focus on some of the limitations of oncolytic viruses and current standard of care therapies, as well as strategies being utilized to overcome these challenges. Due to their strong safety record and unique mechanism of action, OVs have been tested in combination with a variety of cancer therapeutics. Here, we highlight some of the emerging preclinical and clinical data demonstrating the therapeutic potential of OV combination studies.

3.2 Types of Oncolytic Viruses

The anti-tumor response achieved by different OVs depends on the strain of the virus, the oncolytic engineering strategies, and the type of tumor. As a multitude of different viruses have been exploited as oncolytic vectors, this section will provide a brief description of some of the different RNA and DNA viruses used as oncolytic agents that have advanced into patient testing.

3.2.1 Adenovirus

The adenoviral genome is a double-stranded, linear DNA complex. Oncolytic adenoviruses (oAd) are rendered tumor-specific by small deletions of key viral genes or by engineering their expression such that it is under the control of tumor-specific promoters [3]. The *E1B55KD*-deleted adenovirus was initially designed by Dr. Frank McCormick's laboratory to exploit p53 deficiency in cancer cells to allow the virus to replicate and clear malignant cells [4]. While the development of this virus lagged in the United States, Oncorine (H101), an oAd with similar attenuations, was approved by the China State Food and Drug Administration for treating head and neck cancer in combination with chemotherapy [5, 6]. A second generation oAd with improved replication and infection potential is currently being evaluated in patients for safety and efficacy [5]. One of the major pitfalls of oAd is viral entry into neoplastic cells. Adenoviral fiber proteins engage the cell surface coxsackievirus and adenovirus receptor on cells, leading to efficient viral entry; however, in neoplastic cells, coxsackievirus and adenovirus receptor cell surface expression can be downregulated, leading to inefficient viral entry [7]. This challenge can be overcome by utilizing genetically engineered adenovirus (Ad) with fiber protein modifications that permit oAds to recognize tumor cell-specific receptors to facilitate targeted viral entry. For example, Delta-24-RGD (DNX-2401) utilizes an integrin binding motif for efficient coxsackievirus and adenovirus receptor-independent infection of tumor cells and is now being investigated in multiple clinical trials both as a single agent (NCT00805376) and in combination with other agents (NCT02798406).

3.2.2   Herpes Simplex Virus 1 (HSV-1)

The herpes simplex virus 1 (HSV-1) is an enveloped virus with a double-stranded, well characterized genome, that is predicted to contain almost 100 genes, providing ample opportunities for genetic manipulations to enhance tumor selectivity [8]. HSV-1 strains with attenuations in thymidine kinase genes demonstrated decreased neurovirulence and became the first oncolytic HSV prototype to be tested as a therapeutic agent for brain tumors in preclinical studies. Unfortunately, viral thymidine kinase deletion renders the herpes virus resistant to several commonly used anti-herpetic agents. ICP34.5 is a key neurovirulence gene in the HSV-1 genome that is most frequently deleted in oncolytic HSV1-derived vectors (oHSVs) to enhance safety [8]. All oHSVs tested in patients to date have either had deletions or modifications to have tumor selective expression of viral ICP34.5, rendering the virus extremely sensitive to antiviral responses in normal cells. Malignant cells exhibit a disrupted protein kinase R (PKR) response, which compensates for ICP34.5 deletion and facilitates viral replication and oncolysis [8]. Deletion of viral ribonucleotide reductase renders HSV-1 dependent on the cellular counterpart of this gene that is expressed under the tight control of the cell cycle. As malignant cells have dysregulated cell cycle checkpoint controls, this defect is compensated via nucleotide synthesis which facilitates viral genome replication. Deletion of both ICP34.5 and ICP6, the viral counterpart of the large cellular subunit of ribonucleotide reductase, became the backbone of G207, a virus that became the first oncolytic HSV to be tested in patients with malignant brain tumors [9]. Virus-encoded ICP47 functions to block antigen presentation in infected cells, and its deletion is believed to improve anti-tumor immunity [10]. The backbone of Imlygic is deleted for viral genes encoding ICP34.5 and ICP47. This is the first approved oncolytic virus in the USA and EU.

3.2.3   Vaccinia Virus (VV)

The vaccinia virus (VV) is an enveloped, double-stranded DNA virus. In the early 1990s VV-infected tumor cell lysates were administered as vaccines to elicit anti-tumor immune responses [11]. However, this approach was abandoned as there was no significant difference in disease-free survival (DFS) or overall survival (OS). Despite initial setbacks with the tumor vaccination approach, recombinant VVs encoding for tumor antigens or cytokines are currently being tested in numerous clinical trials in combination with chemotherapy [11]. The first replication-competent oncolytic VV (oVV), Pexa Vec, was generated by deleting the viral thymidine kinase gene and engineering the virus to encode for granulocyte-macrophage colony stimulating factor (GM-CSF). Virus-induced immunogenic cell death is postulated to initiate an anti-tumorigenic immune response, which was confirmed in clinical trials where a significant relationship was identified between liver cancer patient survival and increasing viral inoculum [12]. GL-ONC1 is another example of an attenuated oVV that is being tested in patients with peritoneal carcinoma [13]. Patients with ovarian cancer, gastric cancer, mesothelioma, and peritoneal cancer were enrolled in this study. Overall, the oVV was well-tolerated, and viral replication and subsequent tumor cell oncolysis was observed [13].

3.2.4   Reovirus Type 3 Dearing

Reovirus type 3 Dearing is a double-stranded RNA virus that was found to have natural oncolytic properties. The reovirus can infect most human cells effectively but is very sensitive to antiviral signaling. Consequently, most reovirus infections in hosts are asymptomatic [14]. Ras/RAF/MEK signaling is known to negatively regulate cellular antiviral PKR responses. Thus, malignant cells with constitutively activated Ras signaling are particularly sensitive to reovirus infection. Reolysin, developed by Oncolytics Biotech Inc., has been tested as a single agent and in combination in patients with multiple malignancies. It is among the few OVs that can be safely given systemically with doses up to 1^{10} pfu. The combination of Reolysin with gemcitabine is well tolerated with manageable non-hematological toxicities in patients diagnosed with pancreatic ductal adenocarcinoma (PDAC) [15].

3.2.5   Measles Virus (MV)

The measles virus (MV) is a negative-strand RNA virus. An attenuated strain of MV has been harnessed to preferentially kill neoplastic cells. Upon infection, MV induces cell-cell fusion which leads to the formation of large syncytia [16]. The attenuated Edmonston MV strain has been tested in preclinical studies and patients for safety and anti-cancer efficacy [17, 18]. More recently, MV armed with gene therapy such as sodium iodide symporter (NIS), has been used for both the visualization of virally infected tumor cells and for synergy with radioiodine therapy. This virus has also been tested in patients diagnosed with recurrent or refractory multiple myeloma and led to a complete response for one patient enrolled in the trial [17].

3.2.6 Poliovirus (PV)

The poliovirus (PV) is a non-enveloped RNA virus that is associated with a severely debilitating disease. PVSRIPO is a recombinant PV that is attenuated in normal cells and has been utilized as an anti-neoplastic agent for patients diagnosed with glioblastoma (GBM). Intra-tumoral infusion did not show neurovirulent potential of the virus, and patient OS overlapped with historical controls, with patients receiving PVSRIPO reaching a plateau of 21% (95% confidence interval, 11–33) at 24 months, suggesting a possible benefit to a small cohort of patients [19].

3.2.7 Coxsackievirus (CV)

The coxsackievirus (CV) is a non-enveloped RNA virus. CV entry is dependent upon frequently upregulated molecules in cancer, such as ICAM-1 and DAF, making them good oncolytic vectors [20]. Oncolytic CV-A21 is currently undergoing clinical trials for a variety of cancer types including bladder cancer (NCT02043665), melanoma (NCT01227551, NCT00636558, NCT02307149, NCT03408587), non-small cell lung cancer (NCT02043665), breast cancer (NCT00636558), and prostate cancer (NCT00636558). Other oncolytic CVs (oCVs) are also under investigation [21].

3.2.8 Vesicular Stomatitis Virus (VSV)

The vesicular stomatitis virus (VSV) is a negative-strand RNA virus with a small, easily manipulated genome [22]. VSV selectivity is largely based on the reduced type I interferon (IFN) response of tumor cells compared to normal cells. Oncolytic VSV (oVSV) armed with various transgenes including IFN-β [23] and IFN-γ [24] have been tested in several pre-clinical models. oVSV armed with IFN-β was evaluated in mouse models of mesothelioma, where it slowed tumor growth and enhanced overall survival. An oVSV armed with IFN-γ was evaluated in a syngeneic mouse model of breast cancer. The IFN-γ expressing virus induced activation of dendritic cells, slowed tumor growth, and reduced the number and size of lung tumors [24].

A VSV expressing the sodium iodide symporter and IFN-β (VSV-IFN-β-NIS) is undergoing phase I clinical trials for solid tumors (NCT02923466).

3.2.9 Maraba Virus (MRB)

The Maraba virus (MRB) is an enveloped virus with a negative sense, single-stranded RNA genome that is being developed in conjunction with a non-replicating adenovirus as a vaccine strategy. The MG1 strain of Maraba, which is engineered to encode for tumor specific antigen MAGE-3, was found to engage effector immune cell populations without causing unmanageable toxicities in non-human primates [25]. The first human trials with this virus are in progress and will uncover the safety and benefits of this approach.

A recent preclinical study comparing the efficacy of HSV, Reo, VSV, Ad and MRB viruses, concluded that these viruses could also confer long term protection against tumor re-challenge [26]. While exhibiting a strong safety record in clinical trials, OV therapeutic responses administered as monotherapy have been modest. Thus, various efforts to improve OV therapy include the generation of payload armed, second-generation vectors, and combination strategies to exploit tumor or chemotherapy-induced sensitization to improve anti-tumor efficacy.

3.3 Oncolytic Viral Targeting of the Tumor Vasculature

Most solid tumors can only grow a few millimeters before outpacing the oxygen and nutrient supply provided by their existing vasculature. To overcome this, tumors initiate angiogenesis, a critical event in the initiation, progression, and metastasis of malignancies [27, 28]. Tumors are also able to suppress the secretion of endogenous antiangiogenic factors, such as thrombospondin, vasculostatin, angiostatin, endostatin, and IL-12, which antagonize and regulate the growth of new vasculature. Although numerous efforts have been made to modulate key components of angiogenesis, success rates vary [29].

OVs are designed to exploit and hijack the replicative machinery of proliferating tumor cells in order to kill host cells. This oncolytic process has been extended to the tumor endothelium, whereby OVs produce an anti-angiogenic effect during active viral infection and spread in the tumor [29]. Numerous OVs have demonstrated direct cytotoxicity towards growing tumor vasculature. For example, oAd dl922–947 demonstrated antitumor and antiangiogenic properties against anaplastic thyroid carcinoma (ATC). Infection with dl922–947 also decreased potent angiogenic cytokine IL-8, resulting in reduced microvessel density *in vivo* after treatment [29]. Similarly, treatment with engineered OVs in xenograft models of human cancers derived from HSV-1 has been shown to have a direct cytotoxic effect on endothelial cells proliferating *in vitro,* with reduced tumor micro-vessel density in multiple experimental tumors [30, 31]. Intravascular administration of HSV-1716 has been shown to localization to tumor vascular endothelium in a model of ovarian cancer, but not to the vasculature of normal organs [32]. Several OVs have shown vascular disruption *in vivo* after treatment, suggesting that OVs can be harnessed as potent vascular disrupting agents [33]. Collectively, these results suggest that the anti-tumor efficacy of OV is in part due to its antiangiogenic properties.

While numerous reports have uncovered the potent antiangiogenic effect of multiple viruses, this direct oncolytic effect is thought to be transient while the virus persists in the tumor [34]. Temporal studies of changes in tumor vasculature post-treatment have demonstrated both increased vascular permeability and angiogenesis of the residual tumor after clearance of the OV with residual tumor regrowth [35–37]. Increased inflammation and ensuing endothelial cell activation after OV therapy can result in increased vascular permeability and tumor edema that limits overall therapeutic benefit [35, 36]. Thus, combining an OV with an angiostatic therapy or arming OVs with transgenes that can negate the tumoral angiogenic response, appears to be promising.

Not surprisingly, a single dose of an angiostatic cyclic RGD peptide administered before OV therapy in rats bearing intracranial tumors was sufficient to mitigate response and contribute to increased survival of tumour-bearing animals [35]. Consistent with this, blockade of VEGF with avastin in combination with oHSV demonstrated a therapeutic advantage [38]. Second generation armed viruses designed to target the vascular endothelial growth factor (VEGF) pathway by encoding transgenes that block angiogenic responses have also been tested and shown to improve therapeutic response in animals. For example, treatment of mice with an oAd that delivers short hairpin RNA (shRNA) against VEGF slowed tumor xenograft growth and increased OS [39]. Arming strategies to block VEGF have included engineering OVs to secrete soluble VEGFR which functions as a decoy receptor [29, 40]. The therapeutic benefit of blocking angiogenesis is not limited to applications incorporating VEGF. Instead, blockade of other potent angiogenic cytokines, such as fibroblast growth factor (FGF), via arming viruses designed to encode a dominant-negative FGF receptor (dnFGFR) also inhibit angiogenesis and tumor growth to a greater degree than unmodified control viruses [41]. This blockade can also be elicited with expression of potent antiangiogenic genes such as vasculostatin, angiostatin, and endostatin. An oHSV that expresses vasculostatin (Vstat120), reduced tumor microvessel density and significantly improved anti-tumor efficacy in multiple pre-clinical studies [42–44].

Lastly, thrombospondin-1 is another example of a naturally occurring inhibitor of angiogenesis, that can suppress the migration of endothelial cells and stimulate apoptosis. Delivery of thrombospondin-derived anti-angiogenic peptides enhances the efficacy of OVs [45]. Angiostatin and endostatin are two additional endogenous, antiangiogenic proteins that have been shown to improve the efficacy of OVs [46, 47]. This effect is not limited to oHSV but extends to oMV that express a fusion protein of endostatin and angiostatin and has been shown to efficiently decrease tumour-associated blood vessel formation and improve antitumor efficacy [47].

Considering tumors initiate angiogenesis for tumor growth and the implication of angiogenesis in therapeutic resistance, therapeutic options that inhibit this crucial process are necessary. OVs possess inherent antiangiogenic properties and can be armed with additional antiangiogenic payloads, making them promising agents to overcome therapy resistance.

3.4 Targeting Components of the Tumor Extracellular Matrix with Virotherapy to Overcome Therapy Resistance

The extracellular matrix (ECM) is the dynamic network of macromolecules which surrounds cells and tissues and plays a significant role in cancer progression. This dysregulated network is associated with increased cell proliferation [48], angiogenesis [49, 50], and invasion [51]. The quantity and composition of the cancer ECM is also associated with cancer progression and patient prognosis [52–57] and contributes to therapy resistance by acting as a physical barrier, preventing drug dispersion and activating tumor cell signaling [58]. Oncolytic viral therapies are also susceptible to ECM-mediated inhibition, and several strategies that are being developed to overcome this mechanism of resistance will be reviewed.

3.4.1 Tumor Extracellular Matrix Limits Oncolytic Virus Efficacy

Several preclinical studies have identified ECM components as significant factors that limit OV efficacy. Collagen is a common ECM component shown to promote tumor progression [59]. McKee et al. demonstrated that fibrillar collagen significantly reduced viral spread following intra-tumoral injection of oHSV [60]. Multiphoton imaging of human melanoma xenografts treated with OV revealed that viral particles were restricted from collagen-dense areas of tumors. The collagen appeared to exclude the virus based on size, as smaller sized particles were able to penetrate both collagen-rich and collagen-poor regions of the tumor. Treating tumors with collagenase to digest ECM collagen significantly improved the distribution of the virus and enhanced anti-tumor efficacy. A similar study using the collagen type IV degrading enzyme, MMP9, also increased OV spread in mouse brain tumor models [61]. Additionally, hyaluronan (HA) is a large glycosaminoglycan polymer common to many tumor types, with high HA levels associated with metastatic potential and poor OS [56, 62]. HA has been shown to reduce oAd spread within injected tumors [63]. In high HA-containing melanoma and prostate xenograft models, co-injection of OV with hyaluronidase significantly improved virus spread and OS compared to animals treated with virus or hyaluronidase alone [63].

Cumulatively, these early studies suggest that the therapeutic efficacy of OV therapy may be improved by modulating the ECM.

3.4.2   ECM-Modifying OVs Can Overcome ECM-Mediated Resistance

A key advantage of OVs compared to other modalities is that they can be genetically engineered to express therapeutic payloads, with several groups having manufactured OVs encoding ECM degrading enzymes. Compared to frequent and transient injections of ECM modulating molecules, arming OV with ECM modulating enzymes can achieve sustained and robust levels of an ECM-targeted payload. Building on the previous HA study, Guedan et al. created an oAd expressing human sperm hyaluronidase [64]. HA levels were greatly reduced in human melanoma xenograft tumors treated with a hyaluronidase-expressing OV. The authors demonstrated that the hyaluronidase encoding virus could enhance survival in two different mouse tumor models following both intra-tumoral and systemic delivery. Follow-up work demonstrated that the engineered virus-induced CD8+ T-cell infiltration and was efficacious in an immune-competent animal model and indicated that hyaluronidase expression does not suppress systemic anti-tumor immune responses [65]. A version of this virus, VCN-01, is currently in clinical trials for refractory retinoblastoma, pancreatic cancer, and other advanced solid tumors [66, 67]. The use of other ECM modulating factors such as relaxin, DNAse I, Proteinase K, decorin, and MMPs have also demonstrated improved virus spread and enhanced efficacy in preclinical tumor models [68–71]. Together, these reports confirm that OVs can be engineered to overcome ECM mediated resistance to viral spread.

3.4.3   Extracellular Matrix-Modifying Oncolytic Viruses Can Synergize with Existing Therapeutics

Chondroitin sulfate proteoglycans are a family of proteoglycans that are frequently overexpressed in a variety of cancers including glioma, melanoma, and prostate cancer and are associated with tumor invasion and progression [72–74]. Early studies demonstrated engineering an HSV-1 with a bacterial chondroitin-ase to digest these proteoglycans improved virus spread and animal survival in glioblastoma xenograft models [75]. In addition to improving OV-mediated efficacy, the expression of ECM remodeling molecules has the potential to improve the effectiveness of combination therapies by reducing interstitial pressure and overcoming the physical barriers to drug and immune cell penetration. These OVs can work synergistically to improve the delivery and efficacy of chemotherapeutic drugs. The combination of an OV encoding humanized bacterial chondroitinase with the chemotherapeutic temozolomide (TMZ) synergistically improved killing of patient-derived, glioblastoma neurospheres *in vitro*. The combination of the TMZ-modified OV significantly improved survival in an intracranial glioblastoma neurosphere model compared to either treatment alone [76, 77]. It is noteworthy that increased tumor invasion or metastasis has not been reported in any of the preclinical studies testing OV encoding for ECM remodeling enzymes [78]. The safety and efficacy of this approach in patients remains to be tested.

3.4.4 Other Extracellular Matrix Strategies

In addition to enhancing the delivery of small molecules, ECM targeted OVs could potentially synergize with cellular therapies. Concerning the activity of the adaptive immune system, the ECM contributes to the immunosuppressive microenvironment known to inhibit T-cell migration and activity in tumors. As a result, the TME has been one of the limiting factors for chimeric antigen receptor (CAR) T-cell therapies for solid tumors [79]. An OV encoding an ECM modulating molecule could theoretically improve both CAR T-cell penetration and counteract tumor-mediated immunosuppression through lysis of tumor cells and activation of anti-viral responses. The combination of ECM modifying oncolytic OVs to supplement immunologic cell therapies, such as CAR-T-cell therapies, remains to be tested.

The tumor ECM presents as a challenging barrier to cancer therapy. Novel OVs have been engineered to modulate the tumor ECM, and they demonstrate improved anti-tumor efficacy. These viruses can synergize with existing therapeutics to enhance tumor drug delivery and hold significant potential when delivered in combination with emerging immunotherapies.

3.5 Modulating the Anti-Viral Response of the Innate Immune System

The innate immune system is the body's front-line defense pathway that is activated upon infection, leading to the release of cytokines and recruitment of immune cells to the site of infection to clear the pathogen. The innate immune system has proven to be both a useful tool in OV therapy as well as a barrier in successful clinical translation. However, a better understanding of the challenges posed by the innate anti-viral response has led to the development of promising armed OV and combination therapies to circumvent these barriers.

3.5.1 Using Oncolytic Viruses with TNF-α to Target Tumor Growth

Tumor necrosis factor (TNF)-α functions as an effector of host defense by regulating the differentiation of natural killer (NK) cells and has also been implicated in promoting tumor angiogenesis, metastasis, and invasion in multiple solid tumors including ovarian, glioma, and lung cancer [80–82]. Exogenous or macrophage produced TNF-α accelerates epithelial to mesenchymal transition (EMT) and is linked to the acquisition of an invasive phenotype via NF-κB dependent induction of CXCR4, MCP-1, IL-8 and ICAM-1 in cancer cells [83–95]. However, TNF-α can also have anti-tumor properties, by directly engaging tumor cell receptors to induce apoptosis and indirectly through macrophage and NK cell activation in effector cell-mediated tumor cell death [96]. Although TNF-α has cytotoxic and cytostatic effects, many tumors are resistant to its cytotoxic effects [96].

Specifically, the development of OVs armed with TNF-α have demonstrated efficacy in the presence of anti-tumor immune cells. For example, a TNF-α expressing oAd was engineered and evaluated in models of melanoma [97]. Infection with this virus increased secretion of damage associated molecular patterns (DAMPs), adenosine triphosphate (ATP) and High Mobility Group Box Protein 1 (HMGB1). It also slowed tumor xenograft growth in a mouse model of melanoma and increased levels of cytotoxic T- and B-cells within the tumor, highlighting the increased immunogenicity following infection. A second generation of armed oAd expressing both TNF-α and IL-2 increased CD4+ and CD8+ T-cell tumor infiltration *in vivo* and enhanced splenocyte proliferation *ex vivo* [98]. Similarly, an oVSV armed with TNF-α given in combination with a supramolecular activation complex (Smac) mimetic compound to antagonize the inhibitor of apoptosis protein increased anti-tumor efficacy and survival of mice with tumors [99]. Additionally, the vascular permeabilizing effects of TNF-α have been exploited to enhance the delivery of oAd particles within tumor tissue after systemic delivery [100]. However, contrary to these studies, transient blockade of TNF-α with neutralizing antibodies significantly increased viral replication and enhanced survival in tumor-bearing mice [101]. Since different viruses induce different changes in the tumor ECM, the effects of TNF-α on virotherapy likely depend on the type of virus and the tumor site under exploration.

3.5.2 STING and Interferon Signaling

Stimulator of interferon genes (STING) is a transmembrane protein, which controls transcription of type 1 interferon (IFN) and other pro-inflammatory cytokines. In the presence of cytosolic DNA in infected cells, GMP-AMP synthase (cGAS) gets activated and produces cyclic GMP-AMP (cGAMP) [102]. Activation of the cGAS-STING pathway can promote cellular senescence as well as induce production of type I IFN from dendritic cells for anti-tumor priming of CD8+ T-cells. STING agonists have been tested in combination with chemotherapy, radiation, and immune checkpoint inhibitors as anti-cancer regimens [102] and have shown anti-tumor effects in syngeneic mouse models of colon cancer [103]. MK-1454, a cyclic dinucleotide STING agonist is currently being evaluated for safety in a multicenter dose escalation study both as a single agent and in combination with immune checkpoint blocking inhibitors (NCT03010176).

Additionally, the cGAS-STING pathway is important for detecting viral infections and mounting an anti-viral response. Cancers lacking adequate STING signaling responses exhibit increased susceptibility to OV therapy [104–107]. For example, in colorectal cancer, STING signaling is suppressed, limiting the production of type I IFNs, rendering colorectal cancer cells sensitive to OV activity [104]. Additionally, it has been shown that STING signaling is defective in a number of ovarian, melanoma and breast cancer cells and results in sensitivity to oHSV infection both *in vitro* and *in vivo* [104–106, 108]. These data suggest that modulating the STING pathway may enhance OV replication and efficacy through reduction of type I IFNs.

Concerning IFNs, type I IFNs have emerged to have dual characteristics whereby they play inflammatory and anti-tumor roles, while also playing roles in immunosuppression. For example, IFNs can directly inhibit tumor cell proliferation, induce senescence, cell cycle arrest, and apoptosis, suggesting benefit in anti-cancer therapy. However, type I IFNs can also increase expression of checkpoint inhibitors, resulting in stunted anti-tumor T-cell responses [109].

A robust type I IFN response is capable of rapidly clearing viral infections, and its activation has been implicated in acquired resistance to oAd therapy [110]. VSV resistant pancreatic cancer cells exhibit sustained levels of type I IFN production; however, inhibition of JAK/STAT signaling, which is downstream of IFN, rescues OV resistance [111]. Additionally, advanced bladder cancers have been shown express extremely low levels of the type I IFN receptor relative to normal bladder tissue and were exquisitely sensitive to VSV therapy [107]. In cancers with active type I IFN responses that can inhibit OV efficacy through rapid viral clearance, mechanisms to downregulate the type I IFN responses have been employed. For instance, it was shown that the anti-tumor efficacy of VSV is enhanced upon downregulation of IFNR [107]. As a result, siRNA was utilized for IFNR knockdown in bladder cancer cells previously deemed resistant to VSV treatment. Following IFNR knockdown, VSV viral replication was significantly enhanced. VSV in combination with a neutralizing antibody against the IFNR also increased viral replication of VSV in bladder cancer [107]. Collectively, these experiments suggest that tumors with defects in type I IFN production are susceptible to OV therapy.

Type I IFNs can also directly induce tumor cell death and activate an anti-tumor immune response [112, 113] and thus has been investigated in the context of OVs. For example, OVs expressing various forms of type I IFN have been developed to stimulate anti-tumor immune responses. Studies of murine models of non-small cell lung cancer (NSCLC) [114] treated with VSV engineered to express IFN, revealed increased anti-tumor immunity and enhanced survival with similar results observed in mesothelioma models [23]. Additionally, decreased regulatory T-cell infiltration and increased CD8+ T-cell infiltration in the NSCLC model were also identified, highlighting the immune stimulatory function of IFN-β [114]. Chemotherapy and radiation therapy in combination with an IFN-α expressing oAd have also been observed to enhance pancreatic cancer cell death *in vitro* and *in vivo* [115]. Future investigations into methods to tightly regulate TNF-α production in the tumor microenvironment in both spatial and temporal ways will be needed to maximize the therapeutic benefits of the anti-viral and anti-tumor roles of type I IFNs.

Furthermore, in order to exploit the macrophage-mediated anti-cancer effects of IFN-γ, an oncolytic VSV was engineered to express IFN-γ and evaluated in murine models of breast cancer. VSV treatment resulted in increased activation of dendritic cells and increased pro-inflammatory cytokine secretion compared to the parental virus. These anti-tumor immune responses elicited by the oVSV slowed tumor growth, decreased lung metastases and increased overall survival [24]. This pre-clinical study suggests that encoding IFN-y in an OV may initiate potent anti-tumor effects while reducing the toxicity associated with the systemic administration of this cytokine. Cytokines and signaling pathways involved in the innate immune responses, which clear viruses and OVs, are also important for anti-tumor immune responses. OVs have been engineered and combined with other therapeutics to decrease viral clearance while harnessing the anti-tumor properties necessary for maximum therapeutic efficacy.

3.6   Cellular Defenses Impacting Virotherapy

While the immune system plays a critical role in protecting our bodies from pathogens, in the context of OVs, it presents as a double-edged sword. Although OV treatment provides an avenue for the release of tumor peptides from a destroyed cancer cell which can then educate the host immune system to reject neoplasms, immune-mediated viral clearance directly limits virus-mediated destruction of cancer cells. Members of the innate immune system implicated in virus clearance predominantly include macrophages, which can be polarized to a pro-inflammatory M1 phenotype or immunosuppressive M2-like phenotype, and NK cells [116].

3.6.1   *Tumor-Associated Macrophages and Virotherapy*

Tumor-associated macrophages (TAM) induce tumor angiogenesis, are predominantly M2 in phenotype, and can in some cases, account for up to 80% percent of the tumor bulk [117, 118]. TAMs also contribute to an immunosuppressive tumor microenvironment and are associated with resistance to chemotherapy and radiotherapy.

Viral infection has been shown to induce macrophage infiltration and change their polarization to M1 [34, 119]. Multiple studies have demonstrated that macrophages infiltrating tumors after virotherapy can accelerate viral elimination *in vivo* while also secreting tumor promoting cytokine TNF-α [101, 120, 121]. Furthermore, depletion of tumoral myeloid cells has been shown to improve anti-tumor responses in conjunction with OV [122]. Consistent with these observations, transient depletion of macrophages with immunosuppressive high-dose chemotherapy or treatment with immunosuppressive TGF-β prior to administration of oHSV has also been shown to enhance viral replication, spread, and efficacy [121]. This increased therapeutic response was accompanied by decreased infiltration and activation of macrophages and NK cells *in vivo* [123]. In a mouse model of Ewings sarcoma, macrophage depletion achieved through liposomal clodronate and trabectedin has also been used to reduce the amount of M2 macrophages, myeloid derived suppressor cells (MDSC), and NK cell infiltration in the tumor [124]. Recent studies by Delwar et al. have identified phosphorylation of STAT1/3 as a key event in the inhibition of oHSV-1 viral replication by macrophages and microglia in GBM [118]. Inhibition of STAT1/3 phosphorylation using oxindole/imidazole derivative C16, significantly reduced phagocytosis of the oHSV, resulting in tumor regression [118]. OVs engineered to express Vasculostatin (Vstat120), the N-terminal cleavage fragment of brain angiogenesis inhibitor 1 (BAI1) has also shown improved anti-tumor efficacy [42]. Apart from reduced angiogenesis, Vstat120 expression was also found to reduce macrophage and microglia infiltration in GBM and correlated with increased viral replication and altered macrophage TNF-α secretion [118].

As viral infection induces the recruitment of tumor attacking macrophages, some studies have demonstrated efficacy of harnessing virally mediated inflammation to switch TAMs to a tumor attacking M1-like phenotype. A recent report utilizing oncolytic influenza A virus (IAV) infection of lung tumors showed a functional modification of immunosuppressive lung TAMs into a tumor killing M1-like phenotype. This study showed the ability to harness oncolytic IAV to redirect immune cell functions within the TME to destroy tumor cells [125]. Arming of viruses to enhance effector cell function has also been exploited. For example, a recent study uncovered that an IL-12-armed HSV synergized with immune checkpoint blocking antibodies, anti-PD1 and anti-CTLA-4, to increase macrophage and T-cell influx, resulting in tumor rejection. Depletion or inhibition of infiltrating macrophages and/or T-cells reversed the enhanced therapeutic efficacy of the combination of IL-12 expressing oHSV and immune checkpoint blockade [126].

3.6.2 Natural Killer Cells and Their Effects on Virotherapy

NK cells are another critical member of the innate immune cellular defense whose primary function is to destroy virus-infected cells and tumor cells. Unlike cytotoxic T-cells, NK cells can exert their functions without the presence of antibodies or MHC antigens [127]. An increased influx of NK cells in tumors has been shown to impede virotherapy, with their depletion increasing the anti-tumor efficacy of virotherapy [128]. A recent study uncovered that a specific antiviral antibody is not required to link NK cells to HSV-infected tumor cells, as the Fc domain of any human IgG is sufficient to bridge NK cells with HSV infected cells [129]. While innate NK cells result in viral clearance, their increased activation after infection also provides an opportunity to exploit their activity for therapy. Virus-mediated sensitization of tumors to NK cell-mediated killing has been exploited to improve therapeutic responses to CAR-engineered NK cells targeting the epidermal growth factor receptor (EGFR) [130]. Consistent with this concept, an oAd encoding for IL-12 and IL-18 was shown to increase tumor cell infiltration of T- and NK cells with an enhanced therapeutic benefit, which has been associated with improved response to Newcastle disease virus by promoting anti-tumor adaptive immunity [131]. Reovirus treatment of murine melanoma cells has also been shown to activate NK cells via activation of receptors NKp46/NCR on NK cells, and this was found to be essential for its therapeutic response [132]. While NK cells can inhibit OV efficacy through enhanced viral clearance, infiltration of NK cells has also demonstrated increased anti-tumor immunity. Collectively these studies unravel a conundrum wherein both NK cell depletion and NK cell adjuvant therapy appear to improve anti-tumor efficacy of OVs.

Mathematical modelling of this divergent activity uncovered that when the endogenous response to OV infection of infiltrating NK cells is small, the primary effect of endogenous NK cells is to seek out and clear OV infected cells, eliminating the virus. Thus, when few infiltrating NK cells recruited into the tumor, they are incapable of launching an effective anti-tumor response. However, when adjuvant NK cell therapy is provided, the increased effector to target ratio permits exploitation of NK cell activation to more effectively result in tumor clearance [133]. Balancing cellular mediated viral clearance with the anti-tumor properties of macrophages and NK cells is a difficult task. However, by utilizing various treatment regimens including transient cellular depletion and harnessing the unique engineering capabilities of OVs, this task is manageable.

3.7   Application of Virotherapy to Improve Response Rates to Immunotherapy

Immunotherapies have emerged as a powerful strategy for treating cancer with checkpoint inhibitors, bispecific T-cell engagers, and adoptive cellular therapies demonstrating promise in the clinic [134]. However, as the number of patients treated with these modalities increases, so does the variation in patient responses. Additionally, the strongly immunosuppressive TME and the physical barriers imposed by ECM can further restrict the activity, access, and efficacy of many immunotherapies [134]. To overcome these obstacles, researchers are actively pursuing combination studies that come with the challenge of balancing efficacy and toxicity. OVs are being increasingly recognized for their immunotherapeutic potential. This section will review recent advances in the OV field as well as highlight the emerging preclinical and clinical data combining OVs with immunotherapies to overcome some of the challenges associated with cancer treatments.

3.7.1   Oncolytic Viral Therapy: Immune-Mediated Mechanism of Action and Synergy

A complete understanding of how OVs exert their anti-tumor effects is critical for the improvement of this modality and the rational combination of OVs with other immunotherapies. OVs mediate their effects through direct tumor cell killing and by the release of tumor antigens, which can prime systemic, anti-tumor immune responses, which is well characterized by Moesta et al. [135]. In this study, immunocompetent mice bearing bilateral tumors were treated by intratumoral administration of oHSV into one tumor leading to an anti-tumor response in both tumors. Tumor regressions in the non-injected tumors could not be attributed to virus-induced tumor cell destruction but were dependent on tumor-specific CD8+ T-cells such that their depletion inhibited anti-tumor efficacy. These studies suggest that the virus could generate systemic, anti-tumor immune responses with implications for tumor cell rejection in locations distant from the injected tumor site. The critical role of T-cells in mediating OV efficacy has also been demonstrated in immune competent animal models with other OVs including reovirus [136] and adenovirus [137].

While previously limited to pre-clinical evidence, recent clinical trial data have emerged that further support this proposed mechanism of action. Talimogene lapherparevec, a modified oHSV engineered to express GM-CSF to enhance anti-tumor immune responses, represents the first OV approved in the US and the EU. This approval was based largely on a phase III trial with 436 patients for advanced melanoma. Patients receiving talimogene laherparepvec had a 10.8% complete response rate and significantly improved durable responses rates compared to a control arm of patients receiving subcutaneous GM-CSF (16.3% vs. 2.1%, respectively) [10]. As a monotherapy, talimogene laherparepvec performed well, and this study provided one of the first opportunities to investigate OV mechanism of action in a large, clinical setting. A lesion level analysis of talimogene laherparepvec treated patients revealed a strong local response at the site of virus injection with nearly half of injected lesions completely resolved [10]. These data highlight the ability of OVs to potently and preferentially replicate in and destroy tumor cells at the sites of virus infection. In addition to the injected lesions, researchers observed 34% of non-injected, non-visceral lesions and 15% of non-injected, visceral lesions decreased in size by at least half. While these data cannot conclusively exclude the presence of virus in non-injected tumors, they strongly suggest talimogene laherparepvec can prime immune responses capable of mediating anti-tumor effects at distance tumor sites.

In support of these findings, observations of tumor regressions in non-injected lesions have been made in clinical trials with oVV and CV [138, 139]. Additional evidence for the generation of anti-tumor immune responses can be found in a phase I oMV clinical trial for ovarian cancer where OV treatment increased tumor antigen specific T-cell responses in several patients [16]. In a clinical trial with oVV for hepatocellular carcinoma (HCC), investigators found virus administration increased humoral anti-tumor immunity as determined by *ex vivo* complement-dependent cytotoxicity assays with HCC tumor cell lines treated with patient sera [12]. Cumulatively, this pre-clinical and clinical data suggests local destruction of tumor cells at the site of OV infection can prime systemic anti-tumor responses.

3.7.2   Oncolytic Viruses as Delivery Vehicles of Cytokine Payloads

Understanding the processes by which OVs mediate their anti-tumor effects provides opportunities to improve this modality. Many next-generation viruses have been created to encode immune-stimulating molecules as they can lead to robust levels of the desired molecule within the tumor, and localized expression of immunostimulatory payloads, reducing the risk of systemic toxicity. IL-12 is a pleiotropic cytokine capable of stimulating potent NK and T-cell anti-tumor responses and has been evaluated in over 50 clinical trials [140]. The clinical success of IL-12 has been somewhat limited for two reasons:

1. IL-12 can generate severe toxicity following intravenous administration, and
2. The immunosuppressive TME can resist IL-12 mediated anti-tumor activity [141].

OVs expressing IL-12 can potentially overcome both of these barriers as local production of IL-12 can reduce the risk of systemic toxicity. OV-mediated tumor cell death and inflammation can reactivate immunologically "cold" tumors. Markert et al. evaluated an oHSV encoding IL-12 in a syngeneic mouse brain tumor model, which significantly improved survival compared to mice treated with saline or an OV containing no payload [142]. Additionally, no toxicity was observed from this virus when it was injected into the brain of primates. A variant of this virus, M032, is currently in clinical trials for malignant glioma (NCT02062827).

The large packaging capacity of many OVs allows multiple cytokines to be encoded in the viral genome. For instance, Choi et al. generated an oAd expressing IL-12 and IL-18 [131]. IL-18 induces IFNγ expression and is thought to improve anti-tumor immune responses. In a syngeneic B16-F10 murine melanoma model, mice treated with the combination virus survived significantly longer than animals treated with PBS, a no payload control virus, or viruses encoding individual payloads. The authors demonstrated that the combination of cytokine payloads acted synergistically to prime tumor-specific immune responses as seen via IFNγ ELISPOT assays, immune cell infiltration into tumors, and cytokine profiles. OVs encoding various other cytokines and chemokines have been created to manipulate the tumor immune microenvironment and help drive systemic immune responses initiated by OV infection [123, 143, 144].

In addition to cytokines, OVs encoding other transgenes have been generated to modulate inflammation within the tumor microenvironment. PTEN loss is characteristic of a variety of cancers, and mutations are known to increase tumor cell survival and proliferation. Interestingly, PTEN loss also induces the production of immunosuppressive cytokines in the TME, which is associated with resistance to T-cell mediated therapies [145]. Russell et al. created an oHSV encoding a PTEN isoform, PTENα, to counteract the negative impact of PTEN loss in the tumor [146]. In an immune competent mouse model, animals treated with a PTENα-expressing virus lived significantly longer than animals treated with a control virus. Compared to a control virus, this modified virus also enhanced immune cell infiltration and tumor-specific T-cell responses. Interestingly, the authors also found that the PTENα encoding virus reduced the levels of PDL-1 on the surface of infected tumor cells, which is an active target for immunotherapies and normally contributes to tumor immunosuppression. Cumulatively, these studies demonstrate that novel, next-generation OVs that can be engineered to enhance anti-tumor immune responses while maintaining safety.

3.7.3 Oncolytic Viral Therapy to Enhance Immune Checkpoint Blockade

Immune checkpoint blockade is a rapidly growing segment of cancer immunotherapy. The blockade of inhibitory signals present on tumor cells or T-cells can enhance anti-tumor immune responses, and the success of this approach is apparent in the number of trials with checkpoint blockade agents. Clinical data suggest that patients with higher mutational burden, neoantigens, and CD8+ T-cell infiltration in their tumors are the best responders to immune checkpoint inhibitors [147]. Thus, efficacy is limited for many patients with immunologically "cold" tumors. Based on their ability to inflame treated tumors, recruit immune cells, and prime anti-tumor immune responses, OVs are ideally suited for combination with checkpoint inhibitor therapies. The combination with OVs may provide therapeutics benefits to patients who may otherwise not benefit from checkpoint blockade agents. Exciting preclinical [135, 148, 149] and clinical work is emerging supporting the combination of checkpoint inhibitors with OVs.

There are 17 ongoing clinical trials combining OVs with checkpoint inhibitors, and here, we will review the currently published clinical data [150]. Talimogene laherparepvec has been tested in combination with ipilimumab a CTLA-4 inhibitor and pembrolizumab a PD-1 inhibitor in a phase II study for advanced melanoma. Patients were given ipilimumab alone or in combination with talimogene laherparepvec. The objective response rate in the combination group was more than double that of the ipilimumab group (39% vs. 18%, respectively) [151]. Additionally, patients receiving combination treatment had improved responses in non-injected, visceral lesions, with 52% having a decrease in visceral lesion size from baseline compared to 23% of patients in the ipilimumab group. Beyond symptoms associated with viral infection, combination therapy did not result in increased toxicity compared to ipilimumab alone. The combination of talimogene laherparepvec with pembrolizumab has also shown significant promise. In a phase Ib trial for advanced melanoma, patients receiving talimogene laherparepvec and pembrolizumab achieved an objective response rate of 61.9% and a complete response rate of 33.3% [152]. While not directly comparable, pembrolizumab therapy in treatment-naïve patients with advanced melanoma historically results in objective response rates of ~35% [153]. As in the ipilimumab study, the combination of pembrolizumab with talimogene laherparepvec did not increase the toxicities compared to single-agent therapy. Authors found treatment with talimogene laherparepvec increased CD8+ T-cell infiltration into tumors which was associated with responses to the combination treatment. Interestingly, the investigators observed clinical responses in patients with low CD8+ T-cell density in their tumors at baseline suggesting that talimogene laherparepvec may be capable of turning immunologically "cold" tumors "hot", which has resulted in a phase III being underway (NCT02263508).

Systemic administration of checkpoint inhibitors has also been associated with cases of severe toxicity [154, 155], and several investigators have created OVs encoding checkpoint inhibitors or T-cell activators. Viruses encoding PDL-1 inhibitors, CTLA-4 inhibitors, PD-1 inhibitors, CD40L, and other molecules have been created to overcome the potential toxicities associated with the systemic administration of these agents [156]. The oncolytic virus company Replimmune is currently developing an oHSV encoding a CTLA-4 antibody-like molecule for clinical trials in 2019. Together these findings suggest the combination of OVs with checkpoint inhibitors may overcome some of the current obstacles to immune checkpoint therapy.

3.8   Applications of Virotherapy to Chimeric Antigen Receptor T-Cell Therapy

Adoptive cell transfer therapies, such as chimeric antigen receptor (CAR) T-cell therapies, have demonstrated strong efficacy in liquid cancers. However, the TME continues to present challenges typical of an immunosuppressive environment. Significant efforts are underway to overcome these barriers, and combinations with OVs may provide one potential path forward. Several preclinical studies have been conducted to evaluate the therapeutic potential of the combination of OVs. Nishio et al. evaluated the combination of an oAd with CAR-T cells in a neuroblastoma mouse model [157]. The virus was also designed to encode IL-15 and RANTES to promote inflammation at the site of injection. The combination therapy increased CAR-T cell tumor infiltration, persistence, and anti-tumour activity, resulting in an improvement in overall survival compared to either agent alone. Authors also noted that while an oAd expressing no cytokines improved animal survival with CAR-T cell therapy, the inclusion of IL-15 and RANTES payloads further enhanced this effect. This observation highlights the growing potential of next-generation engineered viruses. Other groups have shown the benefits of this combination approach for CAR-T [158, 159] and other adoptive T-cell therapies [160–162], emphasizing the increasing interest in this combination therapy.

In addition to the adoptive transfer of tumor-targeted T-cells, another approach gaining popularity is retargeting existing T-cells using bispecific T-cell engagers (BiTEs) which are antibodies that simultaneously target T-cell surface molecules and tumor antigens. Binding of BiTE molecules to T-cells and tumors triggers the killing of tumor cells [163, 164]. BiTEs are currently in clinical trials for a variety of indications, and Blinatumomab was recently approved for B-cell precursor acute lymphoblastic leukemia. Trafficking of BiTEs is a largely passive process that can make tumor targeting challenging. Encoding oncolytic viruses with BiTE-like molecules could improve tumor delivery and activity especially for solid tumor indications. Feng et al. created an oVV encoding a BiTE-like molecule targeted to tumor antigen EphA2 [165]. In a lung cancer mouse model, researchers demonstrated that the modified virus had enhanced anti-tumor activity and prolonged survival significantly longer than a control virus. In a series of *in vitro* studies, secretion of the BiTE-like molecule could mediate bystander effects and kill uninfected cells when co-cultured with peripheral blood mononuclear cells (PBMCs). These results further highlight the potential of this combination. Additional OVs encoding BiTE-like molecules have been evaluated with similar results, including BiTE-like payloads targeting cancer-associated fibroblasts in the immunosuppressive tumor stromal compartment [166, 167]. The combination of OVs with BiTEs represents a novel approach to improve cancer immunotherapies in certain tumor indications.

Emerging research suggests that these anti-tumor immune responses can be further enhanced by re-engineering OVs to encode potent payloads that can be expressed locally in tumors. Since OV therapy has proven to be safe modality, it is uniquely suited for combination studies with existing immunotherapies. Combination studies with checkpoint inhibitors, adoptive T-cell transfer therapies, BiTE-like molecules, and other agents [168] have shown significant promise in both pre-clinical and clinical settings, demonstrating the ability of OVs to overcome some of the challenges associated with cancer treatments.

3.9 Stem Cells as Trojan Horses for Enhanced Systemic Oncolytic Virus Delivery

One of the key limitations of OV therapy is systemic delivery, and consequently dissemination of virus to distant sites. As such, the idea of harnessing "Trojan horse"-like strategies using stem cells to deliver OV to tumor sites with stealth is exciting, and currently under exploration. This is because unmodified stem cells have the ability to migrate to sites of injury or inflammation, and this property has been exploited for the treatment of stroke [169, 170], degenerative disease [171], trauma [172], and myocardial infarction [173]. The microenvironment of solid tumors is no different from that of non-healing wounds, and thus, can attract stem cells to avidly migrate towards them [174–178].

Neural stem cells (NSCs) for brain tumors was the first utilization of stem cells due to their extensive ability to migrate within the brain [179]. However, the challenges presented by harvesting NSCs lead to interest being refocused to alternative stem cell populations such as mesenchymal stem cells (MSCs) which can more easily be harvested from tissues such as bone marrow, blood, and adipose tissue. MSCs delivered by intravascular injections have demonstrated a significant ability to home to tumors. Their lack of co-stimulatory molecules leads to reduced immunogenicity, and their relative resistance to chemotherapy makes them desirable as carriers for therapeutic payloads [176, 180].

With respect to OVs, the therapeutic efficacy of oAd loaded into menstrual blood derived stem cells was investigated and demonstrated the ability to override virus neutralization and were more effective at inhibiting tumor growth in vivo [181]. Intravascular delivery of MSCs armed with oHSV were also found to effectively home to metastatic melanoma and GBM in the brain and significantly prolong the survival of mice [182, 183]. Adipose-derived MSCs have also been exploited to serve as carriers for an oncolytic measles virus. MSCs could be infected with MV, and MV loaded MSCs could home to tumors in mice, and significantly prolonged survival of mice bearing ovarian cancer [180]. In a recent study, the safety and efficacy of Celyvir (autologous marrow-derived MSCs loaded with an oAd) for treating pediatric neuroblastoma patients was investigated. While the safety profile was excellent, clinical outcome was variable in this small cohort of patients [184]. The ability of MSCs to home to tumors and deliver OVs, makes them an attractive option for overcoming antibody neutralization of OVs and enhancing the feasibility of systemic delivery.

3.10 Interactions Between DNA Damage Response and Oncolytic Viruses

One of the major challenges intrinsic to DNA viruses is their requirement to utilize cellular machinery for DNA synthesis and replication. Therefore, the accessibility of this machinery is important to the therapeutic efficacy of OVs, where some OVs have developed means to increase viral replication and have improved therapeutic potential. For example, HSV has developed a means to usurp the cellular machinery by utilizing components of DNA damage response machinery while also exploiting mechanisms to avoid anti-viral restriction. Typically, HSV manipulates DNA Damage Response (DDR) genes to help promote its replication while concurrently preventing checkpoint blockade to continue cellular and viral replication.

As such, radiation, as well as other DNA damaging chemotherapeutic agents, have been demonstrated to significantly increase oHSV titers in many different cancers both *in vitro* and *in vivo* [185–189]. This synergistic effect is hypothesized to be the result of radiation-mediated increases in cellular growth arrest and DNA damage-inducible protein (GADD34) expression. Radiation-mediated upregulation of GADD34 can functionally compensate for some of the replication deficits of *ICP34.5*, a key neurovirulence gene deleted to improve safety of vectors, deleted viruses leading to increased viral replication. These synergistic properties are seen in multiple clinical models with significantly greater tumor cell killing observed with combination therapy [185–188, 190].

Another virus capable of exploiting DNA damage repair machinery is the adenovirus, where adenovirus-induced host cell DNA damage can potentiate the cytotoxic effects of oAd [191]. oAd mediated disruption of the signaling pathway controlling DNA repair thus renders infected cells sensitive to ionizing radiation *in vitro* and *in vivo* [192]. Additionally, since inhibitors of poly ADP ribose polymerase (PARP) increase sensitivity to DNA damaging agents, oAd induced DNA damage, can also be exploited to synergize with PARP inhibitors to induce cell death [193]. Adenovirus-mediated downregulation of the damage-repair enzyme, O(6)-methylguanine-DNA methyltransferase (MGMT), has also been shown to synergize with TMZ [194].

Apart from increasing DNA damage, chemotherapy-induced changes in cells can also be harnessed to improve viral entry and/or fitness. For example, upregulation of cellular unfolded protein response upon ER stress induced by proteasome inhibitors can augment HSV replication and improve therapeutic outcome [195]. Interestingly, this also sensitized tumor cells to NK cell-mediated killing and a combination of oHSV with a proteasome inhibitor, and adjuvant NK cell therapy improved therapeutic response [196]. Histone deacetylase inhibitors (HDACis) have been shown to induce an upregulation of the Reovirus entry receptor, junctional adhesion molecule 1 (JAM-1), increasing Reolysin-mediated entry and tumor cell killing both *in vitro* and *in vivo* [197].

3.11   Conclusions

OVs are promising agents for anti-cancer therapy that can directly lyse infected cells and induce changes in the tumor microenvironment that impact efficacy (Fig. 3.2). Pre-clinical and clinical evaluation of different OVs has unearthed several barriers that can limit efficacy. However, a systematic understanding of these barriers provides an opportunity for engineering new therapeutic drugs and

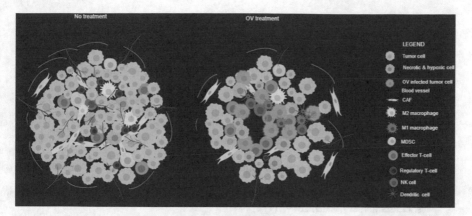

Fig. 3.2 Oncolytic virus infection in a solid tumor. The tumor microenvironment is composed of tumor cells, stromal cells (cancer associated fibroblasts; CAFs), and immune cells (tumor associated macrophages; TAMs, myeloid derived suppressor cells; MDSCs, T-cells, NK cells, and dendritic cells), all of which can be educated by the tumor to aid in tumor growth. Following oncolytic virus (OV) treatment, tumor cells undergo cell death and the surrounding tumor vasculature can also be destroyed. OVs also induce an immune response, resulting in increased infiltration of M1 macrophages, effector T-cells, NK cells and dendritic cells, leading to further tumor cell clearance

treatment regimens that can maximize benefit. The tumor ECM is associated with increased angiogenesis and poor perfusion with a concurrent increase in interstitial pressure, which promotes tumor growth and restricts the delivery of anti-cancer therapies. OVs engineered to express transgenes that directly antagonize angiogenesis have revealed therapeutic benefit. Additionally, OVs encoding for ECM modulating enzymes have also shown improved viral spread and anti-tumor efficacy in multiple preclinical studies. The efficacy of systemic delivery of OVs has been improved by the utilization of "Trojan horse"-like techniques to discreetly deliver viral cargo to "tumor addresses." The obvious "white elephant" in the field is to understand how to control innate defense responses that mediate virus clearance, while also maximizing the development of anti-tumor immunity to induce systemic tumor clearance. Although barriers outlined in this chapter present challenges towards maximizing OV efficacy, multiple innovative approaches advocate for continued pursuit of this very promising anti-cancer therapy.

References

1. Liang M. Oncorine, the world first oncolytic virus medicine and its update in China. Curr Cancer Drug Targets. 2018;18(2):171–6.
2. Fountzilas C, Patel S, Mahalingam D. Review: oncolytic virotherapy, updates and future directions. Oncotarget. 2017;8(60):102617–39.
3. Goradel NH, et al. Oncolytic adenovirus: a tool for cancer therapy in combination with other therapeutic approaches. J Cell Physiol. 2019;234:8636–46.

4. Bischoff JR, et al. An adenovirus mutant that replicates selectively in p53-deficient human tumor cells. Science. 1996;274(5286):373–6.
5. Jiang H, et al. Oncolytic adenovirus research evolution: from cell-cycle checkpoints to immune checkpoints. Curr Opin Virol. 2015;13:33–9.
6. Garber K. China approves world's first oncolytic virus therapy for cancer treatment. J Natl Cancer Inst. 2006;98(5):298–300.
7. Niemann J, Kuhnel F. Oncolytic viruses: adenoviruses. Virus Genes. 2017;53(5):700–6.
8. Kaur B, Chiocca EA, Cripe TP. Oncolytic HSV-1 virotherapy: clinical experience and opportunities for progress. Curr Pharm Biotechnol. 2012;13(9):1842–51.
9. Martuza RL. Conditionally replicating herpes vectors for cancer therapy. J Clin Invest. 2000;105(7):841–6.
10. Andtbacka RH, et al. Talimogene Laherparepvec improves durable response rate in patients with advanced melanoma. J Clin Oncol. 2015;33(25):2780–8.
11. Guo ZS, et al. Vaccinia virus-mediated cancer immunotherapy: cancer vaccines and oncolytics. J Immunother Cancer. 2019;7(1):6.
12. Heo J, et al. Randomized dose-finding clinical trial of oncolytic immunotherapeutic vaccinia JX-594 in liver cancer. Nat Med. 2013;19(3):329–36.
13. Lauer UM, et al. Phase I study of oncolytic vaccinia virus GL-ONC1 in patients with peritoneal carcinomatosis. Clin Cancer Res. 2018;24(18):4388–98.
14. Kim M. Naturally occurring reoviruses for human cancer therapy. BMB Rep. 2015;48(8):454–60.
15. Mahalingam D, et al. A phase II study of Pelareorep (REOLYSIN((R))) in combination with Gemcitabine for patients with advanced pancreatic adenocarcinoma. Cancers (Basel). 2018;10(6).
16. Galanis E, et al. Oncolytic measles virus expressing the sodium iodide symporter to treat drug-resistant ovarian cancer. Cancer Res. 2015;75(1):22–30.
17. Dispenzieri A, et al. Phase I trial of systemic administration of Edmonston strain of measles virus genetically engineered to express the sodium iodide symporter in patients with recurrent or refractory multiple myeloma. Leukemia. 2017;31(12):2791–8.
18. Msaouel P, et al. Clinical trials with oncolytic measles virus: current status and future prospects. Curr Cancer Drug Targets. 2018;18(2):177–87.
19. Desjardins A, et al. Recurrent glioblastoma treated with recombinant poliovirus. N Engl J Med. 2018;379(2):150–61.
20. Newcombe NG, et al. Cellular receptor interactions of C-cluster human group A coxsackieviruses. J Gen Virol. 2003;84(Pt 11):3041–50.
21. Miyamoto S, et al. Coxsackievirus B3 is an oncolytic virus with immunostimulatory properties that is active against lung adenocarcinoma. Cancer Res. 2012;72(10):2609–21.
22. Velazquez-Salinas L, et al. Oncolytic recombinant vesicular stomatitis virus (VSV) is nonpathogenic and nontransmissible in pigs, a natural host of VSV. Hum Gene Ther Clin Dev. 2017;28(2):108–15.
23. Willmon CL, et al. Expression of IFN-beta enhances both efficacy and safety of oncolytic vesicular stomatitis virus for therapy of mesothelioma. Cancer Res. 2009;69(19):7713–20.
24. Bourgeois-Daigneault MC, et al. Oncolytic vesicular stomatitis virus expressing interferongamma has enhanced therapeutic activity. Mol Ther Oncolytics. 2016;3:16001.
25. Pol JG, et al. Preclinical evaluation of a MAGE-A3 vaccination utilizing the oncolytic Maraba virus currently in first-in-human trials. Oncoimmunology. 2019;8(1):e1512329.
26. Martin NT, et al. Pre-surgical neoadjuvant oncolytic virotherapy confers protection against rechallenge in a murine model of breast cancer. Sci Rep. 2019;9(1):1865.
27. Ramjiawan RR, Griffioen AW, Duda DG. Anti-angiogenesis for cancer revisited: is there a role for combinations with immunotherapy? Angiogenesis. 2017;20(2):185–204.
28. Kaur B, et al. Hypoxia and the hypoxia-inducible-factor pathway in glioma growth and angiogenesis. Neuro-Oncology. 2005;7(2):134–53.

29. Angarita FA, et al. Mounting a strategic offense: fighting tumor vasculature with oncolytic viruses. Trends Mol Med. 2013;19(6):378–92.
30. Huszthy PC, et al. Cellular effects of oncolytic viral therapy on the glioblastoma microenvironment. Gene Ther. 2010;17(2):202–16.
31. Mahller YY, et al. Oncolytic HSV and erlotinib inhibit tumor growth and angiogenesis in a novel malignant peripheral nerve sheath tumor xenograft model. Mol Ther. 2007;15(2):279–86.
32. Benencia F, et al. Oncolytic HSV exerts direct antiangiogenic activity in ovarian carcinoma. Hum Gene Ther. 2005;16(6):765–78.
33. Breitbach CJ, et al. Targeted inflammation during oncolytic virus therapy severely compromises tumor blood flow. Mol Ther. 2007;15(9):1686–93.
34. Thorne AH, et al. Role of cysteine-rich 61 protein (CCN1) in macrophage-mediated oncolytic herpes simplex virus clearance. Mol Ther. 2014;22(9):1678–87.
35. Kurozumi K, et al. Effect of tumor microenvironment modulation on the efficacy of oncolytic virus therapy. J Natl Cancer Inst. 2007;99(23):1768–81.
36. Hong B, et al. Suppression of HMGB1 released in the glioblastoma tumor microenvironment reduces tumoral edema. Mol Ther Oncolytics. 2019;12:93–102.
37. Kurozumi K, et al. Oncolytic HSV-1 infection of tumors induces angiogenesis and upregulates CYR61. Mol Ther. 2008;16(8):1382–91.
38. Zhang W, et al. Bevacizumab with angiostatin-armed oHSV increases antiangiogenesis and decreases bevacizumab-induced invasion in U87 glioma. Mol Ther. 2012;20(1):37–45.
39. Yoo JY, et al. VEGF-specific short hairpin RNA-expressing oncolytic adenovirus elicits potent inhibition of angiogenesis and tumor growth. Mol Ther. 2007;15(2):295–302.
40. Guse K, et al. Antiangiogenic arming of an oncolytic vaccinia virus enhances antitumor efficacy in renal cell cancer models. J Virol. 2010;84(2):856–66.
41. Liu TC, et al. Dominant-negative fibroblast growth factor receptor expression enhances antitumoral potency of oncolytic herpes simplex virus in neural tumors. Clin Cancer Res. 2006;12(22):6791–9.
42. Hardcastle J, et al. Enhanced antitumor efficacy of vasculostatin (Vstat120) expressing oncolytic HSV-1. Mol Ther. 2010;18(2):285–94.
43. Bolyard C, et al. Doxorubicin synergizes with 34.5ENVE to enhance antitumor efficacy against metastatic ovarian cancer. Clin Cancer Res. 2014;20(24):6479–94.
44. Meisen WH, et al. Changes in BAI1 and nestin expression are prognostic indicators for survival and metastases in breast cancer and provide opportunities for dual targeted therapies. Mol Cancer Ther. 2015;14(1):307–14.
45. Mirochnik Y, Kwiatek A, Volpert OV. Thrombospondin and apoptosis: molecular mechanisms and use for design of complementation treatments. Curr Drug Targets. 2008;9(10):851–62.
46. Abdollahi A, et al. Endostatin's antiangiogenic signaling network. Mol Cell. 2004;13(5):649–63.
47. Hutzen B, et al. Treatment of medulloblastoma with oncolytic measles viruses expressing the angiogenesis inhibitors endostatin and angiostatin. BMC Cancer. 2014;14:206.
48. Tilghman RW, et al. Matrix rigidity regulates cancer cell growth and cellular phenotype. PLoS One. 2010;5(9):e12905.
49. Good DJ, et al. A tumor suppressor-dependent inhibitor of angiogenesis is immunologically and functionally indistinguishable from a fragment of thrombospondin. Proc Natl Acad Sci U S A. 1990;87(17):6624–8.
50. Fang J, et al. Matrix metalloproteinase-2 is required for the switch to the angiogenic phenotype in a tumor model. Proc Natl Acad Sci U S A. 2000;97(8):3884–9.
51. Brown GT, Murray GI. Current mechanistic insights into the roles of matrix metalloproteinases in tumour invasion and metastasis. J Pathol. 2015;237(3):273–81.
52. Provenzano PP, et al. Collagen density promotes mammary tumor initiation and progression. BMC Med. 2008;6:11.

53. Wang RX, et al. Predictive and prognostic value of matrix metalloproteinase (MMP)-9 in neoadjuvant chemotherapy for triple-negative breast cancer patients. BMC Cancer. 2018;18(1):909.
54. Chen Y, et al. The impact of matrix metalloproteinase 2 on prognosis and clinicopathology of breast cancer patients: a systematic meta-analysis. PLoS One. 2015;10(3):e0121404.
55. Conklin MW, et al. Aligned collagen is a prognostic signature for survival in human breast carcinoma. Am J Pathol. 2011;178(3):1221–32.
56. Ropponen K, et al. Tumor cell-associated hyaluronan as an unfavorable prognostic factor in colorectal cancer. Cancer Res. 1998;58(2):342–7.
57. Whatcott CJ, et al. Desmoplasia in primary tumors and metastatic lesions of pancreatic cancer. Clin Cancer Res. 2015;21(15):3561–8.
58. Munson JM, Shieh AC. Interstitial fluid flow in cancer: implications for disease progression and treatment. Cancer Manag Res. 2014;6:317–28.
59. Fang M, et al. Collagen as a double-edged sword in tumor progression. Tumour Biol. 2014;35(4):2871–82.
60. McKee TD, et al. Degradation of fibrillar collagen in a human melanoma xenograft improves the efficacy of an oncolytic herpes simplex virus vector. Cancer Res. 2006;66(5):2509–13.
61. Hong CS, et al. Ectopic matrix metalloproteinase-9 expression in human brain tumor cells enhances oncolytic HSV vector infection. Gene Ther. 2010;17(10):1200–5.
62. Auvinen P, et al. Hyaluronan in peritumoral stroma and malignant cells associates with breast cancer spreading and predicts survival. Am J Pathol. 2000;156(2):529–36.
63. Ganesh S, et al. Intratumoral coadministration of hyaluronidase enzyme and oncolytic adenoviruses enhances virus potency in metastatic tumor models. Clin Cancer Res. 2008;14(12):3933–41.
64. Guedan S, et al. Hyaluronidase expression by an oncolytic adenovirus enhances its intratumoral spread and suppresses tumor growth. Mol Ther. 2010;18(7):1275–83.
65. Al-Zaher AA, et al. Evidence of anti-tumoral efficacy in an immune competent setting with an iRGD-modified hyaluronidase-armed oncolytic adenovirus. Mol Ther Oncolytics. 2018;8:62–70.
66. Rodriguez-Garcia A, et al. Safety and efficacy of VCN-01, an oncolytic adenovirus combining fiber HSG-binding domain replacement with RGD and hyaluronidase expression. Clin Cancer Res. 2015;21(6):1406–18.
67. Martinez-Velez N, et al. The oncolytic adenovirus VCN-01 as therapeutic approach against pediatric osteosarcoma. Clin Cancer Res. 2016;22(9):2217–25.
68. Tedcastle A, et al. Actin-resistant DNAse I expression from oncolytic Adenovirus Enadenotucirev enhances its intratumoral spread and reduces tumor growth. Mol Ther. 2016;24(4):796–804.
69. Choi IK, et al. Effect of decorin on overcoming the extracellular matrix barrier for oncolytic virotherapy. Gene Ther. 2010;17(2):190–201.
70. Schafer S, et al. Vaccinia virus-mediated intra-tumoral expression of matrix metalloproteinase 9 enhances oncolysis of PC-3 xenograft tumors. BMC Cancer. 2012;12:366.
71. Ganesh S, et al. Relaxin-expressing, fiber chimeric oncolytic adenovirus prolongs survival of tumor-bearing mice. Cancer Res. 2007;67(9):4399–407.
72. Viapiano MS, et al. Novel tumor-specific isoforms of BEHAB/brevican identified in human malignant gliomas. Cancer Res. 2005;65(15):6726–33.
73. Yang J, et al. Melanoma chondroitin sulfate proteoglycan enhances FAK and ERK activation by distinct mechanisms. J Cell Biol. 2004;165(6):881–91.
74. Ricciardelli C, et al. Elevated levels of versican but not decorin predict disease progression in early-stage prostate cancer. Clin Cancer Res. 1998;4(4):963–71.
75. Dmitrieva N, et al. Chondroitinase ABC I-mediated enhancement of oncolytic virus spread and antitumor efficacy. Clin Cancer Res. 2011;17(6):1362–72.
76. Kim Y, et al. Choindroitinase ABC I-mediated enhancement of oncolytic virus spread and anti tumor efficacy: a mathematical model. PLoS One. 2014;9(7):e102499.

77. Jaime-Ramirez AC, et al. Humanized chondroitinase ABC sensitizes glioblastoma cells to temozolomide. J Gene Med. 2017;19(3).
78. Viapiano MS, Matthews RT. From barriers to bridges: chondroitin sulfate proteoglycans in neuropathology. Trends Mol Med. 2006;12(10):488–96.
79. Yan L, Liu B. Critical factors in chimeric antigen receptor-modified T-cell (CAR-T) therapy for solid tumors. Onco Targets Ther. 2019;12:193–204.
80. Kulbe H, et al. The inflammatory cytokine tumor necrosis factor-alpha generates an autocrine tumor-promoting network in epithelial ovarian cancer cells. Cancer Res. 2007;67(2):585–92.
81. Nabors LB, et al. Tumor necrosis factor alpha induces angiogenic factor up-regulation in malignant glioma cells: a role for RNA stabilization and HuR. Cancer Res. 2003;63(14):4181–7.
82. Tomita Y, et al. Spontaneous regression of lung metastasis in the absence of tumor necrosis factor receptor p55. Int J Cancer. 2004;112(6):927–33.
83. Bates RC, DeLeo MJ 3rd, Mercurio AM. The epithelial-mesenchymal transition of colon carcinoma involves expression of IL-8 and CXCR-1-mediated chemotaxis. Exp Cell Res. 2004;299(2):315–24.
84. Chuang MJ, et al. Tumor-derived tumor necrosis factor-alpha promotes progression and epithelial-mesenchymal transition in renal cell carcinoma cells. Cancer Sci. 2008;99(5):905–13.
85. Cheng SM, et al. Interferon-gamma regulation of TNFalpha-induced matrix metalloproteinase 3 expression and migration of human glioma T98G cells. Int J Cancer. 2007;121(6):1190–6.
86. Esteve PO, et al. Protein kinase C-zeta regulates transcription of the matrix metalloproteinase-9 gene induced by IL-1 and TNF-alpha in glioma cells via NF-kappa B. J Biol Chem. 2002;277(38):35150–5.
87. Hagemann T, et al. Enhanced invasiveness of breast cancer cell lines upon co-cultivation with macrophages is due to TNF-alpha dependent up-regulation of matrix metalloproteases. Carcinogenesis. 2004;25(8):1543–9.
88. Hagemann T, et al. Macrophages induce invasiveness of epithelial cancer cells via NF-kappa B and JNK. J Immunol. 2005;175(2):1197–205.
89. Ziprin P, et al. ICAM-1 mediated tumor-mesothelial cell adhesion is modulated by IL-6 and TNF-alpha: a potential mechanism by which surgical trauma increases peritoneal metastases. Cell Commun Adhes. 2003;10(3):141–54.
90. van Grevenstein WM, et al. Inflammatory cytokines stimulate the adhesion of colon carcinoma cells to mesothelial monolayers. Dig Dis Sci. 2007;52(10):2775–83.
91. Choo MK, et al. TAK1-mediated stress signaling pathways are essential for TNF-alpha-promoted pulmonary metastasis of murine colon cancer cells. Int J Cancer. 2006;118(11):2758–64.
92. Kitakata H, et al. Essential roles of tumor necrosis factor receptor p55 in liver metastasis of intrasplenic administration of colon 26 cells. Cancer Res. 2002;62(22):6682–7.
93. Kulbe H, et al. The inflammatory cytokine tumor necrosis factor-alpha regulates chemokine receptor expression on ovarian cancer cells. Cancer Res. 2005;65(22):10355–62.
94. Mochizuki Y, et al. TNF-alpha promotes progression of peritoneal metastasis as demonstrated using a green fluorescence protein (GFP)-tagged human gastric cancer cell line. Clin Exp Metastasis. 2004;21(1):39–47.
95. Alkhamesi NA, et al. ICAM-1 mediated peritoneal carcinomatosis, a target for therapeutic intervention. Clin Exp Metastasis. 2005;22(6):449–59.
96. Josephs SF, et al. Unleashing endogenous TNF-alpha as a cancer immunotherapeutic. J Transl Med. 2018;16(1):242.
97. Hirvinen M, et al. Immunological effects of a tumor necrosis factor alpha-armed oncolytic adenovirus. Hum Gene Ther. 2015;26(3):134–44.
98. Cervera-Carrascon V, et al. TNFa and IL-2 armed adenoviruses enable complete responses by anti-PD-1 checkpoint blockade. Oncoimmunology. 2018;7(5):e1412902.
99. Beug ST, et al. Combination of IAP antagonists and TNF-alpha-armed oncolytic viruses induce tumor vascular shutdown and tumor regression. Mol Ther Oncolytics. 2018;10:28–39.

100. Seki T, et al. Tumour necrosis factor-alpha increases extravasation of virus particles into tumour tissue by activating the Rho A/Rho kinase pathway. J Control Release. 2011;156(3):381–9.
101. Meisen WH, et al. The impact of macrophage- and microglia-secreted TNFalpha on oncolytic HSV-1 therapy in the glioblastoma tumor microenvironment. Clin Cancer Res. 2015;21(14):3274–85.
102. Khoo LT, Chen LY. Role of the cGAS-STING pathway in cancer development and oncotherapeutic approaches. EMBO Rep. 2018;19(12).
103. Ramanjulu JM, et al. Design of amidobenzimidazole STING receptor agonists with systemic activity. Nature. 2018;564(7736):439–43.
104. Xia T, et al. Deregulation of STING signaling in colorectal carcinoma constrains DNA damage responses and correlates with tumorigenesis. Cell Rep. 2016;14(2):282–97.
105. de Queiroz N, et al. Ovarian cancer cells commonly exhibit defective STING signaling which affects sensitivity to viral oncolysis. Mol Cancer Res. 2019;17:974–86.
106. Hummel JL, Safroneeva E, Mossman KL. The role of ICP0-Null HSV-1 and interferon signaling defects in the effective treatment of breast adenocarcinoma. Mol Ther. 2005;12(6):1101–10.
107. Zhang KX, et al. Down-regulation of type I interferon receptor sensitizes bladder cancer cells to vesicular stomatitis virus-induced cell death. Int J Cancer. 2010;127(4):830–8.
108. Xia T, Konno H, Barber GN. Recurrent loss of STING signaling in melanoma correlates with susceptibility to viral oncolysis. Cancer Res. 2016;76(22):6747–59.
109. Snell LM, McGaha TL, Brooks DG. Type I interferon in chronic virus infection and cancer. Trends Immunol. 2017;38(8):542–57.
110. Liikanen I, et al. Induction of interferon pathways mediates in vivo resistance to oncolytic adenovirus. Mol Ther. 2011;19(10):1858–66.
111. Moerdyk-Schauwecker M, et al. Resistance of pancreatic cancer cells to oncolytic vesicular stomatitis virus: role of type I interferon signaling. Virology. 2013;436(1):221–34.
112. Budhwani M, Mazzieri R, Dolcetti R. Plasticity of type I interferon-mediated responses in cancer therapy: from anti-tumor immunity to resistance. Front Oncol. 2018;8:322.
113. Zhang KJ, et al. A potent in vivo antitumor efficacy of novel recombinant type I interferon. Clin Cancer Res. 2017;23(8):2038–49.
114. Patel MR, et al. Vesicular stomatitis virus expressing interferon-beta is oncolytic and promotes antitumor immune responses in a syngeneic murine model of non-small cell lung cancer. Oncotarget. 2015;6(32):33165–77.
115. Salzwedel AO, et al. Combination of interferon-expressing oncolytic adenovirus with chemotherapy and radiation is highly synergistic in hamster model of pancreatic cancer. Oncotarget. 2018;9(26):18041–52.
116. Filley AC, Dey M, System I. Friend or foe of oncolytic virotherapy? Front Oncol. 2017;7:106.
117. Allavena P, et al. The Yin-Yang of tumor-associated macrophages in neoplastic progression and immune surveillance. Immunol Rev. 2008;222:155–61.
118. Delwar ZM, et al. Oncolytic virotherapy blockade by microglia and macrophages requires STAT1/3. Cancer Res. 2018;78(3):718–30.
119. Haseley A, et al. Extracellular matrix protein CCN1 limits oncolytic efficacy in glioma. Cancer Res. 2012;72(6):1353–62.
120. Kober C, et al. Microglia and astrocytes attenuate the replication of the oncolytic vaccinia virus LIVP 1.1.1 in murine GL261 gliomas by acting as vaccinia virus traps. J Transl Med. 2015;13:216.
121. Fulci G, et al. Cyclophosphamide enhances glioma virotherapy by inhibiting innate immune responses. Proc Natl Acad Sci U S A. 2006;103(34):12873–8.
122. Currier MA, et al. VEGF blockade enables oncolytic cancer virotherapy in part by modulating intratumoral myeloid cells. Mol Ther. 2013;21(5):1014–23.
123. Han J, et al. TGFbeta treatment enhances glioblastoma virotherapy by inhibiting the innate immune response. Cancer Res. 2015;75(24):5273–82.

124. Denton NL, et al. Myelolytic treatments enhance oncolytic herpes virotherapy in models of ewing sarcoma by modulating the immune microenvironment. Mol Ther Oncolytics. 2018;11:62–74.
125. Masemann D, et al. Oncolytic influenza virus infection restores immunocompetence of lung tumor-associated alveolar macrophages. Oncoimmunology. 2018;7(5):e1423171.
126. Saha D, Martuza RL, Rabkin SD. Macrophage polarization contributes to glioblastoma eradication by combination immunovirotherapy and immune checkpoint blockade. Cancer Cell. 2017;32(2):253–267 e5.
127. Rezvani K, et al. Engineering natural killer cells for cancer immunotherapy. Mol Ther. 2017;25(8):1769–81.
128. Alvarez-Breckenridge CA, et al. NK cells impede glioblastoma virotherapy through NKp30 and NKp46 natural cytotoxicity receptors. Nat Med. 2012;18(12):1827–34.
129. Dai HS, et al. The Fc domain of immunoglobulin is sufficient to bridge NK cells with virally infected cells. Immunity. 2017;47(1):159–170 e10.
130. Han J, et al. CAR-engineered NK cells targeting wild-type EGFR and EGFRvIII enhance killing of glioblastoma and patient-derived glioblastoma stem cells. Sci Rep. 2015;5:11483.
131. Choi IK, et al. Oncolytic adenovirus co-expressing IL-12 and IL-18 improves tumor-specific immunity via differentiation of T cells expressing IL-12Rbeta2 or IL-18Ralpha. Gene Ther. 2011;18(9):898–909.
132. Bar-On Y, et al. NKp46 recognizes the Sigma1 protein of Reovirus: implications for reovirus-based cancer therapy. J Virol. 2017;91(19).
133. Kim Y, et al. Complex role of NK cells in regulation of oncolytic virus-bortezomib therapy. Proc Natl Acad Sci U S A. 2018;115(19):4927–32.
134. Li Z, et al. Recent updates in cancer immunotherapy: a comprehensive review and perspective of the 2018 China Cancer Immunotherapy Workshop in Beijing. J Hematol Oncol. 2018;11(1):142.
135. Moesta AK, et al. Local delivery of OncoVEX(mGM-CSF) generates systemic antitumor immune responses enhanced by cytotoxic T-lymphocyte-associated protein blockade. Clin Cancer Res. 2017;23(20):6190–202.
136. Prestwich RJ, et al. Immune-mediated antitumor activity of reovirus is required for therapy and is independent of direct viral oncolysis and replication. Clin Cancer Res. 2009;15(13):4374–81.
137. Li X, et al. The efficacy of oncolytic adenovirus is mediated by T-cell responses against virus and tumor in Syrian Hamster model. Clin Cancer Res. 2017;23(1):239–49.
138. Park BH, et al. Use of a targeted oncolytic poxvirus, JX-594, in patients with refractory primary or metastatic liver cancer: a phase I trial. Lancet Oncol. 2008;9(6):533–42.
139. Hwang TH, et al. A mechanistic proof-of-concept clinical trial with JX-594, a targeted multi-mechanistic oncolytic poxvirus, in patients with metastatic melanoma. Mol Ther. 2011;19(10):1913–22.
140. Lasek W, Zagozdzon R, Jakobisiak M. Interleukin 12: still a promising candidate for tumor immunotherapy? Cancer Immunol Immunother. 2014;63(5):419–35.
141. Leonard JP, et al. Effects of single-dose interleukin-12 exposure on interleukin-12-associated toxicity and interferon-gamma production. Blood. 1997;90(7):2541–8.
142. Markert JM, et al. Preclinical evaluation of a genetically engineered herpes simplex virus expressing interleukin-12. J Virol. 2012;86(9):5304–13.
143. Carew JF, et al. A novel approach to cancer therapy using an oncolytic herpes virus to package amplicons containing cytokine genes. Mol Ther. 2001;4(3):250–6.
144. Tosic V, et al. Myxoma virus expressing a fusion protein of interleukin-15 (IL15) and IL15 receptor alpha has enhanced antitumor activity. PLoS One. 2014;9(10):e109801.
145. Peng W, et al. Loss of PTEN promotes resistance to T cell-mediated immunotherapy. Cancer Discov. 2016;6(2):202–16.
146. Russell L, et al. PTEN expression by an oncolytic herpesvirus directs T-cell mediated tumor clearance. Nat Commun. 2018;9(1):5006.

147. Samstein RM, et al. Tumor mutational load predicts survival after immunotherapy across multiple cancer types. Nat Genet. 2019;51(2):202–6.
148. Samson A, et al. Intravenous delivery of oncolytic reovirus to brain tumor patients immunologically primes for subsequent checkpoint blockade. Sci Transl Med. 2018;10(422).
149. Bourgeois-Daigneault MC, et al. Neoadjuvant oncolytic virotherapy before surgery sensitizes triple-negative breast cancer to immune checkpoint therapy. Sci Transl Med. 2018;10(422).
150. LaRocca CJ, Warner SG. Oncolytic viruses and checkpoint inhibitors: combination therapy in clinical trials. Clin Transl Med. 2018;7(1):35.
151. Chesney J, et al. Randomized, open-label phase II study evaluating the efficacy and safety of Talimogene Laherparepvec in combination with Ipilimumab versus Ipilimumab alone in patients with advanced, unresectable melanoma. J Clin Oncol. 2018;36(17):1658–67.
152. Ribas A, et al. Oncolytic virotherapy promotes intratumoral T cell infiltration and improves anti-PD-1 immunotherapy. Cell. 2017;170(6):1109–1119 e10.
153. Robert C, et al. Pembrolizumab versus Ipilimumab in advanced melanoma. N Engl J Med. 2015;372(26):2521–32.
154. Heinzerling L, et al. Cardiotoxicity associated with CTLA4 and PD1 blocking immunotherapy. J Immunother Cancer. 2016;4:50.
155. Bertrand A, et al. Immune related adverse events associated with anti-CTLA-4 antibodies: systematic review and meta-analysis. BMC Med. 2015;13:211.
156. de Graaf JF, et al. Armed oncolytic viruses: a kick-start for anti-tumor immunity. Cytokine Growth Factor Rev. 2018;41:28–39.
157. Nishio N, et al. Armed oncolytic virus enhances immune functions of chimeric antigen receptor-modified T cells in solid tumors. Cancer Res. 2014;74(18):5195–205.
158. Sakkou M, et al. Mesenchymal TNFR2 promotes the development of polyarthritis and comorbid heart valve stenosis. JCI Insight. 2018;3(7).
159. Moon EK, et al. Intra-tumoral delivery of CXCL11 via a vaccinia virus, but not by modified T cells, enhances the efficacy of adoptive T cell therapy and vaccines. Oncoimmunology. 2018;7(3):e1395997.
160. Le Querrec A, et al. Biological criteria for the evaluation of prophylactic treatment with a low molecular weight heparin (Kabi 2165). J Mal Vasc. 1987;12(Suppl B):99–101.
161. Tahtinen S, et al. Adenovirus improves the efficacy of adoptive T-cell therapy by recruiting immune cells to and promoting their activity at the tumor. Cancer Immunol Res. 2015;3(8):915–25.
162. Diaz RM, et al. Oncolytic immunovirotherapy for melanoma using vesicular stomatitis virus. Cancer Res. 2007;67(6):2840–8.
163. Slaney CY, et al. CARs versus BiTEs: a comparison between T cell-redirection strategies for cancer treatment. Cancer Discov. 2018;8(8):924–34.
164. Dahlen E, Veitonmaki N, Norlen P. Bispecific antibodies in cancer immunotherapy. Ther Adv Vaccines Immunother. 2018;6(1):3–17.
165. Yu F, et al. T-cell engager-armed oncolytic vaccinia virus significantly enhances antitumor therapy. Mol Ther. 2014;22(1):102–11.
166. Freedman JD, et al. Oncolytic adenovirus expressing bispecific antibody targets T-cell cytotoxicity in cancer biopsies. EMBO Mol Med. 2017;9(8):1067–87.
167. Freedman JD, et al. An oncolytic virus expressing a T-cell engager simultaneously targets cancer and immunosuppressive stromal cells. Cancer Res. 2018;78(24):6852–65.
168. Bommareddy PK, et al. MEK inhibition enhances oncolytic virus immunotherapy through increased tumor cell killing and T cell activation. Sci Transl Med. 2018;10(471).
169. Chen J, et al. Therapeutic benefit of intracerebral transplantation of bone marrow stromal cells after cerebral ischemia in rats. J Neurol Sci. 2001;189(1–2):49–57.
170. Chen J, et al. Therapeutic benefit of intravenous administration of bone marrow stromal cells after cerebral ischemia in rats. Stroke. 2001;32(4):1005–11.
171. Dezawa M, et al. Bone marrow stromal cells generate muscle cells and repair muscle degeneration. Science. 2005;309(5732):314–7.

172. Lu D, et al. Adult bone marrow stromal cells administered intravenously to rats after traumatic brain injury migrate into brain and improve neurological outcome. Neuroreport. 2001;12(3):559–63.
173. Grinnemo KH, et al. Xenoreactivity and engraftment of human mesenchymal stem cells transplanted into infarcted rat myocardium. J Thorac Cardiovasc Surg. 2004;127(5):1293–300.
174. Gao P, et al. Therapeutic potential of human mesenchymal stem cells producing IL-12 in a mouse xenograft model of renal cell carcinoma. Cancer Lett. 2010;290(2):157–66.
175. Hung SC, et al. Mesenchymal stem cell targeting of microscopic tumors and tumor stroma development monitored by noninvasive in vivo positron emission tomography imaging. Clin Cancer Res. 2005;11(21):7749–56.
176. Nakamura K, et al. Antitumor effect of genetically engineered mesenchymal stem cells in a rat glioma model. Gene Ther. 2004;11(14):1155–64.
177. Studeny M, et al. Bone marrow-derived mesenchymal stem cells as vehicles for interferon-beta delivery into tumors. Cancer Res. 2002;62(13):3603–8.
178. Xiang J, et al. Mesenchymal stem cells as a gene therapy carrier for treatment of fibrosarcoma. Cytotherapy. 2009;11(5):516–26.
179. Aboody KS, et al. Neural stem cells display extensive tropism for pathology in adult brain: evidence from intracranial gliomas. Proc Natl Acad Sci U S A. 2000;97(23):12846–51.
180. Mader EK, et al. Mesenchymal stem cell carriers protect oncolytic measles viruses from antibody neutralization in an orthotopic ovarian cancer therapy model. Clin Cancer Res. 2009;15(23):7246–55.
181. Alfano AL, et al. Oncolytic adenovirus-loaded menstrual blood stem cells overcome the blockade of viral activity exerted by ovarian cancer ascites. Mol Ther Oncolytics. 2017;6:31–44.
182. Duebgen M, et al. Stem cells loaded with multimechanistic oncolytic herpes simplex virus variants for brain tumor therapy. J Natl Cancer Inst. 2014;106(6):dju090.
183. Du W, et al. Stem cell-released oncolytic herpes simplex virus has therapeutic efficacy in brain metastatic melanomas. Proc Natl Acad Sci U S A. 2017;114(30):E6157–65.
184. Melen GJ, et al. Influence of carrier cells on the clinical outcome of children with neuroblastoma treated with high dose of oncolytic adenovirus delivered in mesenchymal stem cells. Cancer Lett. 2016;371(2):161–70.
185. Adusumilli PS, et al. Radiation-induced cellular DNA damage repair response enhances viral gene therapy efficacy in the treatment of malignant pleural mesothelioma. Ann Surg Oncol. 2007;14(1):258–69.
186. Adusumilli PS, et al. Radiation therapy potentiates effective oncolytic viral therapy in the treatment of lung cancer. Ann Thorac Surg. 2005;80(2):409–16; discussion 416-7.
187. Advani SJ, et al. Enhancement of replication of genetically engineered herpes simplex viruses by ionizing radiation: a new paradigm for destruction of therapeutically intractable tumors. Gene Ther. 1998;5(2):160–5.
188. Jarnagin WR, et al. Treatment of cholangiocarcinoma with oncolytic herpes simplex virus combined with external beam radiation therapy. Cancer Gene Ther. 2006;13(3):326–34.
189. Kim SH, et al. Combination of mutated herpes simplex virus type 1 (G207 virus) with radiation for the treatment of squamous cell carcinoma of the head and neck. Eur J Cancer. 2005;41(2):313–22.
190. Blank SV, et al. Replication-selective herpes simplex virus type 1 mutant therapy of cervical cancer is enhanced by low-dose radiation. Hum Gene Ther. 2002;13(5):627–39.
191. Connell CM, et al. Genomic DNA damage and ATR-Chk1 signaling determine oncolytic adenoviral efficacy in human ovarian cancer cells. J Clin Invest. 2011;121(4):1283–97.
192. Kuroda S, et al. Telomerase-dependent oncolytic adenovirus sensitizes human cancer cells to ionizing radiation via inhibition of DNA repair machinery. Cancer Res. 2010;70(22):9339–48.
193. Passaro C, et al. PARP inhibitor olaparib increases the oncolytic activity of dl922-947 in in vitro and in vivo model of anaplastic thyroid carcinoma. Mol Oncol. 2015;9(1):78–92.

194. Jiang H, et al. Oncolytic viruses and DNA-repair machinery: overcoming chemoresistance of gliomas. Expert Rev Anticancer Ther. 2006;6(11):1585–92.
195. Yoo JY, et al. Bortezomib-induced unfolded protein response increases oncolytic HSV-1 replication resulting in synergistic antitumor effects. Clin Cancer Res. 2014;20(14):3787–98.
196. Yoo JY, et al. Bortezomib treatment sensitizes oncolytic HSV-1-treated tumors to NK cell immunotherapy. Clin Cancer Res. 2016;22(21):5265–76.
197. Jaime-Ramirez AC, et al. Reolysin and histone deacetylase inhibition in the treatment of head and neck squamous cell carcinoma. Mol Ther Oncolytics. 2017;5:87–96.

Chapter 4
Novel Methods to Overcome Acquired Resistance to Immunotherapy

Xianda Zhao, Ce Yuan, John Markus Rieth, Dechen Wangmo, and Subbaya Subramanian

Abstract The remarkable success of immunotherapy, including immune checkpoint blockade therapy (ICBT) in clinical settings, such as in melanoma patients and patients with DNA mismatch repair deficient tumors, has shifted the paradigm of cancer treatment. However, immunotherapy continues to face major challenges in controlling malignancy due to both intrinsic and acquired resistance mechanisms. Here, we discuss the mechanisms by which cancer immunotherapy has harnessed the immune system to target tumor progression, as well as the mechanisms of acquired resistance to immunotherapy. We also describe novel approaches in overcoming this resistance, with a particular focus on ICBT. We explore mechanisms by which tumor-intrinsic cues, tumor microenvironmental factors, and the host microbiome might impact the efficacy and resistance often seen during ICBT. Furthermore, we introduce technologies that will identify biomarkers from mouse and human models to predict clinical benefits for ICBT in cancer patients and promising emerging strategies to overcome ICBT resistance.

Keywords Cancer immunotherapy · Immune checkpoint blockade therapy · Resistance · Tumor immunology · Signaling

---

Ce Yuan, John Markus Rieth, and Dechen Wangmo contributed equally to this work.

X. Zhao · C. Yuan · D. Wangmo
Department of Surgery, University of Minnesota Medical School, Minneapolis, MN, USA
e-mail: zhaox714@umn.edu; yuanx236@umn.edu; wangm005@umn.edu

J. M. Rieth
Department of Internal Medicine, Carver College of Medicine, Iowa City, IA, USA
e-mail: john-rieth@uiowa.edu

S. Subramanian (✉)
Department of Surgery, University of Minnesota Medical School, Minneapolis, MN, USA

Masonic Cancer Center, University of Minnesota, Minneapolis, MN, USA
e-mail: subree@umn.edu

© Springer Nature Switzerland AG 2019
M. R. Szewczuk et al. (eds.), *Current Applications for Overcoming Resistance to Targeted Therapies*, Resistance to Targeted Anti-Cancer Therapeutics 20,
https://doi.org/10.1007/978-3-030-21477-7_4

Abbreviations

β2m	Beta-2-microglobulin
A2AR	Adenosine receptor
ADCC	Antibody-dependent cell-mediated cytotoxicity
AKT	Protein kinase B
APC	Antigen-presenting cell
AXL	Tyrosine-protein kinase receptor UFO
BATTLE-1	Biomarker-integrated approaches of targeted therapy for lung cancer elimination
BCG	Bacille Calmette-Guérin
CAF	Cancer-associated fibroblast
CAR	Chimeric antigen receptor
CDK	Cyclin-dependent kinase
CK2	Casein kinase 2
CT	Computed tomography
ctDNA	Circulating tumor DNA
CTLA-4	Cytotoxic T-lymphocyte antigen 4
CTLs	Cytotoxic T-cells
DAMPs	Danger-associated molecular patterns
DC	Dendritic cell
Eomes	Eomesodermin
ERK	Extracellular signal–regulated kinases
FAP	Fibroblast activation protein
Fas	Tumor necrosis factor receptor superfamily, member 6
FasL	Fas ligand
FDA	Food and Drug Administration
GADS	GRB2-related adaptor downstream of Shc
GEM	Genetically engineered mouse
GM-CSF	Granulocyte-macrophage colony-stimulating factor
GRB2	Growth factor receptor-bound protein 2
HMGB1	High-mobility group box 1
ICBT	Immune checkpoint blockade therapy
ICOS	Inducible T-cell co-stimulator
IDO	Indoleamine 2,3-dioxygenase
IFNGR	Interferon-gamma receptor
IFN-α	Interferon-alpha
IFN-γ	Interferon-gamma
IL-2	Interleukin-2
IL-4	Interleukin-4
IRF	Tripartite motif containing 63
JAK	Janus kinases
KIR	Killer cell immunoglobulin-like receptors

LAG-3	Lymphocyte activation gene 3
LCK	Lymphocyte-specific protein tyrosine kinase
LCMV	Lymphocytic choriomeningitis virus
LOXL2	Lysyl oxidase-like 2
MDSC	Myeloid-derived suppressor cell
MHC	Major histocompatibility complex
NCR	Natural cytotoxicity receptors
NK	Natural killer (cell)
PD-1	Programmed death 1
PD-L1	Programmed death-ligand 1
PD-L2	Programmed death-ligand 2
PI3K	Phosphoinositide 3-kinase
PIAS4	Protein inhibitor of activated STAT 4
PIP3	Phosphatidylinositol (3,4,5)-trisphosphate
PKC	Protein kinase C
PROSPECT	Profiling of resistance patterns and oncogenic signaling pathways in evaluation of cancers of the thorax
PTEN	Phosphatase and tensin homolog
RAR	Retinoic acid receptor
RECIST	Response evaluation criteria in solid tumors
ROR2	Receptor tyrosine kinase-like orphan receptor 2
SCF	Skp, Cullin, F-box containing complex
SHP-1	Tyrosine-protein phosphatase non-receptor type 6
SHP-2	Tyrosine-protein phosphatase non-receptor type 11
SMAD3	Mothers against decapentaplegic homolog 3
SOCS1	Suppressor of cytokine signaling 1
SOX3	SRY-box 3
TAGLN	Transgelin
T-bet	T-box transcription factor 21
TCGA	The Cancer Genome Atlas
TCR	T-cell receptors
TGF-β	Transforming growth factor-beta
TIM-3	T-cell immunoglobulin and mucin domain 3
TME	Tumor microenvironment
TNF	Tumor necrosis factor
Tregs	Regulatory T-cells
TWIST2	Twist-related protein 2
VEGF	Vascular endothelial growth factor
VISTA	V-domain immunoglobulin suppressor of T-cell activation
WHO	World Health Organization
WNT5A	Wingless-type MMTV integration site family, member 5A
ZAP70	Zeta-chain-associated protein kinase 70

4.1 Introduction

In recent decades, cancer immunotherapy has joined the ranks of other standard cancer treatments including surgery, radiation, chemotherapy, and targeted therapy. Immunotherapy is not a recent advancement and has existed conceptually, starting in ancient Egypt; however, until the second half of the eighteenth century, no attempt with a scientific explanation for applying immunotherapy to the treatment of cancer was made [1]. It was over 135 years ago when German physicians Fehleisen and Busch observed tumor regression after infection with erysipelas [2, 3]. In the twentieth century, the theory of immune surveillance and the bacille Calmette-Guérin (BCG) tuberculosis vaccine treatment for preventing the recurrence of non–muscle invasive bladder cancer was established [4, 5]. However, in the same era, other treatments such as radiotherapy, chemotherapy, surgery, and targeted therapy quickly developed and prevailed as cancer treatments. In recent decades, a clearer understanding of anti-tumor immunity has led to the development of novel immunotherapy strategies that have been tested in clinical trials.

Unlike other cancer treatments, immunotherapy primarily targets the interactions between malignant cells, immune cells, and other cells in the tumor microenvironment (TME) (Fig. 4.1). Both the innate and adaptive immune systems are involved in anti-tumor immunity through multiple anti-tumor mechanisms. The innate immune system, comprised of eosinophils, basophils, natural killer (NK) cells, macrophages, dendritic cells (DCs), and mast cells, is the first-line of defense against foreign antigens [6]. The professional antigen presenting cells (APCs) of the innate immune system process tumor antigens and prime T-cell activation, while cytotoxic NK cells can directly kill cancer cells through mechanisms including antibody-dependent cell-mediated cytotoxicity (ADCC) or natural cytotoxicity receptors (NCR) and killer cell immunoglobulin-like receptors (KIR)-mediated proteolytic lysis. The antigen-specific T- and B-cells of the adaptive immune system target antigen-specific tumor cells. Tumor-specific T-cells are released into the peripheral blood once primed by APCs in peripheral lymphatic organs and subsequently move to the site of the tumor [7]. The activated tumor-specific T-cells recognize tumor cells presenting tumor-specific or -associated antigens on their major histocompatibility complex (MHC) molecules. Finally, CD8+ tumor-specific T-cells eliminate the cancer cells via cytokine-induced cytotoxicity or mechanisms involving the Fas receptor (FasR) and its ligand (FasL) [7].

Our improved understanding of the mechanisms underlying anti-tumor immunity has significantly advanced the development of cancer immunotherapy. Several immunotherapy strategies have been developed including, antibody-based targeting of oncogenic pathways, tumor antigen vaccines, cytokine treatment, adoptive T-cell therapy, oncolytic virus immunotherapy, and immune checkpoint blockade therapy (ICBT). This chapter introduces mechanisms by which cancer immunotherapy harnesses the effects of the immune system to target malignant progression, mechanisms of acquired resistance to immunotherapy and novel approaches in overcoming this resistance, with a focus on ICBT.

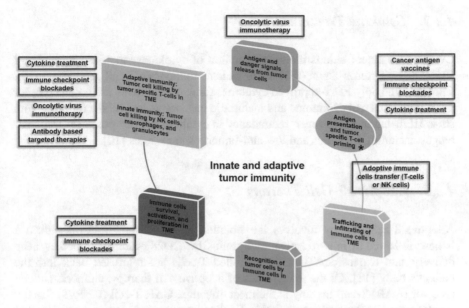

Fig. 4.1 Anti-tumor immunity and tumor immunotherapy. Anti-tumor immunity involves both the innate and adaptive immune responses. (1) Tumor-specific antigens and danger signals released from tumor cells or tumor microenvironment (TME) stimulate anti-tumor immunity. (2) Antigen-presenting cells capture and present tumor antigens to prime tumor-specific T-cells (specific to the adaptive immunity). (3) Innate and adaptive immune cells are trafficked to the TME from the peripheral blood. (4, 5) Recognition of tumor cells and expansion of immune cell population in the TME prepares for the killing of tumor cells. (6) Innate and adaptive immune cells eliminate tumor cells with different mechanisms. Immunotherapy harnesses the innate and adaptive immune system to control tumor development. The primary sites of action of each immunotherapy are summarized. However, it is critical to note that the immune response is under complex, tight regulation. Changes in one of the immune regulatory steps will stimulate feedback regulation and may also alter other steps. Furthermore, one immunotherapy can change several immune regulatory steps simultaneously. *This immune regulatory step is specific to an adaptive immune response. *TME* tumor microenvironment

4.2 Types of Cancer Immunotherapy

4.2.1 Tumor Antigen Vaccines

Tumor antigen vaccines expose patients to tumor antigens that can trigger the body to initiate specific anti-tumor immune responses [8]. In 2010, the first and thus far the only cancer vaccine, sipuleucel-T (Provenge), was approved by the U.S. Food and Drug Administration (FDA) to treat metastatic castration-resistant prostate cancer [8]. Provenge is a DC vaccine that involves harvesting DCs from a patient and exposing them to tumor antigens complexed with granulocyte–macrophage colony-stimulating factor (GM-CSF) [9]. The precursor DCs take in the tumor antigen, and upon maturation, the DCs are reinfused into the patient's body. The mature DCs now present the tumor antigen on their surface, activating T-cells and triggering anti-tumor responses [9].

4.2.2 Cytokine Treatment

Cytokine treatment entails the administration of cytokines, such as interleukin-2 (IL-2) and interferon-alpha (IFN-α), to patients to increase T-cell production [10]. Currently, the only FDA-approved cytokines for cancer patients are bolus IL-2, for those with renal cell carcinoma and metastatic melanoma, and IFN-α for those with stage III melanoma. However, redundancy in cytokine activity poses several challenges, including toxicities and low anti-tumor response rates [10].

4.2.3 Adoptive T-Cell Therapy

Adoptive T-cell therapy involves the isolation of tumor-specific T-cells from a patient, followed by *in vitro* activation by anti-CD3/CD28 beads or antibodies, gene delivery, and expansion. Then the modified T-cells are reinfused back into the patient's body [11]. Of the many kinds of adoptive cell therapy, chimeric antigen receptor (CAR) T-cell therapy is the most effective. CAR T-cell (CAR-T) therapy involves engineering and manipulating T-cells to possess anti-tumor properties that help them recognize and eliminate tumors *in vitro* [11]. CAR-T therapy has been widely tested in young adults and pediatric patients with refractory B-cell lymphoblastic leukemia [12, 13].

4.2.4 Oncolytic Virus Immunotherapy

Oncolytic virus immunotherapy uses genetically engineered attenuated viruses to invade and attack tumor cells [14]. In 2015, the FDA approved a herpes simplex-1 virus, talimogene laherparepvec (T-Vec or Imlygic), for patients with advanced melanoma [15]. Oncolytic viruses can act through different mechanisms. In particular, T-Vec can be directly injected into a melanoma site that cannot be surgically removed [15]. First, T-Vec can selectively invade tumor cells by replicating within tumor cells, causing tumor cell lysis which releases tumor-associated antigens. T-Vec can also produce danger signals or damage-associated molecular patterns (DAMPs), released by damaged cells, to stimulate anti-tumor responses [15]. Second, GM-CSF expressed by T-Vec can further expand anti-tumor immunity [15]. Many oncolytic viruses are now undergoing clinical trials, with some combined with other treatments for patients with different types of cancer [16].

4.2.5 Immune Checkpoint Blockade Therapy

Immune checkpoint blockade therapy (ICBT) inhibits immune checkpoints that suppress T-cell activation [7]. Immune checkpoints are important molecules in the immune system that maintain the balance between co-inhibitory and costimulatory signals that regulate the duration and amplitude of T-cell function [7]. The first-generation co-inhibitory checkpoint receptors to be targeted were cytotoxic T-lymphocyte antigen 4 (CTLA-4) and programmed death 1 (PD-1); where blocking checkpoint receptors showed a higher rate of clinical success, paving the way for additional clinical trials [7]. The first CTLA-4 checkpoint inhibitor, ipilimumab, was approved by the FDA in 2011 for patients with advanced melanoma. Various anti-PD-1 checkpoint inhibitors, such as pembrolizumab (Keytruda) and nivolumab (Opdivo), have been approved by the FDA as adjuvant therapies for patients with multiple types of cancer.

4.3 Development of Resistance to Immune Checkpoint Blockade Therapy

4.3.1 Immune Checkpoint Molecular Biology

Immune checkpoints are formed by T-cell receptors (TCRs) such as CD28, CTLA-4, and PD-1 bound to a ligand such as CD80, CD86, or programmed death-ligand (PD-L) 1/2 on cells in the surrounding microenvironment. Their immunologic synapses are responsible for monitoring and regulating the function of specialized T-cells [7]. Here, we will focus on the CD28/CTLA-4/B7 and the PD-1/PD-L1/PD-L2 system to elucidate the mechanisms of immune checkpoints on tumor immunity.

CD28 and CTLA-4 belong to an immunoglobulin gene superfamily possessing a single extracellular V-like domain [17]. Both CD28 and CTLA-4 are transmembrane proteins primarily expressed by T-cells. When compared with CTLA-4, CD28 expression is elevated on the surface of resting T-cells [17]. The relatively lower CTLA-4 expression on T-cells is due to the interaction of the YVKM motif in the cytoplasmic domain of CTLA-4 with a clathrin-coated pit adaptor complex called AP-50, which causes internalization of CTLA 4 [17, 18]. Phosphorylation of the cytoplasmic domain motif of CTLA-4 can liberate it from AP-50, preventing internalization of CTLA-4 and increasing its expression on cell surfaces [17, 18].

Both CD28 and CTLA-4 bind to ligands CD80 (B7-1) and CD86 (B7-2), which are expressed by APCs and tumor cells [17]. CD86 is generally found on the surface of resting APCs and is expressed at higher levels than CD80, which is induced by the activation of other stimuli. CD28 is constitutively expressed on the surfaces of T-cells. Stimulation by TCRs and co-stimulation by CD28 significantly upregulates CTLA-4 expression in T-cells [17]. Following binding with CD80/CD86, CD28 can recruit proteins, specifically phosphoinositide 3-kinase (PI3K), growth factor receptor-bound protein 2 (GRB2), and GRB2-related adaptor downstream of Shc (GADS), that contain the SH2-domain and SH3-domain. The subsequent downstream events not only promote T-cell activation and proliferation but also help produce cytokines, such as IL-2, IFN-γ, and TNF [17].

In contrast to CD28, CTLA-4 inhibits T-cell activation and has a higher affinity to CD80 and CD86 [17]. Ligation of CD80/CD86 with CTLA-4 seizes the ligands from CD28 and prevents downstream co-stimulatory signalling, resulting in T-cell inactivation. CTLA-4 can also regulate TCR signals by recruiting tyrosine-protein phosphatase non-receptor type 11 (SHP2) via the phosphorylated YVKM motif in its cytoplasmic domain. This interaction causes dephosphorylation of the TCR signalling component and suppresses early-stage action signals [17].

The important, well-understood mechanisms of ICBT involve PD-1 and its ligands PD-L1 and PD-L2. PD-1 is a transmembrane protein that is expressed on activated T-cells after TCR engagement [19]. When stimulated, PD-1 can inhibit downstream TCR signalling pathways facilitating T-cell migration. PD-L1 is primarily expressed on tumor cells, macrophages, fibroblasts, and T-cells whereas PD-L2 is expressed on macrophages and activated DCs. PD-L1 is stimulated by inflammatory IFN-γ, which is secreted by activated T-cells and NK cells and PD-L2 is stimulated by IL-4 [19].

PD-1 inhibitory signalling pathways involve both a direct, proximal inhibitory mechanism and an indirect pathway. When T-cells recognize an antigen, TCR signal transduction is activated, followed by phosphorylation of the ITSM motif by lymphocyte-specific protein tyrosine kinase (LCK) [19]. When PD-L1 is bound to PD-1, tyrosine-protein phosphatase non-receptor type 6 (SHP1) and SHP2 are recruited to ITSM. SHP2 binds to ITSM when T-cells are activated, even though both SHP1 and SHP2 are recruited to ITSM. When recruited to ITSM, SHP2 dephosphorylates zeta-chain-associated protein kinase 70 (ZAP70) and PI3K activates and ultimately blocks the downstream signalling pathways, which include protein kinase C (PKC), protein kinase B (AKT), and extracellular signal-regulated kinases (ERK) [19]. The indirect PD-1 inhibitor mechanism involves cyclin-dependent kinase (CDK)-dependent cellular division and inhibits T-cell proliferation. During T-cell activation, TCR signals increase casein kinase 2 (CK2) expression, which phosphorylates the regulatory domain of phosphatase and tensin homolog (PTEN) [19], leading to activated phosphatidylinositol (3,4,5)-trisphosphate (PIP_3), which then activates AKT. AKT enhances the activity of ubiquitin ligase Skp, Cullin, F-box containing complex (SCF^{skp2}), causing CDK2 to phosphorylate and inactivate mothers against decapentaplegic homolog 3 (SMAD3) [19]. As a result, CDK2 elicits cell cycle progression and proliferation. When PD-1 and PD-L1 are involved, CK2 expression is downregulated, which causes PTEN to dephosphorylate PIP_3 and inhibit its activity. Finally, the CDK2 mediated cell cycle in activated T-cell is inhibited [19].

4.3.2 Resistance to Immune Checkpoint Blockade Therapy

In 1996, the James Allison group reported that in animal models, the use of monoclonal antibodies to block CTLA-4 could treat tumors [20]. In 2011, the first ICBT agent, ipilimumab (anti-CTLA-4), was approved by the FDA to treat patients with stage IV melanoma. In the ensuing years, other ICBT agents were approved to treat patients with various types of cancer [21]. Although ICBT has been used for years, this therapeutic option faces both intrinsic and adaptive resistance that eventually render it ineffective [22].

A large proportion of patients with solid tumors show primary or intrinsic resistance to ICBT [7]. To understand the mechanism of intrinsic resistance, the anti-tumor immune cycle must be reviewed. The anti-tumor immune cycle is comprised of three main steps:

1. Induction of anti-tumor immune responses via recognition of antigens by T-cells.
2. Infiltration and expansion of cancer-specific T- cells into the tumor microenvironment.
3. Recognition and elimination of tumor cells [23].

The number and character (e.g., whether neoantigens, antigens encoded by tumor-specific mutated genes, or non-neoantigens are produced) of mutations in tumor cells determines the initial step of induction. Studies have shown that cancers that have a heavier mutational burden respond better to ICBT because their mutations are more likely to be recognized by immune cells [7]. Therefore, tumors with defective DNA repair mechanisms, are more sensitive to ICBT than tumors with intact DNA repair mechanisms, due to their accumulated mutations [24].

The oncogenic pathways and components (i.e., stromal cells associated with the tumor microenvironment, cytokines and other proteins) in the TME regulate the infiltration, as well as the survival of tumor specific T-cells. Activation or inactivation of certain oncogenes or tumor suppressor genes, such as RAS and PTEN, can impede T-cell infiltration by establishing an immunosuppressive TME [25]. Apoptosis-inducing FasL in the tumor vasculature tends to restrict infiltration of $CD8^+$ T-cells from blood vessels [7]. Myeloid cells in the TME differentiate into myeloid-derived suppressor cells (MDSCs) that inhibit T-cell replication and function [7]. Cancer-associated fibroblasts (CAFs) produce an extracellular matrix that prevents T-cell migration to the tumor site [7]. The recognition and elimination of tumor cells by $CD8^+$ T-cells is largely limited by low expression levels of MHC-I and high expression of multiple inhibitory immune checkpoints on tumor cells. In patients with certain types of cancers, this normal anti-tumor immune response can ultimately lead to intrinsic resistance to ICBT with the detailed mechanisms previously summarized and thoroughly discussed [7, 24, 25].

Conversely, adaptive resistance poses other unique challenges. Although immunotherapy provides long-term anti-tumor responses in the majority of patients, there is a subset of patients in which ICBT initially works, but patients eventually experience a relapse [26]. In particular, 25–30% of patients with metastatic melanoma who at first have a positive response to anti-CTLA-4 or PD-1, deteriorate and relapse over time. Currently, little is understood about the mechanisms that lead to acquired resistance to ICBT, though it likely shares some of the intrinsic resistance mechanisms. In this chapter, we will explore the mechanisms of acquired resistance to ICBT and methods to overcome this resistance.

4.4 Mechanisms of Acquired Resistance to Immune Checkpoint Blockade Therapy

Acquired resistance occurs when tumor cells gain the ability to resist the activity of an anti-cancer agent to which they were previously susceptible. In recent years, multiple mechanisms have been reported on the acquisition of resistance to ICBT, including changes within tumor cells, remodelling of the tumor immune- and micro-environment, and the impact from the gut microbiome. These mechanisms are summarized in Fig. 4.2.

4.4.1 T-Cell Exhaustion

T-cell exhaustion is a state of T-cell dysfunction that occurs during certain chronic infections and cancer progression. Exhausted T-cells have low or no effector function, sustain high expression of inhibitory checkpoints, and exhibit a transcriptional

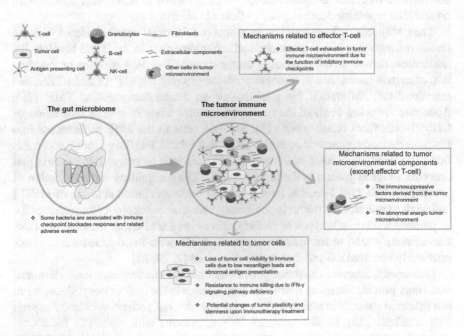

Fig. 4.2 Adaptive resistance to immune checkpoint blockade therapy. Sensitivity to immune checkpoint blockade therapy (ICBT) is regulated by the local tumor microenvironment (TME), as well as by the remote gut microbiome. In the TME, alterations in tumor-specific T-cells, other stromal cells, and tumor cells have shown to have a significant impact on inducing adaptive resistance to ICBT. The association between certain gut bacteria and ICBT response are also observed and may involve an adaptive resistance to ICBT. *ICBT* immune checkpoint blockade therapy; *TME* tumor microenvironment

state that is different from that of functional effector or memory T-cells [27]. T-cell exhaustion starts with loss of function including IL-2 production, high proliferative capacity, and *ex vivo* killing. In the intermediate stages of dysfunction, T-cells lack tumor necrosis factor (TNF) and IFN-γ, are unable to produce β-chemokines and are unable to degranulate. In the final stage of dysfunction, the T-cells specific to the tumor and the virus are physically deleted from the immune microenvironment.

Currently, research is underway to understand how inhibitory immune checkpoints are regulated during T-cell exhaustion and how inhibitory immune checkpoint blockades might help reverse this exhausted state. A genomic region that is specifically associated with chromatin changes during the exhausted state was identified 23.8 kb upstream of the *PDCD1* gene. This region is a potential binding site for the retinoic acid receptor (RAR), T-box transcription factor 21 (T-bet), and SRY-box 3 (SOX3) transcription factors [28]. When the proposed transcription factor binding sites were mutated, PD-1 expression in lymphocytes was suppressed. These results shed light on how inhibitory immune checkpoint expression is upregulated during T-cell exhaustion. However, the upregulation mechanisms of other inhibitory immune checkpoints are still poorly understood.

Targeting PD-1 on tumor-infiltrating T-cells elicited an obvious response by partly reversing T-cell dysfunction. Pauken et al. examined the transcriptional and epigenetic changes that occur over time in exhausted CD8$^+$ T-cells treated by PD-1 pathway inhibitors [29]. They found that based on the expression of eomesodermin (Eomes), T-bet, and PD-1, exhausted T-cells can be divided into two subtypes. The T-bet^{high}Eomes^{low} PD-1^{int} subtype can be reactivated by blocking the PD-1 pathway, whereas the Eomes^{high}PD-1^{high} subtype is more terminally exhausted and responds poorly to PD-1 pathway blockades [29].

Additional epigenetic landscape analyses in mice have suggested that reinvigoration of exhausted T-cells via PD-L1 blockade causes minimal memory development. The reinvigorated exhausted T-cells became exhausted again if the antigen concentration remained high and if they failed to become durable memory T-cells upon antigen clearance in the presence of PD-1 blockades [29]. Thus, although anti-PD-1 treatment can reactivate specific subtypes of exhausted T-cells by reprograming the transcriptional profile, it cannot lead to sustained reversal within the exhausted T-cell epigenetic landscape. The inflexibly dire epigenetic fate of exhausted T-cells provides a possible explanation concerning the subset of patients that initially respond to anti-PD-1 treatment but later relapse. Undoubtedly, T-cell exhaustion is an important mechanism of acquired resistance.

Co-option of alternative inhibitory checkpoints following anti-PD-1 treatment might explain the failure of fully reversing exhausted T-cells to effective T-cells via PD-1 blockade alone. During anti-CTLA-4 and anti-PD-1/PD-L1 treatments, multiple other inhibitory immune checkpoints can be upregulated in tumor-specific T-cells. This may be due to the induction of IFN and other signaling pathways, such as PI3K-AKT [30–32]. For example, T-cell immunoglobulin and mucin domain 3 (TIM-3), a protein encoded by the *HAVCR2* gene, is a cell surface molecule widely expressed on T-cells and innate immune cells, including DCs, NK cells, and monocytes. Functionally, it is activated by galectin-9 and helps stimulate an influx of calcium into the intracellular space and induces programmed cell death [33]. Consequently, activation of TIM-3 on T-cells causes T-cell exhaustion. TIM-3 upregulation has been detected in the resistant lesions of patients with lung adenocarcinoma who initially showed a partial response to anti-PD-1 treatment [34]. More specifically, high expression of TIM-3 predominated on T-cells bound to anti-PD-1 antibody, verifying the role of anti-PD-1 in upregulating TIM-3 [34]. Other inhibitory immune checkpoints have shown a similar effect to TIM-3 in inducing anti-PD-1/anti-CTLA-4 acquired resistance, including lymphocyte activation gene 3 (LAG-3), CD160, and V-domain immunoglobulin suppressor of T-cell activation (VISTA) [30, 32, 34–36]. In preclinical models, co-administration of multiple immune checkpoint blockades has demonstrated improved responses to ICBT [37–39].

Taken together, the understanding of different T-cell exhaustion mechanisms during tumor development and ICBT treatment have expanded our options for treating tumors with combinatory immunotherapies. However, several challenges remain for transforming these cutting-edge concepts from pre-clinical studies to clinical practice. For example, identifying the critical T-cell exhaustion mechanisms in specific tumors and monitoring the involvement of additional T-cell exhaustion mechanisms, such as TIM-3 upregulation, during anti-PD-1/anti-CTLA-4 treatment is still very challenging. Without knowing when and which T-cell exhaustion mechanisms are involved in inducing acquired ICBT resistance, combinatory treatments will be non-specific. Further studies are necessary to develop technologies that can identify tumor-specific T-cell exhaustion mechanisms.

4.4.2   Tumor Microenvironment Remodeling

Additional components of the TME affect the efficacy of immunotherapy [7]. ICBT not only disrupts interactions between tumor-specific T-cells and tumor cells but also blocks interactions between tumor-specific T-cells and other components of the TME. It is now well known that ligands of inhibitory immune checkpoints are highly expressed in the TME and can nullify the impact of inhibitory immune checkpoints on tumor-specific T-cells. Moreover, preclinical studies in mouse tumor models indicated that anti-CTLA-4 antibodies deplete intra-tumoral regulatory T-cells (T_{regs}), primary immunosuppressive cells, via ADCC [40–42]. This function of anti-CTLA-4 antibodies is specific to T_{regs} since CTLA-4 expression is higher on T_{regs} relative to effector T-cells.

Rather than being remodeled by ICBT, the TME actively regulates tumor sensitivity to ICBT. Endothelial cells in tumor capillaries and CAFs restrict CD8+ T-cell infiltration from blood vessels to the tumor cell niche [43–45]. T_{regs} in the TME are known to suppress effector T-cells and APCs via secretion of IL-10 and transforming growth factor-β (TGF-β), or via direct cell-to-cell interactions. MDSCs in the TME secrete inhibitory cytokines and suppress effector T-cell metabolism. Targeting these immunosuppressive mechanisms has been reported to reverse intrinsic resistance to ICBT [7].

In the context of acquired resistance to anti-PD-1 treatment, Zaretsky et al. performed serial biopsies on responsive tumors and ICBT-resistant tumors [46]. The intra-tumoral CD8$^+$ T-cell infiltrate density markedly increased on responsive tumors. However, once those tumors acquired resistance, T-cell infiltration became poor, which resulted in CD8$^+$ T-cells primarily retained in the invasive margin instead of around the tumor cells [46]. This observation suggests that changes in the TME can exclude T-cells from the location of the tumor cells and potentially induce acquired resistance to ICBT.

Furthermore, immune cells undergo complex shifts in metabolic patterns when they are activated. Effector T-cells rely on aerobic glycolysis to fuel their metabolic demands [47]. However, the tumor microenvironment is hypoxic and deprived of glucose and amino acids, which can encumber proper T-cell activation and effector function [47, 48]. ICBT can partially reverse T-cell exhaustion in the TME, but the duration of T-cell reactivation might be shortened by the abnormal TME [49]. Therefore, deprivation of energy supply to reactivated T-cells in the TME is likely one of the reasons that ICBT fails after an initial response.

Although the TME likely contributes to the acquisition of resistance to ICBT, conclusive evidence is lacking, and the precise mechanisms remain poorly understood. Immunotherapy can significantly eliminate tumor cells, leading to a disruption of tumor-stromal cell interactions. However, the consequences of these changes on tumor-stromal cell function, inflammatory and metabolic status, and the physical structure of the microenvironment require further study. Based on our current understanding of mechanisms of resistance to immunotherapy, it is important to further understand the changes in vascular endothelial growth factor (VEGF)-mediated proangiogenic pathways, fibroblast activation protein (FAP)-positive CAF-mediated T-cell exclusion, and tumor and immune cell metabolic profiles.

4.4.3 Tumor Cell Insensitivity to Immune Effectors

Perforin, granzyme, and IFN are the primary immune effectors secreted by CD8$^+$ T-cells when targeting tumor cells. Tumor destruction is conventionally understood to be principally mediated via cell lysis induced by perforin and granzyme. However, IFN-γ can directly help restrict tumor growth by exerting antiproliferative and proapoptotic effects on tumor cells. Most importantly, IFN-γ on tumor cells can directly upregulate the antigen-presenting machinery, including the proteasome subunits, the transporters associated with antigen processing and MHC molecules, ultimately making tumor cells more visible to CD8$^+$ T-cells.

In tumor cells, mutations in the signalling pathways related to IFN-γ can nullify the impact of tumor-specific T-cells. Janus kinases 1 and 2 (JAK1/JAK2) are key molecules in the IFN-γ signalling pathway [50, 51]. Upon exposure to IFN-γ, JAK1/JAK2 are activated and subsequently phosphorylate a tyrosine residue on STATs. Signaling between JAK1/JAK2 and STATs controls downstream cell proliferation, differentiation, migration, and apoptosis [50, 51]. It is noteworthy that the whole-exome sequencing of tumors that developed acquired resistance to anti-PD-1 treatment revealed mutations in JAK1/JAK2 [46]. The wild-type JAK1/JAK2 allele is deleted in tumors with these mutations, leading to the total loss of IFN-induced tumor cell proliferation arrest. Meanwhile, the loss of IFN-γ signalling due to genomic defects has been seen in patients with intrinsic resistance to anti-CTLA-4 treatment [52]. In these patients, inactivating mutations were identified in interferon gamma receptor 1 (IFNGR1), tripartite motif containing 63 (TRIM63), JAK2, and interferon gamma receptor 2 (IFNGR2), as well as amplification of important IFN-γ pathway inhibitors, such as protein inhibitor of activated STAT 4 (PIAS4) and suppressor of cytokine signaling 1 (SOCS1) [52]. Consistent with these findings based on human tumor sample analyses are preclinical studies in mouse models, which have also demonstrated the necessity of the IFN-γ signalling pathway components in a successful anti-PD-1 treatment [53–55].

However, it is noteworthy that the IFN-γ signalling pathway might have dual effects on tumor immunity. In a preclinical melanoma mouse model, inhibiting the JAK1/JAK2 signalling pathway with small molecular inhibitors overcame acquired resistance to ICBT [30]. Conversely, inhibiting the IFN-γ signalling pathway with small inhibitors and small hairpin RNAs targeting JAK1/JAK2 or STAT1 was shown to prevent upregulation of PD-L1. Blocking PD-L1 resulted in increased tumor lysis by NK cells in tumor cell lines [56]. This data revealed the potential tumor-promoting effects of the IFN-γ signalling pathway in certain stages of tumor development. However, the JAK/STAT signalling pathways have broad impacts on immune cell development and function [57]. Systematic inhibition of JAK/STAT signalling has the potential to produce strong off-target (non-tumor related) effects, leading to treatment failure. Meanwhile, systematic inhibition will also cause difficulties in interpreting the mechanisms of JAK/STAT signalling in regulating anti-tumor immunity. Therefore, the differences between systemic JAK1/JAK2 inhibition with chemical inhibitors and tumor-specific loss of JAK1/JAK2 signalling must be considered and differentiated in future studies. Further studies are also needed to confirm whether the tumor-specific IFN-γ signalling pathway has dual effects on acquired resistance to ICBT.

4.4.4   Loss of Tumor Cell Visibility to Immune Cells

Evidence has emerged that tumor cells can become invisible to tumor-specific T-cells following immunotherapy treatment. Among the mechanisms that render tumor cells invisible are mutations in the IFN-γ signalling pathway, which result in decreased MHC-I expression on tumor cells. Additionally, the loss of β-2-microglobulin (β2m), a component of MHC-I that is necessary for the recognition of tumor cells by tumor-infiltrating CD8+ T-cells, was reported in melanoma cell lines isolated from five patients who had been treated with immunotherapy. This resulted in the loss of functional MHC-I expression on tumor cells and subsequently allowed tumor cells to evade immune surveillance by CD8+ T-cells [58]. The analysis of tissues from these patients before immunotherapy treatment indicated positive β2m expression in three of them [58]. Similarly, patients with metastatic melanoma were observed to have decreased β2m expression after dendritic cell-based immunotherapy [59]. These data suggest that the loss of β2m expression can be induced by different types of immunotherapies, which can serve as an important acquired resistance mechanism.

An additional mechanism that renders tumor cells invisible to T-cells is the selection of tumor neoantigens by ICBT [60]. In a study of the evolving landscape of tumor neoantigens during the emergence of acquired resistance to ICBT, the tumors of patients with non–small cell lung cancer underwent matched (i.e., before vs. after ICBT) genomic analyses. The loss of 7 to 18 validated mutation-associated neoantigens was documented in tumors with acquired resistance [61]. Further analysis indicated that the loss of neoantigens was due to the elimination of tumor subclones or the removal of chromosomal regions containing truncated alterations [61]. The neoantigen repertoire is closely related with the T-cell repertoire as the loss of neoantigens will ultimately lead to low diversity of TCR clonality and to inefficient elimination of heterogenous tumor cell populations. In line with this observation, the presence of IFN-γ, which can be induced by ICBT, is associated with the change of tumor antigens. This process is dependent on the presence of antigen-specific cytotoxic T-cells (CTLs), unmasking another paradoxical role of IFN-γ in cancer immunotherapy and a putative mechanism of acquired resistance to ICBT [62].

4.4.5 Tumor Plasticity and Stemness

Tumor progression and resistance to anti-tumor treatments are significantly influenced by the nature of tumor cells themselves. Indeed, the augmented expression of genes involved in epithelial-to-mesenchymal transition (EMT) has been identified as a potential cause of intrinsic resistance to anti-PD-1 treatment. These genes include *FAP*, *tyrosine-protein kinase receptor UFO (AXL)*, *twist-related protein 2 (TWIST2)*, *wingless-type MMTV integration site family member 5A (WNT5A)*, *lysyl oxidase-like 2 (LOXL2)*, *receptor tyrosine kinase-like orphan receptor 2 (ROR2)*, and *transgelin (TAGLN)* [63], all of which are selectively upregulated in aggressive tumor cells. The transcriptional reprogramming of EMT might be driven by TNF-α, a key inflammatory mediator in the TME [64]. Furthermore, in patients with epithelial breast cancer, functional CD8+ T-cells have been shown to induce both EMT and stemness (i.e., stem-cell properties) in tumor cells [65]. Integrated analyses of large, public cancer molecular databases—e.g., The Cancer Genome Atlas (TCGA), the Profiling of Resistance patterns and Oncogenic Signaling Pathways in Evaluation of Cancers of the Thorax (PROSPECT), and the Biomarker-integrated Approaches of Targeted Therapy for Lung Cancer Elimination (BATTLE-1) trial—have demonstrated that inflammatory changes in the TME are positively correlated with the EMT phenotype in patients with lung cancer [66]. This correlation strongly connects the immune changes in the TME with tumor cell aggressiveness. Immunotherapies, like ICBT, regulate the immune TME and therefore, will likely alter tumor plasticity and stemness. Further studies are warranted to confirm the effects of ICBT on tumor EMT and stemness and whether this is a novel mechanism of acquired resistance to immunotherapy.

4.4.6 The Microbiome as a Novel Player in Immune Checkpoint Blockade Therapy Resistance

The human body hosts trillions of microbes, known as the microbiome (or microbiota). Microbes are prevalent throughout the body, including the skin, respiratory tract, urogenital tract, and digestive tract; however, the importance of the microbiome to human health became evident only in the last decade [67–74]. The majority of microbes, both in terms of species and numbers, live in the colon. Studies have shown that the gut microbiome not only affects the local environment (e.g., maintaining the colon's health) but also exerts a systemic effect (e.g., fine-tuning the immune system and maintaining the function of distant organs) [75–80]. Due to their vast numbers and various functions, the microbiome is widely considered to constitute humans' "second genome" [81].

Perturbations to the microbiome (dysbiosis) have been linked with cancers in many anatomic locations, such as the breast, liver, lungs, digestive tract, and reproductive tract [72–74, 82, 83]. Notably, studies in germ-free animals have found reduced tumor development in many locations [84, 85]. A case-control study involving over 600,000 people found that the use of antibiotics was associated with an increased incidence of several types of cancer [86]. As evidenced, the microbiome must play an important role in cancer, but the causality between dysbiosis and many types of cancer remains unclear.

Impact of Microbiome on Immunotherapy Efficacy Functional systemic immunity is as important as local tumor immunity in order for immunotherapy to be effective [87, 88]. Dysbiosis of the gut microbiome can impair immune function, and thus affect immunotherapy. Indeed, several recent studies have shown that the microbiome is essential in maintaining the efficacy of cancer immunotherapy. One species, *Bifidobacterium longum*, was shown to be enriched in the gut microbiome of melanoma patients that responded to anti-PD-1 treatment [89], suggesting systemic immune modulation of the commensal gut microbiome. Interestingly, the gut microbiome transplanted from these anti-PD-1 responders to tumor-bearing mice significantly improved the effectiveness of anti-PD-L1 therapy [89–91].

Similar studies in both human and mice have identified additional specific microbial signatures that are associated with immunotherapy response, whether using anti-PD-1/PD-L1, anti-CTLA-4, or CpG oligodeoxynucleotides [88, 89, 91–94]. Most notably, these studies demonstrate that germ-free or broad-spectrum antibiotics treating tumor-bearing animals significantly reduce responses to immunotherapy. However, these studies were performed by only a small number of research groups. Further validation of their findings in additional animals and human patients will be required to establish the role of bacteria in the anti-PD-1 immunotherapy treatment efficacy.

When the microbiome of patients with metastatic melanoma was enriched with Firmicutes, including *Faecalibacterium prausnitzii*, before they underwent anti-CTLA-4 treatment, they responded well. However, these patients were also susceptible to treatment-related colitis [95, 96]. After their anti-CTLA-4 treatment, responders harboured more *Bacteroides thetaiotaomicron* or *Bacteroides fragilis* in their gut microbiome. Strikingly, resistance to anti-CTLA-4 treatment can be alleviated by *Bacteroides fragilis* gavage, *Bacteroides fragilis* polysaccharide immunization or even the adoptive transfer of *Bacteroides fragilis*–specific T-cells. Zitvogel et al. speculated that antigen sharing might occur between bacteria and tumors, which might explain the effectiveness of *Bacteroides fragilis* polysaccharide immunization and adoptive transfer of *Bacteroides fragilis*–specific T-cells [97].

Moreover, in another metastatic melanoma cohort, both *Faecalibacterium prausnitzii* and *Bacteroides thetaiotaomicron* were associated with responders to combination therapy with anti-PD-1 and anti-CTLA-4 [94]. Currently, two registered clinical trials (NCT03370861 and NCT03353402) involve the microbiome and immunotherapy. Clinical trial NCT03370861 is an observational study with a goal to validate the relationship between the gut microbiome and the activity of the immune system during skin cancer immunotherapy. Clinical trial NCT03353402 is focusing on the microbiome itself as a cancer treatment. Patients with metastatic melanoma who do not respond to immunotherapy will undergo a fecal microbiome transplant (FMT) donated from treatment responders. Table 4.1 summarizes the findings of such studies.

Future Directions for Modulating Microbiota to Improve Immunotherapy Efficacy Our understanding of the microbiome is still rudimentary. Current evidence suggests a beneficial effect of specific microbes in the gut microbiome on immunotherapy, yet the precise mechanisms are unclear. Perhaps the gut microbiome fine tunes distant immune function by enhancing the activation of DCs and the priming of B-cells, T-cells, and NK cells, or by excreting a vast number of microbial metabolites [97, 98], however further validating studies are required.

The methodology of microbiome studies has also been a challenge. So far, most studies have found correlations only in retrospective cohorts. Most importantly, the cohorts have considerably varied between studies, in terms of different sample sizes as well as the heterogeneous background of patients. Another caveat is that the gut microbiome has only been studied in the context of immunotherapy, largely given the ease of gut microbiome sample collection. Finally, the limitations of current high-throughput technologies have also restricted the scope of microbiome studies to-date. As high-throughput technologies become more advanced and the subfields of metatranscriptomics and metabolomics continue to evolve, we will gradually

Table 4.1 Overview of the connection between the microbiome and immunotherapy in mouse and human studies

Cancer	Bacteria	Immunotherapy	Interactions	Refs
Mouse studies				
Melanoma	*Bifidobacterium longum*	Anti-PD-L1	Oral supplementation with this bacterium enhanced immunotherapy	[92]
Sarcoma; Melanoma; Colon carcinoma	*Bacteroides thetaiotaomicron Bacteroides fragilis*	Anti-CTLA-4	Oral supplementation with these bacteria enhanced immunotherapy	[93]
	Bacteroides fragilis	Anti-CTLA-4	Oral supplementation with this bacterium, immunization, and adoptive transfer alleviated resistance to immunotherapy	
Lymphoma; Melanoma; Colon carcinoma	Antibiotics	CpG oligodeoxynucleotides	Antibiotics reduced efficacy of immunotherapy	[144]
Melanoma	FMT from anti-PD1 responders	Anti-PD-L1	FMT improved immunotherapy	[88]
Melanoma	FMT from anti-PD1 responders	Anti-PD-L1	FMT improved immunotherapy	[89]
Melanoma Sarcoma	Antibiotics	Anti-PD-1	Antibiotics reduced response to immunotherapy	[91]
Sarcoma	FMT from anti-PD1 responders		FMT improved immunotherapy	
Melanoma	*Akkermansia muciniphila Enterococcus hirae* 13,144		Oral supplementation with these bacteria enhanced immunotherapy	
Human studies				
Metastatic melanoma	*Dorea formicogenerans Bacteroides caccae*	Anti-PD-1 (pembrolizumab)	Responder microbiome was enriched with these bacteria	[94]
	Faecalibacterium prausnitzii Bacteroides thetaiotaomicron Holdemania filiformis Bacteroides caccae	Anti-CTLA-4 (ipilimumab) + anti-PD-1 (nivolumab)	Responder microbiome was enriched with these bacteria	

(continued)

Table 4.1 (continued)

Cancer	Bacteria	Immunotherapy	Interactions	Refs
Metastatic melanoma	Firmicutes Bacteroidetes	Anti-CTLA-4 (ipilimumab)	Microbiome enriched with Firmicutes was associated with better survival but also colitis Microbiome enriched with Bacteroidetes was associated with no colitis	[96]
Melanoma	Ruminococcaceae	Anti-PD1	Microbiome enriched with Ruminococcaceae had higher alpha diversity	[88]
Metastatic melanoma	*Bifidobacterium longum Collinsella aerofaciens* *Enterococcus faecium*	Anti-PD1	Responder microbiome was enriched with these bacteria	[89]
Metastatic melanoma	Dysbiosis	Anti-CTLA-4	Immunotherapy led to dysbiosis	[93]
Non–small cell lung cancer Renal cell carcinoma Urothelial carcinoma	Antibiotics *Akkermansia muciniphila*	Anti-PD-1	Antibiotics significantly lowered overall survival Responder microbiome was enriched with this bacterium	[91]
Metastatic melanoma	Bacteroidetes	Anti-CTLA-4 ipilimumab)	Microbiome enriched with Bacteroidetes was associated with no colitis	[95]

FMT fecal microbiome transplant

increase our understanding of the role of the microbiome, as a whole, in regulating responses to immunotherapy over time.

4.4.7 Mechanisms of Acquired Resistance to Other Immunotherapy Strategies

Investigations on the mechanisms of acquired resistance to immunotherapy have primarily been focused on ICBT, either in mouse models or human patients. It is believed that some of these mechanisms are at least in part, responsible for the development of resistance to other immunotherapy strategies. Such mechanisms rely on interactions between tumor cells and tumor-infiltrating T-cells. In most of the immunotherapy strategies studied so far, the basic steps of anti-tumor immune responses seem to be the same.

However, exceptions are noticed in two emerging immunotherapy strategies: CAR-T therapy and NK cell-based tumor cell lysis. Both therapies involve genetic modification and infusion of immune cells and have different tumor-killing mechanisms compared to other immunotherapy strategies. For example, CAR-T therapy uses specially engineered patient-derived T-cells to lead an assault on cancer cells that express a specific protein that can be identified by the chimeric antigen receptors on the surface of T-cells [11]. When these CAR-T cells are reinjected into patients, they can identify and attack cancer cells throughout the body [11]. Since the engineered T-cells can usually only identify one antigen, CAR-T cells have been primarily used in blood cancers, which have strong lineage characteristics. Due to the heterogeneity characteristic of solid tumors, CAR-T cell therapy is still limited. NK cells are the major innate immune cell types and the front-line effectors against tumor cells. Currently, both the CAR-expressing NK cells and the bi- and tri-specific killer engagers (BiKEs and TriKEs) modified NK cells were developed and tested in pre-clinical models [99, 100]. Therefore, the tumor targeting mechanisms of current NK cell-based immunotherapies are more like CAR-T therapy, rather than ICBT. However, NK cell-based therapy remains largely untested clinically. A few studies have already reported or summarized some mechanisms of intrinsic and acquired resistance to these two immunotherapy strategies, including genetic mutations in the targeted antigen, alternative splicing of the targeted protein, mutations in the B-cell receptor complex protein CD81, and transduction of unintentionally modified leukemic cell with an anti-CD19 CAR lentivirus during CAR-T cell manufacturing [101–108].

4.5 Detection of Acquired Resistance to Immune Checkpoint Blockade Therapy

Early detection is important to help guide therapy, enhance survival, and avoid complications of futile treatments. New methods of measuring ICBT tumor response are needed as ICBT efficacy is not adequately assessed by the current criteria, which were developed to evaluate cytotoxic chemotherapy in patients with solid tumors. Current criteria includes the objective responses formulated by the World Health Organization (WHO) and Response Evaluation Criteria in Solid Tumors (RECIST) initiative [109]. Unlike conventional therapies, the reduction in tumor burden in patients treated with ICBT frequently occurs after an initial increase in tumor size, possibly due to inflammation or T-cell infiltration; therefore, radiographic imaging may need to be supplemented with additional modes of assessment to evaluate ICBT resistance [110].

Histological analysis of tumors may serve as a better predictor of adaptive resistance to immunotherapy than radiographic evaluation. Following treatment with ICBT, significant differences develop in the tumor microenvironment between responders and non-responders to therapy. The changes following ICBT treatment can be examined via serial biopsies. For example, Chen et al. described an immunologic analysis of longitudinal tumor biopsies in patients with metastatic melanoma who were initially treated with CTLA-4 blockade, followed by PD-1 blockade after serial computed tomography (CT) and documented the progression of tumor size [111]. The biopsies were performed both before and during CTLA-4 blockade therapy, as well as in non-responders whose disease had continued to progress. Before the initiation of CTLA-4 blockade therapy, Chen et al. observed no differences between the measured markers in responders versus non-responders. Early during CTLA-4 blockade therapy, however, responders developed a higher concentration of CD-8+ T-cells when compared with non-responders, suggesting stronger immunologic responses. When the non-responders to CTLA-4 blockade were transitioned to PD-1 blockade, responders to the new therapy experienced a profound increase in T-cell markers CD8, CD4, CD3, in addition to increases in the immunomodulatory markers PD-1, PD-L1, and LAG3. Furthermore, responders to PD-1 blockade also developed the expression of FOXP3 (which forms a transcription complex critical for the development of regulatory T-cells [112]) and of granzyme B (a serine protease secreted by NK cells and cytotoxic T-cells to mediate apoptosis of target cells), giving further evidence of immunological response to therapy. These changes were observed as early as 2 to 3 treatments into PD-1 blockade therapy, demonstrating the potential utility of biopsies in the early assessment of resistance to ICBT.

Researchers continue to develop high-throughput techniques for biopsy samples to measure gene expression signatures in order to identify additional genes associated with acquired ICBT resistance. A total of 411 genes have been identified as potentially correlated with responses to ICBT including cytolytic markers, HLA molecules, IFN-γ pathway effectors, chemokines, and select adhesion molecules, all of which are critical components of the anti-tumor immune response [111]. Furthermore, Anagnostoul et al. explored the utility of neoantigen identification and quantification in biopsy samples to find specific resistance patterns to ICBT in non-small cell lung cancer. Treatment with ICBT was associated with a decline in neoantigen expression, which was eliminated via immunoediting or by the chromosomal loss of neoantigen source DNA [61]. In the tumors of patients who developed resistance to ICBT, Anagnostoul et al. observed an increase in mutations that do not produce neoantigens [61]. This finding could potentially lead to the identification of biomarkers that predict adaptive resistance to ICBT.

Although sequential biopsies of tumors can assist healthcare professionals in monitoring ICBT efficacy, they are expensive and invasive; moreover, they can yield ambiguous results, given the heterogeneous nature of tumors. Biopsies not only cause significant discomfort to patients, but are also associated with several potential risks, including surgical risks such as bleeding, infection, and organ injury. In addition, biopsies have the potential for "seeding" the tumor in other body sites. Finally, the wait time required for tumor evaluation by the pathologist could cause delays in the continuation of treatment, jeopardizing patient survival.

Fortunately, less invasive methods are being studied to monitor tumor response to ICBT. Currently, circulating tumor DNA (ctDNA) is under investigation in cancer patients for both diagnosis and prognosis. Circulating DNA fragments are found in the blood of all individuals, but the levels of circulating DNA tend to be elevated in patients with malignancy [113]. In cancer patients, specific changes can be identified in a percentage of the fragments of ctDNA, including gene mutations [114], cancer-associated microsatellite alterations, and epigenetic DNA-methylation changes [115]. Increases in ctDNA have been associated with increased tumor burden; however, complete surgical resection has been found to decrease the levels of ctDNA [114], demonstrating a potential for monitoring tumor burden.

Gary et al. evaluated ctDNA in 48 patients with BRAS- and NRAS-mutated melanoma, both before the initiation of therapy and after eight weeks of treatment [116]. Of those 48 patients, 19 were treated with ICBT, including 9 with ipilimumab, 3 with nivolumab, 6 with pembrolizumab, and 1 with a combination of ipilimumab and pembrolizumab. In a subgroup of 15 patients, ctDNA was monitored at baseline and at 4 and 8 weeks of ICBT. Responders had either a ten-fold reduction in ctDNA or low baseline ctDNA initially, suggesting that ctDNA is an effective monitoring strategy for melanoma patients on ICBT. However, the study was limited by small sample size and by the heterogeneity of ICBT regimens. Another analysis of ctDNA in 28 patients with non–small cell lung cancer who were on ICBT also showed that in responders, the reduction in ctDNA preceded radiographic evidence of responses to treatment (median time to ctDNA response, 24.5 days; median time to radiographic evidence, 72.5 days) [117]. Similar results have been reported by other studies [118, 119].

In addition to ctDNA measurement, peripheral TCR sequencing is another noninvasive strategy to monitor response to ICBT. TCR sequencing involves deep sequencing of TCR CDR3 regions, which can identify anti-tumor T-cell development and proliferation. Analysis of TCR sequences in patients with various malignancies who responded to pembrolizumab, both before and after treatment revealed that tumor-specific T-cell clones were selectively expanded in the peripheral blood after initiation of ICBT. Moreover, the peak of tumor-specific T-cell expansion occurred earlier than the radiographic responses [120].

4.6   Methods of Overcoming Acquired Resistance to Immune Checkpoint Blockade Therapy

With more robust evidence becoming available on mechanisms of resistance to ICBT, efforts are being made to derive actionable combination strategies to combat such resistance. For reversing intrinsic resistance, the fundamental focus is on transforming immunologically "cold" tumors to "hot" tumors, i.e., to increase immune infiltration and function in the TME. Tactics include enhancing endogenous anti-tumor immunity by treating "cold" tumors with chemotherapy or radiotherapy, thereby inducing tumor antigen release and presentation [7]. However, potential negative consequences, such as the selection of a more aggressive tumor phenotype following chemotherapy, can limit the use of these combinatory strategies to overcome intrinsic resistance.

Intrinsic resistance is primarily due to the nature of tumors; however, acquired resistance is attributed to Darwinian selection and immunoediting induced by ICBT. The heterogeneous genetic and epigenetic traits of tumors, and their various interactions with the microenvironment give rise to the manifestation of diverse immunologic features. Tumor cells that are visible to immune cells are efficiently killed by ICBT, shrinking the tumor. This results in residual tumor cells that have immunosuppressive features or are protected by the surrounding stromal cells. Such tumor cells may eventually regrow and cause disease progression. Therefore, to overcome acquired resistance, an understanding of the dynamic selection mechanisms in specific tumors and targeting both the tumor cells as well as the surrounding stromal cells is required. The revolutionary technologies that were developed in recent years shed light on tumor-specific immunotherapy. Mass cytometry, mass spectrometry imaging, single-cell sequencing, and liquid biopsy tests have been tested to provide a more comprehensive understanding of tumor progression and evolution [121–127]. Further developing and applying these technologies to clinical tests will provide a more precise evaluation of tumor cell and immune microenvironment evolution and consequently reveal valuable targets for immunotherapies.

Chemotherapy is primarily designed to target cancer cells, which proliferate at a higher rate than most normal cells. However, chemotherapy also has significant effects on immune regulation [128]. Traditionally, conventional chemotherapy—even with DNA-damaging agents—has been considered immunosuppressive due to its lymphopenic toxicity. However, an increasing number of experimental studies have suggested that chemotherapy with DNA-damaging agents can promote anti-tumor immunity. In a mouse lung cancer model, oxaliplatin combined with cyclophosphamide significantly induced immunogenicity of tumor cells [129]. Mechanistically, tumor expression and secretion of DAMPs—such as cytosolic DNA, high-mobility group box 1 (HMGB1), calreticulin, hyaluronan, and heat shock protein—are enhanced by DNA-damaging agents [129–131]. The result is that cancer cells and stromal cells increase secretion of type I IFN and other chemokines, to facilitate the function of APCs.

Radiotherapy also enhances MHC class I surface expression and secretion of DAMPs. It activates DCs and enhances cross-presentation of tumor antigens to naïve T-cells for T-cell priming [132–134]. Fas surface expression on tumor cells is also upregulated by radiotherapy, making cells sensitive to programmed cell death induced by the engagement of Fas with FasL on T-cells. Other immunologic targets of radiotherapy include T_{reg} populations and immune checkpoints [135]. Taken together, these mechanisms support the use of immunogenic chemotherapy and radiotherapy to overcome acquired resistance to ICBT due to the loss of T-cell recognition mediated by antigen release/presentation or by the Fas/FasL pathway.

Compensatory upregulation of alternative inhibitory immune checkpoints in response to anti-CTLA-4/anti-PD-1/PD-L1 supports the use of the combination of multiple immune checkpoint inhibitors to overcome acquired resistance [30, 32, 34–36]. Blocking these alternative inhibitory immune checkpoints will probably rescue exhausted T-cells. Meanwhile, efforts have also been made to combine immune-stimulating checkpoints with ICBT. Examples include adding anti-OX40, anti-41BB, anti-CD40, and anti-inducible T-cell co-stimulator (ICOS) to anti-PD-1/PD-L1 therapy. In preclinical models, both strategies have enhanced outcomes in tumor-bearing mice [37–39]. Multiple clinical trials with similar combination strategies are ongoing.

Other combination strategies include adding metabolic inhibitors such as indoleamine 2,3-dioxygenase (IDO) inhibitor and adenosine receptor (A2AR) inhibitor, epigenetic modifiers, and oncogenic targeted therapy to ICBT [25, 136–138]. Doing so could potentially help ameliorate the energy supply to effector T-cells and help reverse epigenetic changes in exhausted T-cells. Oncogenic pathways have numerous interactions with immunosuppressive mechanisms in cancer cells, especially PD-L1 and IL-10 production, CD47 expression, and MHC I reduction [25]. Targeting an oncogenic pathway will probably reduce multiple immunosuppressive mechanisms, making the use of such inhibitors a promising method to overcome acquired resistance to ICBT.

4.7 Conclusion

We are currently at the beginning of a cancer immunotherapy revolution. Decades of solid basic studies have deciphered the key mechanisms of T-cell function regulation and have helped translate at least some of the laboratory findings into clinical practice. However, given the complexity of the human body, the diversity of tumor cell genomes, and the multidimensional interactions of tumors with their microenvironment, enhancing the efficacy and longevity of responses to ICBT in various tumor types remains challenging. Key questions that encompass this complexity require investigation before translating our understanding of resistant mechanisms to treatment strategies to overcome acquired resistance to ICBT.

The greatest challenge is the design of combination therapy. Our experience thus far with anti-CTLA-4 and anti-PD-1/PD-L1 therapy has given us insight into the clinical significance of combining different immune-stimulating mechanisms [139]. For example, CTLA-4 is the competitive inhibitor of CD28. Therefore, inhibiting CTLA-4 will dramatically enhance T-cell priming, stimulating initial anti-tumor immunity [21]. Additionally, the CTLA-4 antibody also binds very efficiently to T_{regs}, inducing depletion of T_{regs} in the tumor microenvironment [21].

Meanwhile, PD-1 is mainly expressed on exhausted T-cells that are usually enriched in the TME. Further analyses of tumors after anti-PD-1 and anti-CTLA-4 therapy have demonstrated that anti-PD-1 predominantly induces the expansion of specific tumor-infiltrating exhausted CD8+ T-cells. In contrast, anti-CTLA-4 induces the expansion of ICOS+ Th1-like CD4+ effector T-cells, in addition to regulating specific subsets of exhausted CD8+ T-cells in the TME [140]. The different immune-stimulating mechanisms make the combination of anti-PD-1 and anti-CTLA-4 more effective than either one alone. However, even with combination therapy, not all patients will respond, and additional strategies will still need to be explored.

Combination strategies are not always more efficient than treatment with a single agent. In mouse models, IDO inhibitors, which regulate tryptophan catabolism in the TME, have shown promising anti-tumor activity [141]. However, in a phase III melanoma clinical trial, the combination of IDO inhibitors and anti-PD-1 failed [142]. Multiple clinical trials with similar targets are currently underway, but conclusive results have yet to be reported. This failure could be because IDO is not the key factor regulating immunosuppression at or because IDO inhibitors only work in a small proportion of tumors, perhaps only when high expression of IDO is the major reason for the failure of anti-PD-1 therapy. The success of anti-CTLA-4 and anti-PD-1 combination and the failure of IDO inhibitors and an anti-PD-1 combination formed a distinct contrast, highlighting the need to understand different combinatory mechanisms and precisely evaluate resistant mechanisms.

Another daunting challenge is the management of toxicity. The combination of anti-CTLA-4 and anti-PD-1/PD-L1 therapy has been successful, in part, because of its role in stimulating T-cell function, but even more so because of its high specificity to tumor-mediated immunosuppression, especially the impact of anti-PD-1/PD-L1. Previous forms of immunotherapy with less specificity have had therapeutic value but have been restricted to only a few tumor types and limited clinical scenarios. Modulating the general immunosuppressive pathways will produce certain anti-tumor immunity, yet strong side effects will significantly restrict the intensity of treatment and neutralize the benefit of tumor regression. Further efforts are needed to identify the immunosuppressive pathways that are selectively upregulated in cancer patients, thereby providing the basis for efficient combination strategies with low toxicity.

Finally, methods by which combination therapy is tested in preclinical settings should be reformed. To thoroughly evaluate the efficacy of combination therapy in overcoming acquired resistance to ICBT, tumor models must mimic real-world clinical conditions. The formation of acquired resistance is primarily due to Darwinian selection and immunoediting in highly heterogeneous human tumors. Thus far, most preclinical studies use tumor models from a single cell line. Not fully mimicking the TME of human tumors [143]. Moreover, most of the current preclinical studies have treated naïve primary tumors, and although this methodology can be used for investigating intrinsic resistance, it cannot be applied to studying acquired resistance. Our group's unpublished data have shown a vast difference in the immune response between a small tumor and an established tumor. Thus, the tumor stage should also be considered and well controlled for when studying acquired resistance in animal models. Patient-derived tumors have provided valuable resources to study acquired resistance, but finding MHC-matched, humanized host animals remains to be a serious obstacle. A genetically engineered mouse (GEM) spontaneous tumor model is an alternative; such tumors, though derived from a uniform mutational pattern, are closer to human lesions than mouse tumors derived from a cell line. Inducing acquired resistance in GEM models and testing novel treatment strategies will dramatically facilitate the translation of combination therapy from the laboratory to clinical settings.

References

1. Oiseth SJ, Aziz MS. Cancer immunotherapy: a brief review of the history, possibilities, and challenges ahead. J Cancer Metastasis Treat. 2017;3:251.
2. Busch W. Aus der Sitzung der medicinischen Section vom 13 November 1867. Berl Klin Wochenschr. 1868;5:137.
3. Coley WB. The treatment of malignant tumors by repeated inoculations of erysipelas. With a report of ten original cases. 1893. Clin Orthop Relat Res. 1991;(262):3–11.
4. Ribatti D. The concept of immune surveillance against tumors. The first theories. Oncotarget. 2017;8(4):7175–80. https://doi.org/10.18632/oncotarget.12739.
5. Herr HW, Morales A. History of bacillus Calmette-Guerin and bladder cancer: an immunotherapy success story. J Urol. 2008;179(1):53–6. https://doi.org/10.1016/j.juro.2007.08.122.
6. de Visser KE, Eichten A, Coussens LM. Paradoxical roles of the immune system during cancer development. Nat Rev Cancer. 2006;6(1):24–37. https://doi.org/10.1038/nrc1782.
7. Zhao X, Subramanian S. Intrinsic resistance of solid tumors to immune checkpoint blockade therapy. Cancer Res. 2017;77(4):817–22. https://doi.org/10.1158/0008-5472.can-16-2379.
8. Cheever MA, Higano CS. PROVENGE (Sipuleucel-T) in prostate cancer: the first FDA-approved therapeutic cancer vaccine. Clin Cancer Res. 2011;17(11):3520–6. https://doi.org/10.1158/1078-0432.ccr-10-3126.
9. Higano CS. Sipuleucel-T: autologous cellular immunotherapy for metastatic castration-resistant prostate cancer. New York: Springer; 2010.
10. Lee S, Margolin K. Cytokines in cancer immunotherapy. Cancers (Basel). 2011;3(4):3856–93. https://doi.org/10.3390/cancers3043856.
11. Baruch EN, Berg AL, Besser MJ, Schachter J, Markel G. Adoptive T cell therapy: an overview of obstacles and opportunities. Cancer. 2017;123(S11):2154–62. https://doi.org/10.1002/cncr.30491.
12. Maude SL, Frey N, Shaw PA, Aplenc R, Barrett DM, Bunin NJ, et al. Chimeric antigen receptor T cells for sustained remissions in leukemia. N Engl J Med. 2014;371(16):1507–17. https://doi.org/10.1056/NEJMoa1407222.
13. Maude SL, Teachey DT, Porter DL, Grupp SA. CD19-targeted chimeric antigen receptor T-cell therapy for acute lymphoblastic leukemia. Blood. 2015;125(26):4017–23. https://doi.org/10.1182/blood-2014-12-580068.
14. Fukuhara H, Ino Y, Todo T. Oncolytic virus therapy: a new era of cancer treatment at dawn. Cancer Sci. 2016;107(10):1373–9. https://doi.org/10.1111/cas.13027.
15. Kohlhapp FJ, Kaufman HL. Molecular pathways: mechanism of action for Talimogene Laherparepvec, a new oncolytic virus immunotherapy. Clin Cancer Res. 2016;22(5):1048–54. https://doi.org/10.1158/1078-0432.ccr-15-2667.
16. Lawler SE, Speranza MC, Cho CF, Chiocca EA. Oncolytic viruses in cancer treatment: a review. JAMA Oncol. 2016;3(6):841.
17. Sansom DM. CD28, CTLA-4 and their ligands: who does what and to whom? Immunology. 2000;101(2):169–77.
18. Shiratori T, Miyatake S, Ohno H, Nakaseko C, Isono K, Bonifacino JS, et al. Tyrosine phosphorylation controls internalization of CTLA-4 by regulating its interaction with clathrin-associated adaptor complex AP-2. Immunity. 1997;6(5):583–9.
19. Zuazo M, Gato-Canas M, Llorente N, Ibanez-Vea M, Arasanz H, Kochan G, et al. Molecular mechanisms of programmed cell death-1 dependent T cell suppression: relevance for immunotherapy. Ann Transl Med. 2017;5(19):385. https://doi.org/10.21037/atm.2017.06.11.
20. Leach DR, Krummel MF, Allison JP. Enhancement of antitumor immunity by CTLA-4 blockade. Science. 1996;271(5256):1734–6.
21. Ribas A, Wolchok JD. Cancer immunotherapy using checkpoint blockade. Science. 2018;359(6382):1350–5.
22. Syn NL, Teng MWL, Mok TSK, Soo RA. De-novo and acquired resistance to immune checkpoint targeting. Lancet Oncol. 2017;18(12):e731–e41. https://doi.org/10.1016/s1470-2045(17)30607-1.

23. Chen DS, Mellman I. Oncology meets immunology: the cancer-immunity cycle. Immunity. 2013;39(1):1–10. https://doi.org/10.1016/j.immuni.2013.07.012.
24. Zhao X, May A, Lou E, Subramanian S. Genotypic and phenotypic signatures to predict immune checkpoint blockade therapy response in patients with colorectal cancer. Transl Res. 2018;196:62–70. https://doi.org/10.1016/j.trsl.2018.02.001.
25. Zhao X, Subramanian S. Oncogenic pathways that affect antitumor immune response and immune checkpoint blockade therapy. Pharmacol Ther. 2018;181:76–84. https://doi.org/10.1016/j.pharmthera.2017.07.004.
26. Restifo NP, Smyth MJ, Snyder A. Acquired resistance to immunotherapy and future challenges. Nat Rev Cancer. 2016;16(2):121–6. https://doi.org/10.1038/nrc.2016.2.
27. Wherry EJ, Kurachi M. Molecular and cellular insights into T cell exhaustion. Nat Rev Immunol. 2015;15(8):486–99. https://doi.org/10.1038/nri3862.
28. Sen DR, Kaminski J, Barnitz RA, Kurachi M, Gerdemann U, Yates KB, et al. The epigenetic landscape of T cell exhaustion. Science. 2016;354(6316):1165–9. https://doi.org/10.1126/science.aae0491.
29. Pauken KE, Sammons MA, Odorizzi PM, Manne S, Godec J, Khan O, et al. Epigenetic stability of exhausted T cells limits durability of reinvigoration by PD-1 blockade. Science. 2016;354(6316):1160–5. https://doi.org/10.1126/science.aaf2807.
30. Benci JL, Xu B, Qiu Y, Wu TJ, Dada H, Twyman-Saint Victor C, et al. Tumor interferon signaling regulates a multigenic resistance program to immune checkpoint blockade. Cell. 2016;167(6):1540–54.e12. https://doi.org/10.1016/j.cell.2016.11.022.
31. Spranger S, Spaapen RM, Zha Y, Williams J, Meng Y, Ha TT, et al. Up-regulation of PD-L1, IDO, and T(regs) in the melanoma tumor microenvironment is driven by CD8(+) T cells. Sci Transl Med. 2013;5(200):200ra116. https://doi.org/10.1126/scitranslmed.3006504.
32. Shayan G, Srivastava R, Li J, Schmitt N, Kane LP, Ferris RL. Adaptive resistance to anti-PD1 therapy by Tim-3 upregulation is mediated by the PI3K-Akt pathway in head and neck cancer. Oncoimmunology. 2017;6(1):e1261779. https://doi.org/10.1080/2162402x.2016.1261779.
33. Zhu C, Anderson AC, Kuchroo VK. TIM-3 and its regulatory role in immune responses. Curr Top Microbiol Immunol. 2011;350:1–15. https://doi.org/10.1007/82_2010_84.
34. Koyama S, Akbay EA, Li YY, Herter-Sprie GS, Buczkowski KA, Richards WG, et al. Adaptive resistance to therapeutic PD-1 blockade is associated with upregulation of alternative immune checkpoints. Nat Commun. 2016;7:10501. https://doi.org/10.1038/ncomms10501.
35. Huang RY, Francois A, McGray AR, Miliotto A, Odunsi K. Compensatory upregulation of PD-1, LAG-3, and CTLA-4 limits the efficacy of single-agent checkpoint blockade in metastatic ovarian cancer. Oncoimmunology. 2017;6(1):e1249561. https://doi.org/10.1080/21624 02x.2016.1249561.
36. Gao J, Ward JF, Pettaway CA, Shi LZ, Subudhi SK, Vence LM, et al. VISTA is an inhibitory immune checkpoint that is increased after ipilimumab therapy in patients with prostate cancer. Nat Med. 2017;23(5):551–5. https://doi.org/10.1038/nm.4308.
37. Curran MA, Montalvo W, Yagita H, Allison JP. PD-1 and CTLA-4 combination blockade expands infiltrating T cells and reduces regulatory T and myeloid cells within B16 melanoma tumors. Proc Natl Acad Sci U S A. 2010;107(9):4275–80. https://doi.org/10.1073/pnas.0915174107.
38. Allard B, Pommey S, Smyth MJ, Stagg J. Targeting CD73 enhances the antitumor activity of anti-PD-1 and anti-CTLA-4 mAbs. Clin Cancer Res. 2013;19(20):5626–35. https://doi.org/10.1158/1078-0432.ccr-13-0545.
39. Chen S, Lee LF, Fisher TS, Jessen B, Elliott M, Evering W, et al. Combination of 4-1BB agonist and PD-1 antagonist promotes antitumor effector/memory CD8 T cells in a poorly immunogenic tumor model. Cancer Immunol Res. 2015;3(2):149–60. https://doi.org/10.1158/2326-6066.cir-14-0118.
40. Du X, Tang F, Liu M, Su J, Zhang Y, Wu W, et al. A reappraisal of CTLA-4 checkpoint blockade in cancer immunotherapy. Cell Res. 2018;28(4):416–32. https://doi.org/10.1038/s41422-018-0011-0.

41. Arce Vargas F, Furness AJS, Litchfield K, Joshi K, Rosenthal R, Ghorani E, et al. Fc effector function contributes to the activity of human anti-CTLA-4 antibodies. Cancer Cell. 2018;33(4):649–663.e4. https://doi.org/10.1016/j.ccell.2018.02.010.

42. Romano E, Kusio-Kobialka M, Foukas PG, Baumgaertner P, Meyer C, Ballabeni P, et al. Ipilimumab-dependent cell-mediated cytotoxicity of regulatory T cells ex vivo by nonclassical monocytes in melanoma patients. Proc Natl Acad Sci U S A. 2015;112(19):6140–5. https://doi.org/10.1073/pnas.1417320112.

43. Motz GT, Santoro SP, Wang LP, Garrabrant T, Lastra RR, Hagemann IS, et al. Tumor endothelium FasL establishes a selective immune barrier promoting tolerance in tumors. Nat Med. 2014;20(6):607–15. https://doi.org/10.1038/nm.3541.

44. Feig C, Jones JO, Kraman M, Wells RJ, Deonarine A, Chan DS, et al. Targeting CXCL12 from FAP-expressing carcinoma-associated fibroblasts synergizes with anti-PD-L1 immunotherapy in pancreatic cancer. Proc Natl Acad Sci U S A. 2013;110(50):20212–7. https://doi.org/10.1073/pnas.1320318110.

45. Chen L, Qiu X, Wang X, He J. FAP positive fibroblasts induce immune checkpoint blockade resistance in colorectal cancer via promoting immunosuppression. Biochem Biophys Res Commun. 2017;487(1):8–14. https://doi.org/10.1016/j.bbrc.2017.03.039.

46. Zaretsky JM, Garcia-Diaz A, Shin DS, Escuin-Ordinas H, Hugo W, Hu-Lieskovan S, et al. Mutations associated with acquired resistance to PD-1 blockade in melanoma. N Engl J Med. 2016;375(9):819–29. https://doi.org/10.1056/NEJMoa1604958.

47. Kouidhi S, Elgaaied AB, Chouaib S. Impact of metabolism on T-cell differentiation and function and cross talk with tumor microenvironment. Front Immunol. 2017;8:270. https://doi.org/10.3389/fimmu.2017.00270.

48. Kouidhi S, Noman MZ, Kieda C, Elgaaied AB, Chouaib S. Intrinsic and tumor microenvironment-induced metabolism adaptations of T cells and impact on their differentiation and function. Front Immunol. 2016;7:114. https://doi.org/10.3389/fimmu.2016.00114.

49. Delgoffe GM. Filling the tank: keeping antitumor T cells metabolically fit for the Long Haul. Cancer Immunol Res. 2016;4(12):1001–6. https://doi.org/10.1158/2326-6066.cir-16-0244.

50. Buchert M, Burns CJ, Ernst M. Targeting JAK kinase in solid tumors: emerging opportunities and challenges. Oncogene. 2016;35(8):939–51. https://doi.org/10.1038/onc.2015.150.

51. O'Shea JJ, Schwartz DM, Villarino AV, Gadina M, McInnes IB, Laurence A. The JAK-STAT pathway: impact on human disease and therapeutic intervention. Annu Rev Med. 2015;66:311–28. https://doi.org/10.1146/annurev-med-051113-024537.

52. Gao J, Shi LZ, Zhao H, Chen J, Xiong L, He Q, et al. Loss of IFN-gamma pathway genes in tumor cells as a mechanism of resistance to anti-CTLA-4 therapy. Cell. 2016;167(2):397–404.e9. https://doi.org/10.1016/j.cell.2016.08.069.

53. Peng W, Liu C, Xu C, Lou Y, Chen J, Yang Y, et al. PD-1 blockade enhances T-cell migration to tumors by elevating IFN-gamma inducible chemokines. Cancer Res. 2012;72(20):5209–18. https://doi.org/10.1158/0008-5472.can-12-1187.

54. Wang X, Schoenhals JE, Li A, Valdecanas DR, Ye H, Zang F, et al. Suppression of type I IFN signaling in tumors mediates resistance to anti-PD-1 treatment that can be overcome by radiotherapy. Cancer Res. 2017;77(4):839–50. https://doi.org/10.1158/0008-5472.can-15-3142.

55. Manguso RT, Pope HW, Zimmer MD, Brown FD, Yates KB, Miller BC, et al. In vivo CRISPR screening identifies Ptpn2 as a cancer immunotherapy target. Nature. 2017;547(7664):413–8. https://doi.org/10.1038/nature23270.

56. Bellucci R, Martin A, Bommarito D, Wang K, Hansen SH, Freeman GJ, et al. Interferon-gamma-induced activation of JAK1 and JAK2 suppresses tumor cell susceptibility to NK cells through upregulation of PD-L1 expression. Oncoimmunology. 2015;4(6):e1008824. https://doi.org/10.1080/2162402x.2015.1008824.

57. Villarino AV, Kanno Y, Ferdinand JR, O'Shea JJ. Mechanisms of Jak/STAT signaling in immunity and disease. J Immunol. 2015;194(1):21–7. https://doi.org/10.4049/jimmunol.1401867.

58. Restifo NP, Marincola FM, Kawakami Y, Taubenberger J, Yannelli JR, Rosenberg SA. Loss of functional beta 2-microglobulin in metastatic melanomas from five patients receiving immunotherapy. J Natl Cancer Inst. 1996;88(2):100–8.

59. del Campo AB, Kyte JA, Carretero J, Zinchencko S, Mendez R, Gonzalez-Aseguinolaza G, et al. Immune escape of cancer cells with beta2-microglobulin loss over the course of metastatic melanoma. Int J Cancer. 2014;134(1):102–13. https://doi.org/10.1002/ijc.28338.

60. McGranahan N, Furness AJ, Rosenthal R, Ramskov S, Lyngaa R, Saini SK, et al. Clonal neoantigens elicit T cell immunoreactivity and sensitivity to immune checkpoint blockade. Science. 2016;351(6280):1463–9. https://doi.org/10.1126/science.aaf1490.

61. Anagnostou V, Smith KN, Forde PM, Niknafs N, Bhattacharya R, White J, et al. Evolution of neoantigen landscape during immune checkpoint blockade in non-small cell lung cancer. Cancer Discov. 2017;7(3):264–76. https://doi.org/10.1158/2159-8290.cd-16-0828.

62. Takeda K, Nakayama M, Hayakawa Y, Kojima Y, Ikeda H, Imai N, et al. IFN-gamma is required for cytotoxic T cell-dependent cancer genome immunoediting. Nat Commun. 2017;8:14607. https://doi.org/10.1038/ncomms14607.

63. Hugo W, Zaretsky JM, Sun L, Song C, Moreno BH, Hu-Lieskovan S, et al. Genomic and transcriptomic features of response to anti-PD-1 therapy in metastatic melanoma. Cell. 2017;168(3):542. https://doi.org/10.1016/j.cell.2017.01.010.

64. Falletta P, Sanchez-Del-Campo L, Chauhan J, Effern M, Kenyon A, Kershaw CJ, et al. Translation reprogramming is an evolutionarily conserved driver of phenotypic plasticity and therapeutic resistance in melanoma. Genes Dev. 2017;31(1):18–33. https://doi.org/10.1101/gad.290940.116.

65. Santisteban M, Reiman JM, Asiedu MK, Behrens MD, Nassar A, Kalli KR, et al. Immune-induced epithelial to mesenchymal transition in vivo generates breast cancer stem cells. Cancer Res. 2009;69(7):2887–95. https://doi.org/10.1158/0008-5472.can-08-3343.

66. Lou Y, Diao L, Cuentas ER, Denning WL, Chen L, Fan YH, et al. Epithelial-mesenchymal transition is associated with a distinct tumor microenvironment including elevation of inflammatory signals and multiple immune checkpoints in lung adenocarcinoma. Clin Cancer Res. 2016;22(14):3630–42. https://doi.org/10.1158/1078-0432.ccr-15-1434.

67. Gevers D, Knight R, Petrosino JF, Huang K, McGuire AL, Birren BW, et al. The human microbiome project: a community resource for the healthy human microbiome. PLoS Biol. 2012;10(8):e1001377. https://doi.org/10.1371/journal.pbio.1001377.

68. Ley RE, Turnbaugh PJ, Klein S, Gordon JI. Microbial ecology: human gut microbes associated with obesity. Nature. 2006;444(7122):1022–3. https://doi.org/10.1038/4441022a.

69. Turnbaugh PJ, Ley RE, Mahowald MA, Magrini V, Mardis ER, Gordon JI. An obesity-associated gut microbiome with increased capacity for energy harvest. Nature. 2006;444(7122):1027–31. https://doi.org/10.1038/nature05414.

70. Turnbaugh PJ, REL MH, Fraser-Liggett C, Knight R, Gordon JI. The human microbiome project: exploring the microbial part of ourselves in a changing world. Nature. 2007;449(7164):804.

71. Turnbaugh PJ, Gordon JI. The core gut microbiome, energy balance and obesity. J Physiol. 2009;587(Pt 17):4153–8. https://doi.org/10.1113/jphysiol.2009.174136.

72. Zackular JP, Baxter NT, Iverson KD, Sadler WD, Petrosino JF, Chen GY, et al. The gut microbiome modulates colon tumorigenesis. MBio. 2013;4(6):e00692–13. https://doi.org/10.1128/mBio.00692-13.

73. Hieken TJ, Chen J, Hoskin TL, Walther-Antonio M, Johnson S, Ramaker S, et al. The microbiome of aseptically collected human breast tissue in benign and malignant disease. Sci Rep. 2016;6:30751. https://doi.org/10.1038/srep30751.

74. Tsay JJ, Wu BG, Badri MH, Clemente JC, Shen N, Meyn P, et al. Airway microbiota is associated with up-regulation of the PI3K pathway in lung cancer. Am J Respir Crit Care Med. 2018;198:1188–98. https://doi.org/10.1164/rccm.201710-2118OC.

75. Tremaroli V, Backhed F. Functional interactions between the gut microbiota and host metabolism. Nature. 2012;489(7415):242–9. https://doi.org/10.1038/nature11552.

76. Belkaid Y, Hand TW. Role of the microbiota in immunity and inflammation. Cell. 2014;157(1):121–41.

77. Candon S, Perez-Arroyo A, Marquet C, Valette F, Foray AP, Pelletier B, et al. Antibiotics in early life alter the gut microbiome and increase disease incidence in a spontaneous mouse

model of autoimmune insulin-dependent diabetes. PLoS One. 2015;10(5):e0125448. https://doi.org/10.1371/journal.pone.0125448.

78. Sender R, Fuchs S, Milo R. Revised estimates for the number of human and bacteria cells in the body. PLoS Biol. 2016;14(8):e1002533. https://doi.org/10.1371/journal.pbio.1002533.

79. Abdollahi-Roodsaz S, Abramson SB, Scher JU. The metabolic role of the gut microbiota in health and rheumatic disease: mechanisms and interventions. Nat Rev Rheumatol. 2016;12(8):446–55. https://doi.org/10.1038/nrrheum.2016.68.

80. Yuan C, Burns MB, Subramanian S, Blekhman R. Interaction between host micrornas and the gut microbiota in colorectal cancer. mSystems. 2018;3(3). https://doi.org/10.1128/mSystems.00205-17.

81. Zhu B, Wang X, Li L. Human gut microbiome: the second genome of human body. Protein Cell. 2010;1(8):718–25. https://doi.org/10.1007/s13238-010-0093-z.

82. Yoshimoto S, Loo TM, Atarashi K, Kanda H, Sato S, Oyadomari S, et al. Obesity-induced gut microbial metabolite promotes liver cancer through senescence secretome. Nature. 2013;499(7456):97–101. https://doi.org/10.1038/nature12347.

83. Sheflin AM, Whitney AK, Weir TL. Cancer-promoting effects of microbial dysbiosis. Curr Oncol Rep. 2014;16(10):406. https://doi.org/10.1007/s11912-014-0406-0.

84. Goodman B, Gardner H. The microbiome and cancer. J Pathol. 2018;244:667–76.

85. Schwabe RF, Jobin C. The microbiome and cancer. Nat Rev Cancer. 2013;13(11):800–12. https://doi.org/10.1038/nrc3610.

86. Boursi B, Mamtani R, Haynes K, Yang YX. Recurrent antibiotic exposure may promote cancer formation—another step in understanding the role of the human microbiota? Eur J Cancer. 2015;51(17):2655–64. https://doi.org/10.1016/j.ejca.2015.08.015.

87. Spitzer MH, Carmi Y, Reticker-Flynn NE, Kwek SS, Madhireddy D, Martins MM, et al. Systemic immunity is required for effective cancer immunotherapy. Cell. 2017;168(3):487–502.e15. https://doi.org/10.1016/j.cell.2016.12.022.

88. Gopalakrishnan V, Spencer CN, Nezi L, Reuben A, Andrews MC, Karpinets TV, et al. Gut microbiome modulates response to anti-PD-1 immunotherapy in melanoma patients. Science. 2018;359(6371):97–103. https://doi.org/10.1126/science.aan4236.

89. Matson V, Fessler J, Bao R, Chongsuwat T, Zha Y, Alegre ML, et al. The commensal microbiome is associated with anti-PD-1 efficacy in metastatic melanoma patients. Science. 2018;359(6371):104–8. https://doi.org/10.1126/science.aao3290.

90. Gopalakrishnan V, Helmink BA, Spencer CN, Reuben A, Wargo JA. The influence of the gut microbiome on cancer, immunity, and cancer immunotherapy. Cancer Cell. 2018;33(4):570–80. https://doi.org/10.1016/j.ccell.2018.03.015.

91. Routy B, Le Chatelier E, Derosa L, Duong CPM, Alou MT, Daillere R, et al. Gut microbiome influences efficacy of PD-1-based immunotherapy against epithelial tumors. Science. 2018;359(6371):91–7. https://doi.org/10.1126/science.aan3706.

92. Sivan A, Corrales L, Hubert N, Williams JB, Aquino-Michaels K, Earley ZM, et al. Commensal Bifidobacterium promotes antitumor immunity and facilitates anti-PD-L1 efficacy. Science. 2015;350(6264):1084–9. https://doi.org/10.1126/science.aac4255.

93. Vetizou M, Pitt JM, Daillere R, Lepage P, Waldschmitt N, Flament C, et al. Anticancer immunotherapy by CTLA-4 blockade relies on the gut microbiota. Science. 2015;350(6264):1079–84. https://doi.org/10.1126/science.aad1329.

94. Frankel AE, Coughlin LA, Kim J, Froehlich TW, Xie Y, Frenkel EP, et al. Metagenomic shotgun sequencing and unbiased metabolomic profiling identify specific human gut microbiota and metabolites associated with immune checkpoint therapy efficacy in melanoma patients. Neoplasia. 2017;19(10):848–55. https://doi.org/10.1016/j.neo.2017.08.004.

95. Dubin K, Callahan MK, Ren B, Khanin R, Viale A, Ling L, et al. Intestinal microbiome analyses identify melanoma patients at risk for checkpoint-blockade-induced colitis. Nat Commun. 2016;7:10391. https://doi.org/10.1038/ncomms10391.

96. Chaput N, Lepage P, Coutzac C, Soularue E, Le Roux K, Monot C, et al. Baseline gut microbiota predicts clinical response and colitis in metastatic melanoma patients treated with ipilimumab. Ann Oncol. 2017;28(6):1368–79. https://doi.org/10.1093/annonc/mdx108.

97. Zitvogel L, Ayyoub M, Routy B, Kroemer G. Microbiome and anticancer immunosurveil-lance. Cell. 2016;165(2):276–87. https://doi.org/10.1016/j.cell.2016.03.001.
98. Ganal SC, Sanos SL, Kallfass C, Oberle K, Johner C, Kirschning C, et al. Priming of natural killer cells by nonmucosal mononuclear phagocytes requires instructive signals from commensal microbiota. Immunity. 2012;37(1):171–86. https://doi.org/10.1016/j.immuni.2012.05.020.
99. Felices M, Lenvik TR, Davis ZB, Miller JS, Vallera DA. Generation of BiKEs and TriKEs to improve NK cell-mediated targeting of tumor cells. Methods Mol Biol. 2016;1441:333–46. https://doi.org/10.1007/978-1-4939-3684-7_28.
100. Rezvani K, Rouce R, Liu E, Shpall E. Engineering natural killer cells for cancer immuno-therapy. Mol Ther. 2017;25(8):1769–81. https://doi.org/10.1016/j.ymthe.2017.06.012.
101. Sotillo E, Barrett DM, Black KL, Bagashev A, Oldridge D, Wu G, et al. Convergence of acquired mutations and alternative splicing of CD19 enables resistance to CART-19 immunotherapy. Cancer Discov. 2015;5(12):1282–95. https://doi.org/10.1158/2159-8290.cd-15-1020.
102. Fischer J, Paret C, El Malki K, Alt F, Wingerter A, Neu MA, et al. CD19 isoforms enabling resistance to CART-19 immunotherapy are expressed in B-ALL patients at initial diagnosis. J Immunother. 2017;40(5):187–95. https://doi.org/10.1097/cji.0000000000000169.
103. Pardoll DM. Distinct mechanisms of tumor resistance to NK killing: of mice and men. Immunity. 2015;42(4):605–6. https://doi.org/10.1016/j.immuni.2015.04.007.
104. Lowry LE, Zehring WA. Potentiation of natural killer cells for cancer immunotherapy: a review of literature. Front Immunol. 2017;8:1061. https://doi.org/10.3389/fimmu.2017.01061.
105. Ruella M, Xu J, Barrett DM, Fraietta JA, Reich TJ, Ambrose DE, et al. Induction of resistance to chimeric antigen receptor T cell therapy by transduction of a single leukemic B cell. Nat Med. 2018;24(10):1499–503. https://doi.org/10.1038/s41591-018-0201-9.
106. Braig F, Brandt A, Goebeler M, Tony HP, Kurze AK, Nollau P, et al. Resistance to anti-CD19/CD3 BiTE in acute lymphoblastic leukemia may be mediated by disrupted CD19 membrane trafficking. Blood. 2017;129(1):100–4. https://doi.org/10.1182/blood-2016-05-718395.
107. van Zelm MC, Smet J, Adams B, Mascart F, Schandene L, Janssen F, et al. CD81 gene defect in humans disrupts CD19 complex formation and leads to antibody deficiency. J Clin Invest. 2010;120(4):1265–74. https://doi.org/10.1172/JCI39748.
108. Orlando EJ, Han X, Tribouley C, Wood PA, Leary RJ, Riester M, et al. Genetic mecha-nisms of target antigen loss in CAR19 therapy of acute lymphoblastic leukemia. Nat Med. 2018;24(10):1504–6. https://doi.org/10.1038/s41591-018-0146-z.
109. Ribas A, Chmielowski B, Glaspy JA. Do we need a different set of response assessment cri-teria for tumor immunotherapy? Clin Cancer Res. 2009;15:7116–8.
110. Wolchok JD, Hoos A, O'Day S, Weber JS, Hamid O, Lebbé C, et al. Guidelines for the evaluation of immune therapy activity in solid tumors: immune-related response criteria. Clin Cancer Res. 2009;15:7412–20.
111. Chen PL, Roh W, Reuben A, Cooper ZA, Spencer CN, Prieto PA, et al. Analysis of immune signatures in longitudinal tumor samples yields insight into biomarkers of response and mech-anisms of resistance to immune checkpoint blockade. Cancer Discov. 2016;6(8):827–37.
112. Rudra D, deRoos P, Chaudhry A, Niec RE, Arvey A, Samstein RM, et al. Transcription factor Foxp3 and its protein partners form a complex regulatory network. Nat Immunol. 2012;13(10):1010–9. https://doi.org/10.1038/ni.2402.
113. van der Vaart M, Pretorius PJ. Circulating DNA. Its origin and fluctuation. Ann N Y Acad Sci. 2008;1137:18–26. https://doi.org/10.1196/annals.1448.022.
114. Diehl F, Schmidt K, Choti MA, Romans K, Goodman S, Li M, et al. Circulating mutant DNA to assess tumor dynamics. Nat Med. 2008;14(9):985–90. https://doi.org/10.1038/nm.1789.
115. Ma M, Zhu H, Zhang C, Sun X, Gao X, Chen G. "Liquid biopsy"-ctDNA detection with great potential and challenges. Ann Transl Med. 2015;3(16):235. https://doi.org/10.3978/j.issn.2305-5839.2015.09.29.
116. Gray ES, Rizos H, Reid AL, Boyd SC, Pereira MR, Lo J, et al. Circulating tumor DNA to monitor treatment response and detect acquired resistance in patients with metastatic mela-noma. Oncotarget. 2015;6(39):42008–18. https://doi.org/10.18632/oncotarget.5788.

117. Goldberg SB, Narayan A, Kole AJ, Decker RH, Teysir J, Carriero NJ, et al. Early assessment of lung cancer immunotherapy response via circulating tumor DNA. Clin Cancer Res. 2018;24(8):1872–80. https://doi.org/10.1158/1078-0432.ccr-17-1341.

118. Lee JH, Long GV, Boyd S, Lo S, Menzies AM, Tembe V, et al. Circulating tumour DNA predicts response to anti-PD1 antibodies in metastatic melanoma. Ann Oncol. 2017;28(5):1130–6. https://doi.org/10.1093/annonc/mdx026.

119. Lipson EJ, Velculescu VE, Pritchard TS, Sausen M, Pardoll DM, Topalian SL, et al. Circulating tumor DNA analysis as a real-time method for monitoring tumor burden in melanoma patients undergoing treatment with immune checkpoint blockade. J Immunother Cancer. 2014;2(1):42. https://doi.org/10.1186/s40425-014-0042-0.

120. Le DT, Durham JN, Smith KN, Wang H, Bartlett BR, Aulakh LK, et al. Mismatch repair deficiency predicts response of solid tumors to PD-1 blockade. Science. 2017;357(6349):409–13. https://doi.org/10.1126/science.aan6733.

121. Behrmann J, Etmann C, Boskamp T, Casadonte R, Kriegsmann J, Maass P. Deep learning for tumor classification in imaging mass spectrometry. Bioinformatics. 2018;34(7):1215–23. https://doi.org/10.1093/bioinformatics/btx724.

122. Mao X, He J, Li T, Lu Z, Sun J, Meng Y, et al. Application of imaging mass spectrometry for the molecular diagnosis of human breast tumors. Sci Rep. 2016;6:21043. https://doi.org/10.1038/srep21043.

123. Leelatian N, Doxie DB, Greenplate AR, Mobley BC, Lehman JM, Sinnaeve J, et al. Single cell analysis of human tissues and solid tumors with mass cytometry. Cytometry B Clin Cytom. 2017;92(1):68–78. https://doi.org/10.1002/cyto.b.21481.

124. Bendall SC, Simonds EF, Qiu P, Amir el AD, Krutzik PO, Finck R, et al. Single-cell mass cytometry of differential immune and drug responses across a human hematopoietic continuum. Science. 2011;332(6030):687–96. https://doi.org/10.1126/science.1198704.

125. Navin N, Kendall J, Troge J, Andrews P, Rodgers L, McIndoo J, et al. Tumour evolution inferred by single-cell sequencing. Nature. 2011;472(7341):90–4. https://doi.org/10.1038/nature09807.

126. Crowley E, Di Nicolantonio F, Loupakis F, Bardelli A. Liquid biopsy: monitoring cancer-genetics in the blood. Nat Rev Clin Oncol. 2013;10(8):472–84. https://doi.org/10.1038/nrclinonc.2013.110.

127. Heitzer E, Ulz P, Geigl JB. Circulating tumor DNA as a liquid biopsy for cancer. Clin Chem. 2015;61(1):112–23. https://doi.org/10.1373/clinchem.2014.222679.

128. Bracci L, Schiavoni G, Sistigu A, Belardelli F. Immune-based mechanisms of cytotoxic chemotherapy: implications for the design of novel and rationale-based combined treatments against cancer. Cell Death Differ. 2014;21(1):15–25. https://doi.org/10.1038/cdd.2013.67.

129. Pfirschke C, Engblom C, Rickelt S, Cortez-Retamozo V, Garris C, Pucci F, et al. Immunogenic chemotherapy sensitizes tumors to checkpoint blockade therapy. Immunity. 2016;44(2):343–54. https://doi.org/10.1016/j.immuni.2015.11.024.

130. Aoto K, Mimura K, Okayama H, Saito M, Chida S, Noda M, et al. Immunogenic tumor cell death induced by chemotherapy in patients with breast cancer and esophageal squamous cell carcinoma. Oncol Rep. 2018;39(1):151–9. https://doi.org/10.3892/or.2017.6097.

131. Hernandez C, Huebener P, Schwabe RF. Damage-associated molecular patterns in cancer: a double-edged sword. Oncogene. 2016;35(46):5931–41. https://doi.org/10.1038/onc.2016.104.

132. Sharabi AB, Lim M, DeWeese TL, Drake CG. Radiation and checkpoint blockade immunotherapy: radiosensitisation and potential mechanisms of synergy. Lancet Oncol. 2015;16(13):e498–509. https://doi.org/10.1016/s1470-2045(15)00007-8.

133. Gupta A, Probst HC, Vuong V, Landshammer A, Muth S, Yagita H, et al. Radiotherapy promotes tumor-specific effector CD8+ T cells via dendritic cell activation. J Immunol. 2012;189(2):558–66. https://doi.org/10.4049/jimmunol.1200563.

134. Gameiro SR, Jammeh ML, Wattenberg MM, Tsang KY, Ferrone S, Hodge JW. Radiation-induced immunogenic modulation of tumor enhances antigen processing and calreticulin

exposure, resulting in enhanced T-cell killing. Oncotarget. 2014;5(2):403–16. https://doi.org/10.18632/oncotarget.1719.

135. Park B, Yee C, Lee KM. The effect of radiation on the immune response to cancers. Int J Mol Sci. 2014;15(1):927–43. https://doi.org/10.3390/ijms15010927.

136. Prendergast GC, Malachowski WP, DuHadaway JB, Muller AJ. Discovery of IDO1 inhibitors: from bench to bedside. Cancer Res. 2017;77(24):6795–811. https://doi.org/10.1158/0008-5472.can-17-2285.

137. Leone RD, Lo YC, Powell JD. A2aR antagonists: next generation checkpoint blockade for cancer immunotherapy. Comput Struct Biotechnol J. 2015;13:265–72. https://doi.org/10.1016/j.csbj.2015.03.008.

138. Terranova-Barberio M, Thomas S, Munster PN. Epigenetic modifiers in immunotherapy: a focus on checkpoint inhibitors. Immunotherapy. 2016;8(6):705–19. https://doi.org/10.2217/imt-2016-0014.

139. Chae YK, Arya A, Iams W, Cruz MR, Chandra S, Choi J, et al. Current landscape and future of dual anti-CTLA4 and PD-1/PD-L1 blockade immunotherapy in cancer; lessons learned from clinical trials with melanoma and non-small cell lung cancer (NSCLC). J Immunother Cancer. 2018;6(1):39. https://doi.org/10.1186/s40425-018-0349-3.

140. Wei SC, Levine JH, Cogdill AP, Zhao Y, Anang NAS, Andrews MC, et al. Distinct cellular mechanisms underlie anti-CTLA-4 and anti-PD-1 checkpoint blockade. Cell. 2017;170(6):1120–33.e17. https://doi.org/10.1016/j.cell.2017.07.024.

141. Liu X, Shin N, Koblish HK, Yang G, Wang Q, Wang K, et al. Selective inhibition of IDO1 effectively regulates mediators of antitumor immunity. Blood. 2010;115(17):3520–30. https://doi.org/10.1182/blood-2009-09-246124.

142. Lowe D. IDO inhibitors hit a wall. Science. 2018. http://blogs.sciencemag.org/pipeline/archives/2018/04/09/ido-inhibitors-hit-a-wall. Accessed 9 Jul 2018.

143. Olson B, Li Y, Lin Y, Liu ET, Patnaik A. Mouse models for cancer immunotherapy research. Cancer Discov. 2018;8(11):1358–65. https://doi.org/10.1158/2159-8290.CD-18-0044.

144. Iida N, Dzutsev A, Stewart CA, Smith L, Bouladoux N, Weingarten RA, et al. Commensal bacteria control cancer response to therapy by modulating the tumor microenvironment. Science. 2013;342(6161):967–70. https://doi.org/10.1126/science.1240527.

Chapter 5
Therapies to Overcome Multidrug-Resistant Receptors

Noura Al-Zeheimi and Sirin A. Adham

Abstract ATP-binding cassette (ABC) transporters are a type of multidrug-resistant (MDR) receptor present on the surface of cancer cells that function to pump out toxic agents including those that exert therapeutic effects. Given the role of MDR receptors, they significantly contribute to conferring resistance to cytotoxic chemotherapies. Thus, inhibition of the MDR receptor activity can potentially improve patient response to treatment. Current research is heavily focused on discovering novel therapeutic options that inhibit or alter MDR activity or expression. Present therapies that attempt to overcome MDR exert their therapeutic effects by killing cancer cells, indirectly having an inhibitory effect on MDR receptors. In this chapter, we review therapies that are designed to directly target and overcome MDR receptors in several types of cancer. The strategies employed by these therapies to overcome the challenges associated with MDR receptors include regulating MDR receptor expression through epigenetic modifications, inhibiting MDR receptor activity through the use of tyrosine kinase inhibitors or active secondary metabolites, and finally using nanotechnology to improve drug delivery specificity. This new generation of therapies explicitly designed to overcome MDR receptors in cancer show promise, with many being tested and awaiting results from clinical trials for future FDA approval.

Keywords Multidrug-resistant receptors · ABC transporters · Cancer · Chemotherapy · Tyrosine kinases · Active secondary metabolites · Nanomedicine · Nanocarrier drug delivery

N. Al-Zeheimi · S. A. Adham (✉)
Department of Biology, College of Science, Sultan Qaboos University, Muscat, Oman
e-mail: p081878@student.squ.edu.om; sadham@squ.edu.om

© Springer Nature Switzerland AG 2019
M. R. Szewczuk et al. (eds.), *Current Applications for Overcoming Resistance to Targeted Therapies*, Resistance to Targeted Anti-Cancer Therapeutics 20,
https://doi.org/10.1007/978-3-030-21477-7_5

Abbreviations

ABC	ATP-binding cassette
ADR	Adriamycin
AMPK	AMP kinase
BCR-ABL	Breakpoint cluster region protein—Abelson murine leukemia
BCRP	Breast cancer resistant protein
BNL	Borneol
CML	Chronic myeloid leukemia
CSCs	Cancer stem cells
DFS	Disease-free survival
EGCG	Epigallocatechin-3-gallate
EGFR	Epidermal growth factor receptor
EMT	Epithelial-to-mesenchymal transition
ER- α	Estrogen-α
FDA	Food and Drug Administration
FTC	Fumitremorgin C
GSH	Glutathione
HA	Hyaluronic acid
HCC	Hepatocellular carcinoma
JAK/STAT	Janus kinase and signal transducer and activator of transcription
LRP1	Lipoprotein receptor-related protein 1
MAPK	Mitogen-activated protein kinase
MDR	Multidrug-resistant
MDR1	Multidrug-resistant protein-1
miRNA	Micro RNA
MMIC	Malignant melanoma-initiating cells
MMP	Matrix metalloproteinases
MRP	Multidrug resistance-associated protein
MSNP	Mesoporous silica nanoparticle
MTO	Mitoxantrone dihydrochloride
NBD	Nucleotide-binding domains
NRP-1	Neuropilin-1
NSCLC	Non-small cell lung cancer
OS	Overall survival
PDGFR	Platelet-derived growth factor receptor
P-gp	P-glycoprotein
Plk1	Polo-like kinase 1
PP2	Pyrazolo [3,4-d]pyrimidine
PTEN	Phosphatase and Tensin homolog
RCC	Renal cell carcinoma
ROS	Reactive oxygen species
RTK	Receptor tyrosine kinase
siRNA	Small interfering RNA
THC	Tetrahydrocurcumin

TKI   Tyrosine kinase inhibitor
TK   Tyrosine kinase
TMD   Transmembrane domain
TME   Tumor microenvironment
VEGFR   Vascular endothelial growth factor receptor

5.1   Introduction

The development of multidrug resistance presents as a significant scientific and clinical challenge, particularly, concerning cancer. Understanding the mechanisms of multidrug resistance on cellular and molecular levels is an area of active research that will ultimately lead to better control of this clinical challenge. Multidrug resistance can be classified as intrinsic or acquired resistance, categories which can be applied to general resistance as well. Intrinsic resistance occurs innately in individual tumours and is characteristic in patients who do not respond to initial treatment exposure [1].

Conversely, acquired resistance appears during or following treatment, with patients typically relapsing and experiencing disease recurrence [2]. Development of resistance is further complicated because resistance to a single drug can lead to resistance to structurally as well as non-structurally related drugs, causing the development of multidrug resistance [3]. The mechanisms of cross-resistance to non-structurally related chemotherapy drugs (cisplatin, paclitaxel, doxorubicin and topotecan) were identified in an *in vitro* model using ovarian cancer cells, in which overexpression of multidrug-resistant transporters was capable of pumping out different unrelated chemotherapy drugs [4].

The differential response of cancer cells and the development of resistance to chemotherapy is thought to be a result of several factors, including tumour heterogeneity [5], microenvironment fluctuations [6], epigenetic modifications [7], and genomic instability [8]. Mechanisms of development of multidrug resistance can be classified as kinetic, pharmacological, or biochemical [9]. This chapter will focus on the biochemical mechanism of drug resistance with an emphasis on the overexpression of drug efflux pumps, particularly ATP Binding Cassette (ABC) transporters, and potential therapeutic targets to overcome resistance acquired as a result of these drug efflux pumps.

5.2   Multidrug-Resistant Receptors: The ABC Transporter Superfamily

ABC transporters are a class of drug efflux pumps that comprise a large proportion of multidrug-resistant (MDR) receptors. ABC transporters can be divided into seven groups (A to G) and consist of 48 genes (and their associated protein products) and three pseudogenes [10]. Structurally, each ABC transporter consists of a total of four domains: two nucleotide-binding domains (NBD) and two transmembrane domains (TMD). The NBD of ABC genes can be distinguished from other ATPases through the presence of consensus motifs Walker A and Walker B in addition to a C motif [10]. The 12 α helices of the TMDs are the key structural component of the transporter, as this is the site of substrate recognition and binding.

ABC transporters move substrates against their concentration-gradients, making transportation energy-dependent. Once a substrate binds to the TMD, a pore-like structure is formed and accompanied by ATP hydrolysis, opens up to the extracellular space [11]. Different compounds are transported depending on which specific ABC transporter is expressed. For example, ABCB1 (P-glycoprotein (P-gp) or multidrug resistant protein-1; MDR1) carries large hydrophobic compounds such as anthracyclines, taxanes and alkaloids, while ABCC1 (multidrug resistance-associated protein 1; MRP1) and ABCG2 (breast cancer resistant protein; BCRP) can transport hydrophobic drugs and large anionic compounds such as mitoxantrone and anthracyclines [3, 12]. Given the cargo that can be transported by ABC transporters, pumping out chemotherapeutic agents provides a means for tumour cells to escape the cytotoxic effects of chemotherapy by decreasing their intracellular accumulation, which ultimately reduces cell sensitivity [12]. Given the effects of ABC transporters, it is perhaps not surprising that overexpression of ABCB1, ABCC1, ABCC2 (MRP2), ABCC3 (MRP3) and ABCG2 has been associated with the development of resistance [13]. However, the expression of extrusion pumps in tumour cells varies depending on the cell type and the drug used. For example, ovarian cancer cells were found to overexpress ABCB1 primarily, and its inhibition resulted in sensitization of cells to paclitaxel [14]. However, in malignant melanoma-initiating cells (MMIC), which are characterized by the expression of cell surface marker CD144, ABCB5 was found to be expressed and responsible for resistance to Vemurafenib (PLX4032) [15].

Cancer stem cells (CSCs) are cells that have the indefinite potential for self-renewal and remain a challenge in the clinical treatment of cancer [16]. Unsurprisingly, CSCs also have a high expression of various ABC transporters [11]. The development of resistance can be attributed to tumor stem cells expressing ABC transporters that have been shown to protect cancer stem cells from chemotherapeutic agents [17]. For example, breast cancer stem cells are characterized by surface antigen CD44+/ CD24- expression and are also known to overexpress the ABCG2 transporter which plays a significant role in conferring chemotherapy resistance [18]. Currently, there is no standard therapy available that has been shown to target specific proteins and other components exclusively expressed on CSCs. Therefore, targeting ABC transporters in CSCs presents as a promising option in the treatment of cancer [11, 16].

Given the complex role played by MDRs in the development of chemoresistance coupled with the overexpression of these receptors on malignant cells, notably CSCs, targeting MDR receptors presents as an effective way to overcome resistance in tumours that are unresponsive to the conventional therapeutic agents. The US Food and Drug Administration (FDA) website (https://www.fda.gov/drugs/developmentapprovalprocess/developmentresources/druginteractionslabeling/ucm093664. htm) lists examples of *in vitro* inhibitors for MDR receptors. Currently, Cabazitaxel is the only FDA approved drug efflux inhibitor. Cabazitaxel is typically administered in combination with Prednisone and has shown efficacy in the treatment of patients with refractory metastatic prostate cancer who were initially treated with a docetaxel-based regimen [19]. However, there is active research underway evaluating the efficacy of other potential inhibitors of these receptors and will be discussed in detail below. Most studies report on indirect MDR receptor inhibition by currently used therapeutic agents. However, several *in vitro* and *in vivo* studies have shown different mechanisms of ABC transporter inhibition, which have resulted in more effective drug treatment due to their increased intracellular accumulation.

5.3 Tyrosine Kinase Inhibitors Indirectly Modulate Multidrug-Resistant Receptor Activity

Tyrosine kinases (TKs) transfer a phosphate group from ATP to target proteins within a cell, playing a crucial role in signal transduction. TKs activate the mitogen-activated protein kinase (MAPK), Janus kinase and signal transducer and activator of transcription (JAK/STAT) or PI3K/AKT pathways to transduce signals. These pathways modulate proliferation, survival, differentiation and anti-apoptotic signalling, implicating TKs in cancer progression [20, 21]. Tyrosine kinases can be classified as receptor and non-receptor kinases. Generally, when a ligand binds to the extracellular domain of receptor tyrosine kinases (RTKs), downstream signalling is activated through serine/threonine kinases. However, non-receptor kinases, which do not have a transmembrane domain, are activated by oligomerization or autophosphorylation or by other kinases to mediate signal transduction [22]. In this section, we will focus on RTKs, the most well-known TKs. There are 58 members of RTKs, including the epidermal growth factor receptors (EGFRs), vascular endothelial growth factor receptors (VEGFRs), and platelet-derived growth factor receptors (PDGFRs), all of which are well-known tumour markers [23].

Given the role of TKs in cancer progression, many tyrosine kinase inhibitors (TKIs) have been approved as therapeutic agents for cancer [24]. These inhibitors act by preventing the binding of ATP to the ATP binding sites on the kinases or by blocking the kinase binding site or dimerization, which subsequently blocks TK signalling [22]. Accumulating evidence has suggested that tyrosine kinase inhibitors (TKIs) can act as inhibitors for MDR receptors as blocking the ATP binding site of the ABC transporters interferes with their functionality [25–27]. For example, Src kinase inhibitor 4-amino-5(4-chlorophenyl)-7-(t-butyl) pyrazolo [3,4-d]pyrimidine (PP2) and verapamil, an ABC transporter inhibitor, demonstrated synergy in restoring paclitaxel sensitivity in ABCB1 overexpressing paclitaxel-resistant human CaOV3TaxR and mouse ID8TaxR ovarian cancer cells, resulting in subsequent cell death [28].

Given the broad role of tyrosine kinases, there are multiple targets for TKIs depending on the target TK and its associated signalling pathway. TKIs targeting the EGFR, VEGFR, and BCR-ABL, have been the most heavily studied and will be the focus of the remainder of this section. Table 5.1 provides a comprehensive list of tyrosine kinase inhibitors used to target MDR receptors.

Table 5.1 Tyrosine kinase inhibitors that indirectly target multidrug-resistant receptors

Tyrosine kinase inhibitors (TKIs)	Cancer type	Targeted ABC receptor	Reference
(PP2) 4-amino-5(4-chlorophenyl)-7-(t-butyl) pyrazolo[3,4-d] pyrimidine-Src inhibitor	Paclitaxel resistant human (CaOV3TaxR) and mouse (ID8TaxR) ovarian cancer cells	ABCB1	[28]
EGFR TKIs			
Gefitinib and Vandetanib	Colon cancer cells HT-29	ABCG2	[25]
Lapatinib analogues (GW583340 and GW2974)	ABCG2 overexpressing cells and ABCB1 overexpressing cells	ABCB1 and ABCG2	[26]
Lapatinib and Trastuzumab combination	Nude mouse model	ABCB1	[33]
Pelitinib (EKB-569)	Lung cancer cells	ABCB1 and ABCG2	[36]
Osimertinib (AZD9291)		ABCB1	[37, 38]
Tyrphostin AG-1478 (AG1478)	KB-C2 an ABCB1-overexpressing cells and cells overexpressing ABCG2	ABCB1and ABCG2	[39]
Afatinib	Multidrug resistance in ABCG2 overexpressing cancer cells and ABCG2- overexpressing cell xenograft tumors	ABCG2	[40]
Dacomitinib	*In vitro* and *in vivo* models	ABCG2	[42]
Gefitinib	Human myelomonocytic cells	ABCB1, ABCC1 and ABCG2	[9, 43]
BCR-ABL TKIs			
Imatinib (Gleevec)		ABCB1, ABCC1, ABCC10 and ABCG2	[9]
Imatinib mesylate and AG957 combination	Multidrug-resistant chronic myelogenous leukemia (CML) K562 cell line	ABCB1	[46]
Asciminib (ABL001)	Refractory chronic myeloid Leukemia (CML)	ABCB1 and ABCG,	[47]
Nilotinib (AMN107)	Cells overexpressing the ABCB1 and ABCG2 -HEK293/MRP7 cells- HEK/MDR-1 cells- ABCB1, ABCC10 and ABCG2 xenograft models and K562-ABCG2 cells	ABCB1, ABCG2, MRP7and ABCC10	[48–50]
Ponatinib		ABCB1, ABCC10 and ABCG2	[52]

(continued)

Table 5.1 (continued)

Tyrosine kinase inhibitors (TKIs)	Cancer type	Targeted ABC receptor	Reference
VEGFR TKIs			
Sunitinib	Cells overexpressing ABCB1 and ABCG2, RCC with *VHL* gene mutation	ABCB1, ABCG2, ABCC2 and ABCC4	[56, 57]
Sorafenib		ABCB1, ABCG2, ABCC2 and ABCC4	[60]
Other TKIs			
Voruciclib	Cells overexpressing ABCC-10, ABCB1or ABCG2	ABCC-10, ABCB1 and ABCG2	[61]
Ribociclib	MCF-7 breast carcinoma cell lines	ABCB1 and ABCG2	[62]
Ceritinib	Leukemia cells (ex-vivo model)	ABCB1	[63]
Polo-like kinase 1 inhibitor (BI 2536) and ABCB1 and ABCG2 inhibitors, nilotinib and lapatinib	Cells overexpressing ABCB1 and ABCG2 in cervical carcinoma KB-V-1 and human colon carcinoma S1-M1-80 sublines	ABCB1 and ABCG2	[64]
Ibrutinib	ABCC1 overexpressing HEK293/ MRP1 and HL60/ADR cells	ABCC1	[69]

5.3.1   Overcoming Multidrug-Resistant Receptors as a Secondary Action of EGFR Tyrosine Kinase Inhibitors

TKIs targeting the EGFR have been shown to inhibit MDR receptor activity, in addition, to inhibiting EGFR signalling directly [29, 30]. For example, first-generation EGFR inhibitors gefitinib and erlotinib and new TKI lapatinib, have been approved for the treatment of non-small cell lung cancer (NSCLC) [31]. Although gefitinib, lapatinib and erlotinib share a similar chemical structure, they exhibit a somewhat controversial pattern of interaction with ABC transporters, behaving as inhibitors, substrates or modulators depending the on cellular context and concentrations [32].

Biochemical characterization of gefitinib, neratinib, vandetanib and pelitinib demonstrated these EGFR TKIs closely interact with ABCG2. The concentration of the EGFR TKI determines whether these small molecule inhibitors enhance or suppress the ATPase activity of ABCG2 [32]. For example, a short period of exposure to gefitinib or vandetanib restored sensitivity to anti-neoplastic agent SN-38 in HT-29 colon cancer cells by binding to ABCG2/BCRP [25].

Lapatinib and Analogues Lapatinib analogues GW583340 and GW2974 inhibit the EGFR and HER2 activity by binding to the ATP binding site on tyrosine, preventing phosphorylation. Lapatinib and its analogues have been shown to reduce the drug efflux activity of ABCB1 and ABCG2 and increase cellular concentrations of drugs, particularly [3H]- mitoxantrone in ABCG2 overexpressing cells and [3H]-paclitaxel in cells overexpressing ABCB1. The lapatinib analogues also demonstrated the ability to inhibit the function of both wild type ABCG2-482-R2 and its mutant variant ABCG2-482-T7 derived from HEK293 embryonic kidney cells [26]. As a consequence of drug resistance in breast cancer cells overexpressing ABCB1, molecules involved in migration and invasion such as EGFR/HER2 were also upregulated and thus promoted the expression of CD147 and matrix metalloproteinase-2 and -9 (MMP2/9) [33]. CD147 is a multifunctional protein involved in the induction of MMP2/9 enzymes that are involved in the degradation of type IV collagen of the basement membrane and therefore induce invasion and metastasis of tumor cells [34, 35]. Using lapatinib as an inhibitor of EGFR/HER2 and trastuzumab as an inhibitor of HER2 decreased expression of EGFR, HER2, CD147 and MMP2/9, reversing the drug resistance [33].

Pelitinib Pelitinib (EKB-569) alters ATPase activity and is a competitive inhibitor for ABCB1 and ABCG2 [32, 36]. Hyperthermia is known to increase the expression of both ABCB1 and ABCG2, which would promote the development of resistance. However, pelitinib has been shown to sensitize lung cancer cells exposed to hypothermia [36].

Osmertinib Irreversible EGFR inhibitor osimertinib (AZD9291) is a third generation TKI specific to EGFR active mutations and resistance-associated T790M point mutations [37]. Docking and molecular dynamics simulations demonstrated a strong interaction between osimertinib and ABCB1, with osimertinib enhancing ATPase activity. However, western blots demonstrated no change in ABCB1 protein expression levels following osmertinib treatment. These results demonstrate that osimertinib inhibits the ABCB1 function by modulating ATPase activity and inhibiting the paclitaxel efflux in ABCB1 overexpressing cells without altering the protein expression level [37, 38].

Tyrphostin Tyrphostin (AG1478) is an EGFR TKI that exhibits a chemosensitizing role in the ABCB1 overexpressing KB-C2 cancer cell line and in the ABCG2 overexpressing cells [39]. Tyrphostin had a more significant effect in restoring sensitivity in ABCG2 overexpressing cells compared to wildtype variants. Additionally, tyrphostin was found to promote intracellular accumulation of [3H]-paclitaxel and [3H]-mitoxantrone in cells overexpressing ABCB1 or ABCG2, respectively. Similar to osmertinib, tyrphostin inhibited transporter activity without altering ABCB1 or ABCG2 gene or protein expression [39].

Afatinib Afatinib is an FDA approved small molecule TKI that has demonstrated chemosensitizing functions, particularly in reversing multidrug resistance in ABCG2 overexpressing cancer cells [40, 41]. An *in vivo* experiment showed that co-treatment of xenograft tumours overexpressing ABCG2 with afatinib and topotecan actively prevented tumour growth [40]. This is possibly due to afatinib restoring chemosensitivity of ABCG2 overexpressing cancer cells by acting as a competitive inhibitor of ABCG2 to block ATPase activity in a concentration-dependent manner. At higher concentrations, afatinib suppresses ABCG2 expression, underscoring its importance as a therapeutic agent in the treatment of MDR cancers [40].

Dacomitinib Dacomitinib is a known pan-ErbB TKI and shown to inhibit ABCG2 efflux ability and increase accumulation of intracellular anti-cancer agents *in vitro* and *in vivo* [42]. As outlined, ABCG2 acts as the general target for most EGFR TKIs such as gefitinib, erlotinib, lapatinib, neratinib, vandetanib, and pelitinib. Additional to ABCG2, the EGFR TKIs were found to interact with different ABC transporters, with some acting as a general substrate for multiple ABC transporters [9]. For example, neratinib, vandetanib and pelitinib interact with ABCG2 whereas gefitinib binds to ABCB1, ABCC1 and ABCG2 [9, 43]. These findings underscore the overlapping mechanisms of action of TKIs that could have broad clinical applications depending on the type of receptor overexpressed in the cancer being treated.

5.3.2 BCR-ABL Tyrosine Kinase Inhibitors as Therapeutic Agents to Overcome Multidrug-Resistant Receptors

Inhibition of oncogenic tyrosine kinase product BCR-ABL of the Philadelphia chromosome by small molecule inhibitor imatinib (Gleevec®) was a breakthrough for the treatment of chronic myeloid leukemia (CML) [44]. Imatinib is a selective competitive inhibitor of deregulated BCR-ABL enzymatic activity [45], binding to the ATP binding site. Interestingly, imatinib has also been shown to inhibit the activity of multiple MDR receptors including ABCB1, ABCC1, ABCC10 and ABCG2 [9]. For example, the combination of imatinib mesylate and EGFR TKI tyrphostin (AG957) was used to enhance the chemosensitivity to doxorubicin on K562 MDR CML cells [46].

Following the clinical success of BCR-ABL inhibitors in the treatment of CML, other inhibitors began to be evaluated for clinical efficacy. For example, kinase inhibitor asciminib (ABL001) is currently undergoing phase I clinical trials for the treatment of refractory CML. So far, asciminib and has shown promising results in *in vitro* settings, successfully overcoming drug resistance through the inhibition of ABCB1 and ABCG2 [47].

Second generation TKI nilotinib (AMN107), has been shown to enhance paclitaxel and mitoxantrone sensitivity in cells overexpressing the ABCB1 and ABCG2, respectively. Nilotinib has also been shown to reverse the action of ABCC10 (MRP7) and restore sensitivity to paclitaxel in ABCC10 overexpressing HEK293 embryonic kidney cells [48]. Interestingly, nilotinib also inhibits the activity of ABCB1 and ABCG2 at the blood-brain barrier in rat brain capillaries, and the combination of nilotinib and doxorubicin enhanced sensitivity in ABCB1-mediated drug-resistant HEK cells [49]. In MDR xenograft models, nilotinib stimulated the anti-cancer activity of paclitaxel and doxorubicin in ABCB1, ABCC10 and ABCG2 models [50]. Of several BCR-ABL TKIs, nilotinib was the most potent ABCB1 and ABCG2 inhibitor; however, nilotinib and dasatinib both decreased ABCG2 surface expression in ABCG2 overexpressing K562 cells [51]. Additionally, ponatinib is another approved BCR-ABL inhibitor that also inhibits VEGFR and EGFR activity [52]. Thus BCR-ABL TKIs, present as a promising area of research and a potential therapeutic option for several patients.

5.3.3   *VEGFR Tyrosine Kinase Inhibitors as Therapeutic Agents to Overcome Multidrug-Resistant Receptors*

Small molecule inhibitors targeting angiogenic tyrosine kinase VEGFR have also been approved for the treatment of several cancers, including renal cell carcinoma (RCC), advanced pancreatic neuroendocrine tumours and imatinib-resistant gastrointestinal stromal tumours [53–55]. The interaction of sunitinib, a VEGFR TKI, with MDR-associated ABC transporters was first reported in 2009. Low micromolar concentrations of sunitinib affect the cellular bioavailability of co-administered MDR-substrate drugs as a result of conformational changes that occur due to its attachment to the transporter substrate binding pocket in ABCB1 and ABCG2 overexpressing cells [56]. Sunitinib was shown to prevent MDR in RCC with mutated *VHL*. Co-treatment of ABCG2 overexpressing cells with elacridar, an ABCB1 and ABCG2 inhibitor enhanced the cytotoxic effect of sunitinib [57]. Sorafenib is another VEGFR TKI approved for the treatment of unresectable hepatocellular carcinoma (HCC), advanced RCC, and progressive differentiated thyroid carcinoma [58]. Sorafenib RAF serine/threonine kinase isoforms of several RTKs, including VEGFR, FLT-3, PDGFRs, c-KIT and RET [59]. Both VEGF TKIs sunitinib and sorafenib were shown to act as inhibitors for different MDR receptors such as ABCB1, ABCG2, ABCC2 and ABCC4 [60].

5.3.4 Other Tyrosine Kinase Inhibitors as Therapeutic Agents to Overcome Multidrug-Resistant Receptors

Given the broad range of tyrosine kinases, it is unsurprising that there are several other TKIs that are active agents to overcome MDR, with several undergoing clinical trials including voruciclib [61], ribociclib [62], and ceritinib [63]. Voruciclib is currently in phase I clinical trials to be used to overcome MDR. Voruciclib is a small molecular weight inhibitor which sensitized ABCC10 overexpressing cells to paclitaxel and enhanced the intracellular accumulation of cytotoxic drugs by decreasing the efflux potential of both ABCB1 and ABCG2-overexpressing cells [61]. Ribociclib is a cyclin-dependent kinase inhibitor was found to be a substrate for ABCB1 which inhibited the activity of ABCB1, ABCG2 and cytochrome P450; this inhibition was able to reverse the action of both daunorubicin and mitoxantrone resistance in human MCF-7 breast carcinoma cell lines [62]. Ceritinib is anaplastic lymphoma kinase (ALK), blocked the effect of ABCB1 function in leukemia cells which led to the accumulation of doxorubicin inside the cells in an ex-vivo model [63].

Polo-Like Kinase 1 Polo-like kinase 1 (Plk1) is overexpressed in many cancer cells. Inhibition of Plk1 by BI 2536 promoted G2/M cell cycle arrest in human OVCAR8 ovarian cancer cells, MCF7 breast cancer cells and KB-3-1 epidermoid carcinoma cells. However, BI 2536 did not have any effect in resistant ABCB1 or ABCG2 overexpressing cell lines. The use of BI 2536 and tariquidar, an ABCB1 inhibitor, Fumitremorgin C (FTC), an ABCG2 inhibitor, along with nilotinib, an ABCB1 and ABCG2 substrate, and lapatinib enhanced chemosensitivity of resistant cells overexpressing ABCB1 and ABCG2 in KB-V-1 cervical carcinoma and S1-M1-80 colon carcinoma sublines, restoring cell cycle arrest at G2/M in both cell lines [64].

Verapamil Verapamil is a calcium channel blocker. Verapamil exerts a chemosensitivity role in ABCB1 overexpressing cells by downregulating ABCB1 and survivin and upregulating Bim expression by preventing Src activation. These effects of verapamil were tested in several multidrug resistant cells, including RPMI8226, RPMI8226/ADM, RPMI8226/VCR, RPMI8226/DEX and RPMI8226/L-PAM. Verapamil restored chemosensitivity in resistant MCF7/ADR breast cancer cells by binding to the ABCB1 and downregulating anti-apoptotic survivin [65]. Src inhibitor dasatinib was also shown to enhance drug sensitivity by inhibiting ABCB1 and stimulating Bim expression in doxorubicin-resistant cells [66].

Ibrutinib Ibrutinib is an FDA-approved TKI that inhibits tyrosine kinase activity in Bruton's cell lymphoma and chronic lymphoid leukemia [67, 68]. Ibrutinib treatment of ABCC1 overexpressing HEK293 cells and HL60/ADR resulted in the accumulation of ABCC1 substrates and promoted the chemosensitivity by antagonizing the efflux activity of the ABCC1 [69]. Ibrutinib demonstrated a superior inhibitory effect in ABCC1 overexpressing cells compared to MK571, a known ABCC1 inhibitor. Additionally, an ABCC1 overexpressing HEK29 tumour xenograft model demonstrated a chemosensitizing effect of vincristine [69].

Westover and Fengzhi have reviewed different strategies of inhibiting ABCG2 in oncology and revised the literature to include advancements in methods to overcome ABCG2-mediated resistance [70]. The study concluded that, despite all of the efforts to either inhibit ABCG2 activity or its expression, outcomes are not yet reflected on improvements in patients care.

5.4 Targeting Multidrug-Resistant Receptor Activity Through the Use of Secondary Active Metabolites and Natural Compounds

Several studies have reported on the chemosensitizing effect of active secondary compounds from plants such as alkaloids, phenolics, and terpenoids. These agents have been able to sensitize cells to chemotherapy even when the chemotherapeutics were not effective at high concentrations [71].

Active compounds capsaicin and piperine act as substrates for ABCB1. The concurrent use of both compounds inhibited doxorubicin efflux and increased its cytotoxicity in Caco-2 colon cancer and CEM/ADR 5000 lymphoblastic leukemia cell lines [71]. Modified low molecular weight piperine analogs Pip1 and Pip2 had significantly greater interaction with ABCB1 than piperine and also altered ABCB1 efflux. These analogs exhibited superior chemosensitivity effects compared to piperine, reducing resistance to vincristine, colchicine or paclitaxel in ABCB1-overexpressing KB cervical and SW480 colon cancer cells [72].

Curcumin is a metabolite found in turmeric which has been reported to have several anti-cancer effects [73, 74]. Curcumin has been shown to inhibit the expression and activity of ABCB1 in KB-V1 cervical carcinoma cells, increasing vinblastine sensitivity [72]. GO-Y030, GO-Y078, GO-Y168, and GO-Y172 are analogs of curcumin that were shown to directly inhibit the function of the ABCG2/BCRP without affecting its expression level. The naturally bioavailable active curcumin compounds GO-Y030 and GO-Y078 also enhanced the sensitivity of ABCG2-overexpressing K562 myelogenous leukemia cells to anti-neoplastic drug SN-38 [75]. Through ATPase assays and photoaffinity labelling, a study demonstrated that tetrahydrocurcumin (THC) inhibited the efflux activity of ABCB1, ABCG2 and ABCC1 by interacting with the substrate binding sites [76]. THC demonstrated an enhanced intracellular accumulation and sensitivity to anti-cancer metabolites including vinblastine, etoposide and mitoxantrone in resistant KB-V-1 cervical carcinoma cells, MCF-7 breast cancer cells, and ABCG2 overexpressing

MCF7ADRVp3000 cells, respectively with no effect observed on the wildtype parental cancer cell lines [76].

Berberine treatment of hypoxia-induced doxorubicin resistance in MCF7 cells reversed chemoresistance caused by hypoxia through inhibition of AMP kinase (AMPK), which is essential for glucose activation and fatty acid uptake and oxidation when cellular energy is low, HIF-1α and ABCB1 at low dosages [77]. *Scutellaria baicalensis* increased sensitivity to cisplatin by reducing the expression of HIF-1α, ABCG1, and ABCG2 in ovarian cancer cells [78]. The polyphenolic component in the catechins of the green tea, (−)-Epigallocatechin-3-gallate (EGCG), showed dual inhibition of ABCB1 and ABCG2 activity in tamoxifen-resistant MCF7 cells by two different mechanisms of action. ABCG2 activity was inhibited by EGCG alone, whereas ABCB1 was downregulated by EGCG and proteasome inhibitor MG132 [79]. Additionally, the flavonoid compound Vitxen suppressed ABCB1 in HCT-116 colorectal cancer cells, inhibited autophagy and induced apoptosis, suggesting that Vitxen is a promising agent to overcome chemoresistance in colorectal cancer [80].

There are several other multidrug-resistant inhibitors for ABCB1, including PSC833 (valspodar), VX710 and XR9576. These compounds have demonstrated a chemosensitizing ability to vincristine in the RD rhabdomyosarcoma cell line [81]. Acridone, which is known for its anti-malaria activity [82], was found to be promising for chemotherapy as it promoted apoptosis and inhibited ABCG2 in a breast cancer mouse model [83]. Similarly, emodin, a natural chemical that acts as an anticancer agent, and doxorubicin on A594 lung adenocarcinoma and HCT-15 colorectal carcinoma cell lines modulated endocytic receptor, low-density lipoprotein receptor-related protein 1 (LRP1) expression and promoted accumulation of doxorubicin [84]. Lignins are secondary metabolites produced by Arctium lappa including arctigenin, matairesinol, arctiin, (iso) lappaol A and lappaol C and have shown inhibitory effects in MDR on cancer cells. For example, co-treatment of CaCo-2 and CEM/ADR5000 cells with lignins promoted cytotoxicity in MDR cells overexpressing ABCB1 [85].

Secondary metabolites from citrus have also been shown to be natural ABCB1 inhibitors. The extracts from *Citrus jambhiri* (Lush) and *Cirus pyriformis* (Hassk) such as limonin and other flavonoids and sterols have demonstrated the ability to reduce drug efflux of CEM/ADR5000 drug-resistant human leukemia cells and increased sensitivity of doxorubicin to resistant Caco-2 cells [86]. Limonin demonstrated a superior sensitizing effect in doxorubicin-resistant CEM/ADR5000 cells compared to other citrus compounds [86].

Plant metabolites can inhibit the function of the ABC transporters by acting as competitive inhibitors affecting the phosphorylation of the transporters or reduce their expression. Collectively, these natural compounds can reverse MDR by inhibiting the ABC transporter activity. Secondary metabolites as a therapeutic option to overcome MDR receptors are listed in Table 5.2.

Table 5.2 Secondary metabolites as a therapeutic option to overcome multidrug-resistant receptors

Secondary metabolites	Cancer type	Targeted ABC receptor	Reference
Capsaicin and Piperine	Colon cancer (Caco-2) Lymphoblastic leukemia (CEM/ADR)	ABCB1	[71]
Piperine analogs (Pip1 and Pip2)	ABCB1 overexpressing Cervical KB and Colon SW480 cancer cells	ABCB1	[72]
Curcumin	Cervical carcinoma KB-V1 cells	ABCB1	[72]
Curcumin analogs (GO-Y030, GO-Y078, GO-Y168, GO-Y172)	Myelogenous leukemia-K562 cells and ABCG2 overexpressing K562 cells	ABCG2	[75]
Curcumins tetrahydrocurcumin (THC)	Cervical carcinoma (KB-V -1) cells, resistant breast cancer MCF-7MDR cells and ABCG2 overexpressing cells (MCF7FL1000)	ABCB1, ABCG2 and ABCC1	[76]
Beberine	Doxorubicin resistant MCF7 cells	ABCB1	[77]
Scutellaria baicalensis	Ovarian cancer cell lines	ABCG1 and ABCG2	[78]
(−)-Epigallocatechin-3-gallate (EGCG)	Tamoxifen resistant MCF7 cells	ABCB1and ABCG2	[79]
Vitxen	Colorectal cancer cells HCT-116	ABCB1	[80]
PSC833 (Valspodar), VX710 and XR9576	Rhabdomyosarcoma RD cell line	ABCB1	[81]
Acridone	Breast cancer mouse model	ABCG2	[83]
Emodin	Lung adenocarcinoma (A549) and Colorectal carcinoma (HCT-15) cell lines	LRP1	[84]
Lignins	CaCo2 and CEM/ADR5000	ABCB1	[85]
Citrus/limonin	Resistant human leukaemia CEM/ADR5000 cells and doxorubicin resistant Caco-2	ABCB1	[86]

5.5 Epigenetic Regulators as Potential Therapeutic Targets

Epigenetics are posttranscriptional modifications that take place at the chromatin level, such as DNA methylation, histone acetylation and deacetylation that affect gene expression [87, 88]. Epigenetic regulation has been of increasing research interest and has been implicated in regulating gene expression that contributes to cancer progression. Recent studies have shown that MDR expression is modulated at the epigenetic level [89–91]. Unmethylated and methylated *ABCG2* genes show differential response to their substrates. For example, RCC cell lines with different *ABCG2* methylation demonstrated varying responses to known ABCG2 substrates including mitoxantrone, topotecan and SN-38. UOK121 and UOK143, the methylated cell lines, were more sensitive than the UOK181 unmethylated cell line to all three drugs [92]. These findings suggest that methylation-mediated ABCG2 expression sensitized the resistant RCC cells to mitoxantrone, topotecan and SN-38, all of which act as ABCG2 substrates. In a different type of cancer, the evidence of epigenetic regulation of ABCG2 has shown supporting results. For instance, in glioblastoma, the use of melatonin demonstrated a synergistic toxic effect along with temozolomide in treating BTSCs and A172 malignant glioma cells. Interestingly, melatonin acted as a methylating agent for the ABCG2/BCRP promoter in glioma cells and inhibited the expression of ABCG2 and hence prevented efflux of the cytotoxic drugs, showing much promise for the use of melatonin in the treatment of this malignant form of brain cancer [93]. Although our understanding of epigenetic regulation of MDR gene expression is in a state of infancy, preliminary data has provided evidence for further research in understanding MDR expression through epigenetics.

5.5.1 Targeting Multidrug-Resistant Receptor Expression Through miRNA and siRNA Regulation

MicroRNAs (miRNAs) are gene regulators involved in MDR. Recent studies have shown that regulating the expression of MDR proteins through epigenetic modifications, small interfering RNA (siRNA) or miRNA enhances drug efficacy and restores sensitivity in MDR cells. For example, ABCB1, ABCC5 and ABCG1 were demonstrated to be the primary targets for miRNA-129-5p in gastric cancer cells. Due to the hypermethylation of miRNA-129-5p in MDR cells (SGC7901/ADR) compared to parental cells (SGC7901/VCR), 5-Aza-2′-deoxycytidine (5-AZA-dc) was used to demethylate miRNA-129-5p to restore doxorubicin sensitivity to resistant cells [94].

Furthermore, differential expression of miR-34a, miR-222, miR-452 and miR-29a in docetaxel or adriamycin resistant MCF7 breast cancer cells was also directly related to MDR expression. However, treatment of resistant MCF7 cells with anti-proliferative agent β-elemene influenced MDR miRNA expression to significantly increase *PTEN*, which in turn significantly reduced *ABCB1* expression [95]. Similarly, knocking down *ABCG2/BCRP* expression using siRNA in MCF7 cells in the presence of the PI3K inhibitor LY294002 increased MCF7 chemosensitivity to mitoxantrone [96]. *ABCG2* expression was inhibited by the action of anti-estrogen toremifene in estrogen-α (ER- α) positive breast cancer MCF7 cells, improving intracellular accumulation of mitoxantrone by ABCG2 efflux inhibition and multidrug resistance reversal [97].

More recently, we found that neuropilin-1 (NRP-1) overexpressing BT-474 breast cancer cells (BT-474 NRP-1) were associated with a reduction in ABCG2/BCRP expression and sensitized cancer cells to a combination treatment of adriamycin/cyclophosphamide by inactivating the NRP-1/ITGB3/FAK/Akt/NF-κB p65 signalling pathway [98]. This suggests that the expression of specific essential proteins may alter the expression of efflux pumps and ultimately change the way cells respond to cytotoxic drugs, a facet of research that requires more attention. Regulating the expression of the MDR proteins through epigenetic modifications, siRNA or mi-RNA is promising as it results in the enhancement of drug efficacy and restoring sensitivity in MDR cells.

5.6 Nanomedicine as a Potential Therapy to Overcome the Limitations of Multidrug-Resistant Receptor Therapies

5.6.1 Mechanisms of Nanodelivery to Overcome Multidrug-Resistant Receptors

Conventional therapies used to overcome MDR receptors are limited in their benefits due to toxicity and associated adverse side effects affecting the heart, liver and bones [99]. Novel applications of nanomedicine are a promising innovative approach to treat MDR tumours. Unlike traditional modes of therapeutic administration, nanocarriers have demonstrated enhanced drug uptake and selective intracellular accumulation in MDR cancer cells. Advanced delivery systems using active transport have been gaining interest as this form of technology is based on ligands that preferentially bind to highly expressed receptors in MDR tumours. The nanocarriers can exploit this expression by delivering drugs directly to MDR cancer cells, reducing the toxic side effects in normal cells [100].

Additionally, nanocarriers have been shown to reduce the toxic effects observed in nonmalignant tissues due to their tumour-targeting specificity when delivering therapies [101]. These nanocarriers are referred to as "smart" drug delivery systems as they overcome MDR by relying on specific physical properties characteristic of tumours and modulating bio-distribution and pharmacokinetics to enhance therapeutic efficacy with reduced drug toxicity [102]. The five main classes of nanocarriers used to treat MDR cancers include lipid-based nanoparticles (liposomes), polymer-based nanoparticles (micelles), dendrimers, and metallic and magnetic nanoparticles [103].

For example, doxorubicin encapsulated in hydrophobic polymeric micelles caused indirect inhibition of ABCB1 efflux and enhanced the intracellular drug concentration without affecting ABCB1 expression in a cell culture model [104]. Dextran-based polymeric nanoparticles encapsulating doxorubicin were tested in sensitive and resistant KHOS, KHOSR2, U-2OS, and U-2OSR2 osteosarcoma cell lines and showed doxorubicin nuclear uptake, enhanced apoptosis and drug distribution in the resistant cells, comparable to that of sensitive cells. Overcoming MDR receptors may be due to the nuclear accumulation of doxorubicin that causes an epigenetic modification in the *ABCB1* transcription region [105]. Additionally, encapsulating the siMDR1 in dextran-based nanocarrier suppresses the expression of resistant glycoprotein ABCB1 in KHOSR2 cancer cells [106]. In addition to doxorubicin delivery using nanocarriers, liposome nanocarriers have also been used to load mitoxantrone (LPG-MX) for the treatment of Huh-7 human HCC cells which express high levels of ABCG2 [107]. Collectively, using nanocarriers for single drug delivery showed improvement in drug efficacy and low toxicity in normal cells, all of which are desirable features for a drug delivery system.

5.6.2 CD44-Based Tumour Targeting Nanocarriers to Overcome Multidrug-Resistant Receptors

Another mode of targeting MDR tumours is through targeting cancer cells in which CD44, an MDR marker, is upregulated. When hyaluronic acid (HA) binds to CD44, proliferation and invasion pathways are activated to promote cancer progression [108, 109]. HA attached to a nanocarrier carrying a drug was used in a CD44-based tumour targeting system and showed enhanced uptake by CD44 overexpressing cells and increased drug toxicity [110]. MDR Colo-320 and HT-29 colon cancer cell lines are known to overexpress CD44 and ABCB1, and delivery of imatinib using hyaluronan-coated liposomes showed an increase in intracellular imatinib uptake [111]. These results reveal a previously untested promising method to preferentially target MDR cells that overexpress membrane receptors as a novel therapy.

5.6.3 Folate Receptor-Based Tumour Targeting Nanocarrier to Overcome Multidrug-Resistant Receptors

There is a significant need to modify chemotherapy drugs so they do not act as substrates for MDR receptors and can continue to exert their therapeutic effects on cancer cells. A proposed method to overcome MDR drug efflux is to conjugate therapeutics to folate to bypass MDR receptors and effectively deliver therapeutics to the intended cell and sites of action. Folate cofactors play an essential role in nucleotide synthesis which necessary for DNA replication, and folate receptors are highly upregulated in solid tumours, and MDR cells and thus are considered an excellent active transport target [112]. In addition to folate being a target for nano delivery, liposomal nanocarriers to transfer anti-folate drug (Pemetrexed) were used to overcome MDR in resistant MCF7/ABCC5 cells and xenograft models. These nanocarriers increased the permeability, retention and efficacy of Pemetrexed, thereby enhancing its cytotoxicity, and decreased the IC_{50} by 6.4-fold in MCF7 cells and 2.2-fold in resistant MCF7/ABCC5 compared to free Pemetrexed [113]. Folate micelles loaded with paclitaxel and verapamil to overcome ABCB1 in carboxymethylated chitosan modified with deoxycholic acid enhanced the drug cytotoxicity in resistant ABCB1 overexpressing MCF7/ADR cells through promoting drug delivery via folate receptor-mediated endocytosis [114].

5.6.4 Using Dual Drug Delivery to Enhance Drug Efficacy to Overcome Multidrug-Resistant Receptors

Co-targeting or combination drug delivery system using nanocarriers is a modern delivery system focused on targeting multidrug resistance. Treating the MDR cancer cells with a combination of chemotherapy and tyrosine kinase inhibitors in a nanocarrier has an excellent inhibitory effect on MDR pumps than using a single chemotherapy drug [115, 116]. Similarly, codelivery of siRNA with chemotherapy to downregulate MDR receptors showed a promising effect on sensitizing the MDR cells to drugs [99, 117].

Liposomes are potential nanocarriers that have been used to deliver antiangiogenic bevacizumab and doxorubicin in MDR HER2 positive BT474 (BT474/MDR) cells [118]. These nanocarriers enhanced drug sensitivity in ABCB1 overexpressing BT47 cells, by promoting growth inhibition and decreased cellular toxicity in the normal cells [118]. Furthermore, codelivery of doxorubicin and paclitaxel, both of which are considered to be ABCB1 substrates, in resistant MCF7 breast cancer cells, using polymeric mixed micelles (PF–DP) enhanced drug uptake and cytotoxicity, relative to the use of free drugs or single drug encapsulated by micelles. This codelivery *in vivo* also showed significant growth inhibition, higher tissue uptake and prolonged circulation in the blood but low uptake in cardiac tissues [119]. Additionally, codelivery of miR-375 and doxorubicin-HCl using lipid-coated hollow mesoporous silica nanocarrier in resistant HepG2/ADR HCC cells enhanced the accumulation of doxorubicin in the resistant cells and the xenograft model, increasing the anti-tumour activity of doxorubicin by miR-375-mediated suppression of ABCB1 [120].

Co-delivery of cytotoxic drugs and MDR efflux pump inhibitors (siRNA/shRNA/ MDR inhibitors) have been widely investigated and show promising responses and increase drug sensitivity in MDA resistant cancer cells [121]. *In vitro* experiments in gefitinib-resistant HeLa cells showed that dual delivery of gefitinib and *ABCB1*-targeting *shMDR-1* using nanocarrier chitosan, enhanced apoptosis and restored gefitinib sensitivity by silencing *ABCB1* expression [122]. Another study showed that combining paclitaxel and siRNA for *ABCB1* in PEO-PbAE nanoparticles sensitized MDR human SKOV3TR ovarian adenocarcinoma cells by increasing intracellular accumulation of paclitaxel, promoting cytotoxicity and apoptosis [123]. The dual delivery of a chemotherapeutic agent and siRNA for the treatment of MDR cancer cells was further supported by a group that treated MDR human A594/DPP lung adenocarcinoma cells using generation 5 polyamidoamine (PAMAM) dendrimers (G5.NH2)-modified selenium nanoparticles (G5@Se NPs) encapsulating the siRNA for *ABCB1* and cisplatin (DDP). This dual drug delivery resulted in the inhibition of *ABCB1* expression and improved cytotoxicity and apoptosis in the resistant cells [124]. Additionally, the use of G5@Se-DDP NPs in an A549/DDP lung tumour xenograft model reduced the cytotoxicity in vital organs [124]. Codelivery of doxorubicin and siRNA inhibiting *ABCB1* expression using a multifunctional mesoporous silica nanoparticle (MSNP) carrier in the MCF-7/MDR xenograft model in nude mice improved tumour growth inhibition and induced apoptosis [125].

Furthermore, it has been shown that co-delivery of doxorubicin and secondary active metabolite curcumin (ABCB1 inhibitor) in pegylated polymeric micelles (DOX+Cur)-PM reversed MDR in drug-resistant MCF7/ADR breast cancer cells by increasing cellular uptake, significantly reducing tumour growth in 4T1-bearing mice compared to free DOX+Cur or DOX-PM [126]. Loading the PEG-PAMAM polymers with paclitaxel and natural compound Borneol (BNL), an ABCB1 inhibitor enhanced intracellular accumulation of paclitaxel in paclitaxel-resistant A2780/PTX ovarian cancer cells compared to free drug delivery and reduced the tumour growth *in vivo* [127]. The use of nanoparticle polymers loaded with mitoxantrone dihydrochloride (MTO) and quercetin, an inhibitor of ABCB1, in MCF7 breast cancer cells, A2780 sensitive ovarian carcinoma cells (sensitive) and A2780 adriamycin resistant cells reduced the IC_{50} due to the ABCB1 inhibitor which blocked drug efflux and therefore reversed MDR [128].

Collectively, robust inhibition of tumour resistance has been achieved through dual delivery of chemotherapy and compounds such as siRNA, natural compounds and TKIs that block MDR receptor activity by nanocarriers.

5.6.5   Targeted Release as a Strategy to Overcome Multidrug-Resistant Receptors

To improve nanomedicine specificity, selectivity and toxicity, the time and site of the drug release as a function of biological, chemical and physical stimuli need to be determined. Currently, several stimuli to enhance MDR sensitivity have been studied, including, pH, redox, magnetic and photodynamic or combination of the two, and will be discussed in the remainder of this section [99].

pH-Responsive Nanocarrier Drug Release to Overcome Multidrug-Resistant Receptors The tumour microenvironment (TME) is more acidic (pH of 6.5 to 7.2) when compared to healthy tissue (pH of 7.4) [129, 130]. With this pH difference, it is a useful chemical stimulus to enhance the selectivity and safety of drug encapsulation by nanocarriers [129]. For example, codelivery of doxorubicin and siRNA against ABCB1 by chitosan-coated mixed micellar nanocarriers that polyplex as pH-responsive, was shown to enhance doxorubicin intracellular accumulation, increase toxicity, and prolong circulation in the blood and was associated with better survival compared to the free doxorubicin group when tested in MDR 4T1 breast cancer cells *in vivo* [131]. Due to the specificity of the polyplexes, the spleen and kidney were not affected by doxorubicin, and their structures remained similar to that of the control group whereas free doxorubicin resulted in red and white pulp structures in the spleen and kidneys [131]. Using pH-responsive nanogels peptide-Dox and Verapamil (PD/VER) containing both doxorubicin and ABCB1 inhibitor (Verapamil, VER) for the treatment of Adriamycin resistant ovarian cancer cells A2780ADR improves the cellular uptake. Both drugs synergistically enhanced the cytotoxicity and increased the anti-MDR by 6.5–folds using PD/VER nano-gels relative to the treatment with free doxorubicin [132]. Moreover, the pH-responsive cyclodextrin (Ac-aCD) can promote the anti-tumour activity of paclitaxel, docetaxel, cis-diamminedichloroplatinum, camptothecin, and doxorubicin. Delivery of Ac-aCD to resistant MCF7 and MDA-MB-231 breast cancer cells reduced ABCB1 expression and activity and increased MDR cell sensitivity to the drugs mentioned [133].

Redox-responsive Nanocarrier Drug Release to Overcome Multidrug-Resistant Receptors Tumour cells, particularly those that are drug resistant, have abnormal metabolism, and in attempts to balance intracellular redox, cells express high concentrations of glutathione (GSH), which plays a critical role as an antioxidant in addition to other metabolic activities [117, 134]. Intracellular GSH concentration is over 100 times higher compared to extracellularly, making GSH a potential stimulus for tumour tissues [134]. For example, nanocarriers with disulphide bond linkers can undergo conformational changes at the target site because the disulphide bond is reduced by GSH through thiolysis, resulting in the drugs being integrated inside the cells [134, 117]. A redox-responsive micelle containing a single disulphide bond-bridged block polymer of poly (ε-caprolactone) and poly (ethyl ethylene phosphate) (PCL-SS-PEEP) carrying doxorubicin for the treatment of ABCB1 overexpressing MCF7/ADR cells increased cellular doxorubicin retention by reduction of intracellular GSH [135].

Enzyme-Responsive Nanocarriers to Overcome Multidrug-Resistant Receptors Multidrug-resistant and metastatic cells overexpress proteins that are involved in epithelial-to-mesenchymal transition (EMT) including enzymes involved in extracellular matrix degradation such as MMPs, proteases, phospholipases and glycosidases [136]. In light of this, MMP-peptide sensitive linkers attached to copolymers such as PEG2k-pp-PE have shown inhibition of ABCB1 and subsequently lead to increased paclitaxel sensitivity in MDR NCI/ADR-RES ovarian and breast cancer cells [136].

External Stimuli-Responsive Nanocarrier Drug Release to Overcome Multidrug-Resistant Receptors Physical targets such as photodynamic, hyperthermia and ultrasound are considered to be external stimuli that enhance drug delivery to the site of the tumour. Photosensitizers promote the formation of reactive oxygen species (ROS) and enhance cell permeability to promote drug unloading inside MDR cells, acting as selective molecules for MDR cells. Combination of photodynamics using polymers (MIT-PEP-PPP) mixed with micelles encapsulating mitoxantrone effectively reversed resistance in MCF7 breast cancer cells mediated by the increase of ROS, reduced ABCB1 function and improved drug accumulation [137].

As outlined above, introducing nanomedicine as a component of MDR treatment facilitates improved drug uptake, localization, and selectivity while reducing toxicity in healthy cells. FDA approval of nanomedicine-based therapies will reduce the burden associated with MDR tumours. With advancements in nanocarrier specificity, nanomedicine can potentially lead to more successful outcomes in treating cancer by employing precision medicine.

5.7 Conclusions

Increased mortality as a result of multidrug resistance has called for improved treatment options that preferentially target MDR receptors with the intention of decreasing disease burden. Reducing MDR receptor expression is a critical step towards enhancing intracellular drug accumulation that is regulated by genetic or epigenetic modifications. Targeting MDR receptor function through the use of secondary active metabolites and tyrosine kinase inhibitors in combination with chemotherapy is another method of overcoming MDR. Secondary metabolites and tyrosine kinase inhibitors both effectively increase MDR cancer cell sensitivity to treatment by blocking the receptor substrate binding site, reducing the efflux activity of the pumps, and in some cases, decreasing MDR receptor expression. The mechanisms discussed to overcome MDR receptors are summarized in Fig. 5.1. Although current therapeutic options to decrease MDR receptor expression and activity

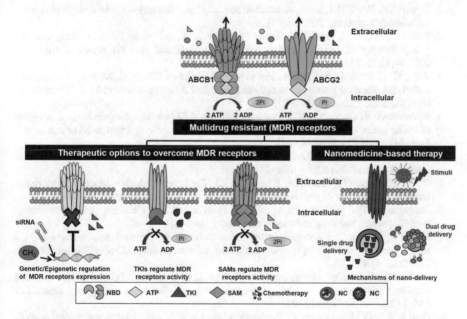

Fig. 5.1 Schematic representation of therapies used to overcome multidrug-resistant receptors. Multidrug resistance can be acquired through the overexpression of ABC transporters as either full transporters such as P-glycoprotein (ABCB1) or half transporters such as the breast cancer resistant protein (BCRP/ABCG2). Inhibition of multidrug-resistant (MDR) receptor expression by siRNA or epigenetic regulation such as methylation (CH_3) as well as the use of secondary active metabolites (SAM) or tyrosine kinase inhibitors (TKIs) has demonstrated efficacy in modulated MDR. Application of these strategies has demonstrated reduced the MDR receptor activity through binding to the nucleotide binding domain (NBD). The use of nanocarriers employing specific drug release strategies for intracellular drug delivery and prevention of MDR receptor drug efflux is a promising therapy to overcome limitations associated with conventional therapies overcoming MDR receptors. *ABCB1* P-glycoprotein; *BCRP/ABCG2* breast cancer resistant protein; *CH₃* methylation; *SAM* secondary active metabolites; *TKIs* tyrosine kinase inhibitors; *MDR* multidrug resistant receptors; *NBD* nucleotide binding domain

effectively reduce MDR, they are also associated with several adverse effects in normal tissues. This has led to the use of nanotechnology to overcome the adverse effects. Targeting MDR receptors with modified nanoparticle conjugates holds promise in the development of therapies that overcome acquired resistance to chemotherapy and targeted therapy. The recent introduction of multi-stimuli-responsive nanocarriers has resulted in improved specificity and selectivity of drugs, taking a significant step forward in precision medicine while adverse effects in normal cells. Although the future of targeting MDR receptors seems promising, we have a long way to go as Cabazitaxel is currently the only FDA-approved drug which inhibits MDR receptors to increase chemotherapy sensitivity.

References

1. Lippert TH, Ruoff H-J, Volm M. Intrinsic and acquired drug resistance in malignant tumors. Arzneimittelforschung. 2008;58(06):261–4.
2. Tsuruo T, Naito M, Tomida A, Fujita N, Mashima T, Sakamoto H, et al. Molecular targeting therapy of cancer: drug resistance, apoptosis and survival signal. Cancer Sci. 2003;94(1):15–21.
3. Wang H, Hajar A, Li S, Chen X, Parissenti AM, Brindley DN, et al. Multiple mechanisms underlying acquired resistance to taxanes in selected docetaxel-resistant MCF-7 breast cancer cells. BMC Cancer. 2014;14(1):37.
4. Januchowski R, Sterzyńska K, Zaorska K, Sosińska P, Klejewski A, Brązert M, et al. Analysis of MDR genes expression and cross-resistance in eight drug resistant ovarian cancer cell lines. J Ovarian Res. 2016;9(1):65.
5. Burrell RA, Swanton C. Tumour heterogeneity and the evolution of polyclonal drug resistance. Mol Oncol. 2014;8(6):1095–111.
6. Barker HE, Paget JT, Khan AA, Harrington KJ. The tumour microenvironment after radiotherapy: mechanisms of resistance and recurrence. Nat Rev Cancer. 2015;15(7):409.
7. Easwaran H, Tsai H-C, Baylin SB. Cancer epigenetics: tumor heterogeneity, plasticity of stem-like states, and drug resistance. Mol Cell. 2014;54(5):716–27.
8. Huang S. Genetic and non-genetic instability in tumor progression: link between the fitness landscape and the epigenetic landscape of cancer cells. Cancer Metastasis Rev. 2013;32(3-4):423–48.
9. Beretta GL, Cassinelli G, Pennati M, Zuco V, Gatti L. Overcoming ABC transporter-mediated multidrug resistance: the dual role of tyrosine kinase inhibitors as multitargeting agents. Eur J Med Chem. 2017;142:271–89.
10. Gatti L, Cossa G, L Beretta G, Zaffaroni N, Perego P. Novel insights into targeting ATP-binding cassette transporters for antitumor therapy. Curr Med Chem. 2011;18(27):4237–49.
11. Begicevic R-R, Falasca M. ABC Transporters in cancer stem cells: beyond chemoresistance. Int J Mol Sci. 2017;18(11):2362.
12. Rivera E, Gomez H. Chemotherapy resistance in metastatic breast cancer: the evolving role of ixabepilone. Breast Cancer Res. 2010;12(Suppl 2):S2.
13. Huang J, Li H, Ren G. Epithelial-mesenchymal transition and drug resistance in breast cancer. Int J Oncol. 2015;47(3):840–8.
14. Eyre R, Harvey I, Stemke-Hale K, Lennard TW, Tyson-Capper A, Meeson AP. Reversing paclitaxel resistance in ovarian cancer cells via inhibition of the ABCB1 expressing side population. Tumor Biol. 2014;35(10):9879–92.
15. Xiao J, Egger ME, McMasters KM, Hao H. Differential expression of ABCB5 in BRAF inhibitor-resistant melanoma cell lines. BMC Cancer. 2018;18(1):675.

16. Agliano A, Calvo A, Box C. The challenge of targeting cancer stem cells to halt metastasis. Semin Cancer Biol. 2017;44:25–42.
17. Dean M, Fojo T, Bates S. Tumour stem cells and drug resistance. Nat Rev Cancer. 2005;5(4):275.
18. Chuthapisith S, Eremin J, El-Sheemey M, Eremin O. Breast cancer chemoresistance: emerging importance of cancer stem cells. Surg Oncol. 2010;19(1):27–32.
19. Galsky MD, Dritselis A, Kirkpatrick P, Oh WK. Cabazitaxel. Nat Rev Drug Discov. 2010;9:677–8.
20. Lemmon MA, Schlessinger J. Cell signaling by receptor tyrosine kinases. Cell. 2010;141(7):1117–34.
21. Cargnello M, Roux PP. Activation and function of the MAPKs and their substrates, the MAPK-activated protein kinases. Microbiol Mol Biol Rev. 2012;76(2):496.
22. Anreddy N, Gupta P, Kathawala RJ, Patel A, Wurpel JN, Chen Z-S. Tyrosine kinase inhibitors as reversal agents for ABC transporter mediated drug resistance. Molecules. 2014;19(9):13848–77.
23. Setia S, Nehru B, Sanyal SN. Upregulation of MAPK/Erk and PI3K/Akt pathways in ulcerative colitis-associated colon cancer. Biomed Pharmacother. 2014;68(8):1023–9.
24. Arora A, Scholar EM. Role of tyrosine kinase inhibitors in cancer therapy. J Pharmacol Exp Therapeut. 2005;315(3):971–9.
25. Azzariti A, Porcelli L, Simone GM, Quatrale AE, Colabufo NA, Berardi F, et al. Tyrosine kinase inhibitors and multidrug resistance proteins: interactions and biological consequences. Cancer Chemother Pharmacol. 2010;65(2):335.
26. Sodani K, Tiwari AK, Singh S, Patel A, Xiao Z-J, Chen J-J, et al. GW583340 and GW2974, human EGFR and HER-2 inhibitors, reverse ABCG2-and ABCB1-mediated drug resistance. Biochem Pharmacol. 2012;83(12):1613–22.
27. Wu S, Fu L. Tyrosine kinase inhibitors enhanced the efficacy of conventional chemotherapeutic agent in multidrug resistant cancer cells. Mol Cancer. 2018;17(1):25.
28. George JA, Chen T, Taylor CC. SRC tyrosine kinase and multidrug resistance protein-1 inhibitions act independently but cooperatively to restore paclitaxel sensitivity to paclitaxel-resistant ovarian cancer cells. Cancer Res. 2005;65(22):10381–8.
29. Fan Y-F, Zhang W, Zeng L, Lei Z-N, Cai C-Y, Gupta P, et al. Dacomitinib antagonizes multidrug resistance (MDR) in cancer cells by inhibiting the efflux activity of ABCB1 and ABCG2 transporters. Cancer Lett. 2018;421:186–98.
30. Butti R, Das S, Gunasekaran VP, Yadav AS, Kumar D, Kundu GC. Receptor tyrosine kinases (RTKs) in breast cancer: signaling, therapeutic implications and challenges. Mol Cancer. 2018;17(1):34.
31. Cohen MH, Williams GA, Sridhara R, Chen G, Pazdur R. FDA drug approval summary: gefitinib (ZD1839)(Iressa®) tablets. Oncologist. 2003;8(4):303–6.
32. Hegedüs C, Truta-Feles K, Antalffy G, Várady G, Német K, Özvegy-Laczka C, et al. Interaction of the EGFR inhibitors gefitinib, vandetanib, pelitinib and neratinib with the ABCG2 multidrug transporter: implications for the emergence and reversal of cancer drug resistance. Biochem Pharmacol. 2012;84(3):260–7.
33. Jin Y, Zhang W, Wang H, Zhang Z, Chu C, Liu X, et al. EGFR/HER2 inhibitors effectively reduce the malignant potential of MDR breast cancer evoked by P-gp substrates in vitro and in vivo. Oncol Rep. 2016;35(2):771–8.
34. Dong W, Li H, Zhang Y, Yang H, Guo M, Li L, et al. Matrix metalloproteinase 2 promotes cell growth and invasion in colorectal cancer. Acta Biochim Biophys Sin. 2011;43(11):840–8.
35. Han Y-H, Gao B, Huang J-H, Wang Z, Guo Z, Jie Q, et al. Expression of CD147, PCNA, VEGF, MMPs and their clinical significance in the giant cell tumor of bones. Int J Clin Exp Pathol. 2015;8(7):8446.
36. To KK, Poon DC, Wei Y, Wang F, Lin G, Fu L. Pelitinib (EKB-569) targets the up-regulation of ABCB1 and ABCG2 induced by hyperthermia to eradicate lung cancer. Br J Pharmacol. 2015;172(16):4089–106.

37. Zhang X-Y, Zhang Y-K, Wang Y-J, Gupta P, Zeng L, Xu M, et al. Osimertinib (AZD9291), a mutant-selective EGFR inhibitor, reverses ABCB1-mediated drug resistance in cancer cells. Molecules. 2016;21(9):1236.
38. Chen Z, Chen Y, Xu M, Chen L, Zhang X, To KKW, et al. Osimertinib (AZD9291) enhanced the efficacy of chemotherapeutic agents in ABCB1-and ABCG2-overexpressing cells in vitro, in vivo, and ex vivo. Mol Cancer Ther. 2016;15:1845–58.
39. Shi Z, Tiwari AK, Shukla S, Robey RW, Kim I-W, Parmar S, et al. Inhibiting the function of ABCB1 and ABCG2 by the EGFR tyrosine kinase inhibitor AG1478. Biochem Pharmacol. 2009;77(5):781–93.
40. Wang X-K, To KKW, Huang LY, Xu J-H, Yang K, Wang F, et al. Afatinib circumvents multidrug resistance via dually inhibiting ATP binding cassette subfamily G member 2 in vitro and in vivo. Oncotarget. 2014;5(23):11971.
41. Wang S-q, S-t L, B-x Z, Yang F-h, Wang Y-t, Liang Q-y, et al. Afatinib reverses multidrug resistance in ovarian cancer via dually inhibiting ATP binding cassette subfamily B member 1. Oncotarget. 2015;6(28):26142.
42. Guo X, To KKW, Chen Z, Wang X, Zhang J, Luo M, et al. Dacomitinib potentiates the efficacy of conventional chemotherapeutic agents via inhibiting the drug efflux function of ABCG2 in vitro and in vivo. J Exp Clin Cancer Res. 2018;37(1):31.
43. Özvegy-Laczka C, Hegedűs T, Várady G, Ujhelly O, Schuetz JD, Varadi A, et al. High-affinity interaction of tyrosine kinase inhibitors with the ABCG2 multidrug transporter. Mol Pharmacol. 2004;65(6):1485–95.
44. Pray LA. Gleevec: the breakthrough in cancer treatment. Nat Educ. 2008;1(1):37.
45. Druker BJ, Tamura S, Buchdunger E, Ohno S, Segal GM, Fanning S, et al. Effects of a selective inhibitor of the Abl tyrosine kinase on the growth of Bcr–Abl positive cells. Nat Med. 1996;2(5):561.
46. Yeheskely-Hayon D, Regev R, Eytan GD, Dann EJ. The tyrosine kinase inhibitors imatinib and AG957 reverse multidrug resistance in a chronic myelogenous leukemia cell line. Leuk Res. 2005;29(7):793–802.
47. Eadie LN, Saunders VA, Branford S, White DL, Hughes TP. The new allosteric inhibitor asciminib is susceptible to resistance mediated by ABCB1 and ABCG2 overexpression in vitro. Oncotarget. 2018;9(17):13423.
48. Shen T, Kuang Y-H, Ashby CR Jr, Lei Y, Chen A, Zhou Y, et al. Imatinib and nilotinib reverse multidrug resistance in cancer cells by inhibiting the efflux activity of the MRP7 (ABCC10). PLoS One. 2009;4(10):e7520.
49. Shukla S, Skoumbourdis AP, Walsh MJ, Hartz AM, Fung KL, Wu C-P, et al. Synthesis and characterization of a BODIPY conjugate of the BCR-ABL kinase inhibitor Tasigna (nilotinib): evidence for transport of Tasigna and its fluorescent derivative by ABC drug transporters. Mol Pharm. 2011;8(4):1292–302.
50. Tiwari AK, Sodani K. Dai C-l, Abuznait AH, Singh S, Xiao Z-J et al. Nilotinib potentiates anticancer drug sensitivity in murine ABCB1-, ABCG2-, and ABCC10-multidrug resistance xenograft models. Cancer Lett. 2013;328(2):307–17.
51. Dohse M, Scharenberg C, Shukla S, Robey RW, Volkmann T, Deeken JF, et al. Comparison of ATP-binding cassette transporter interactions with the tyrosine kinase inhibitors imatinib, nilotinib and dasatinib. Drug Metab Dispos. 2010;38:1371–80.
52. Prasad V, Mailankody S. The accelerated approval of oncologic drugs: lessons from ponatinib. JAMA. 2014;311(4):353–4.
53. Chow LQ, Eckhardt SG. Sunitinib: from rational design to clinical efficacy. J Clin Oncol. 2007;25(7):884–96.
54. Goodman VL, Rock EP, Dagher R, Ramchandani RP, Abraham S, Gobburu JV, et al. Approval summary: sunitinib for the treatment of imatinib refractory or intolerant gastrointestinal stromal tumors and advanced renal cell carcinoma. Clin Cancer Res. 2007;13(5):1367–73.
55. Blumenthal GM, Cortazar P, Zhang JJ, Tang S, Sridhara R, Murgo A, et al. FDA approval summary: sunitinib for the treatment of progressive well-differentiated locally advanced or metastatic pancreatic neuroendocrine tumors. Oncologist. 2012;17:1108–13.

56. Shukla S, Robey RW, Bates SE, Ambudkar SV. Sunitinib (Sutent, SU11248), a small-molecule receptor tyrosine kinase inhibitor, blocks function of the ATP-binding cassette (ABC) transporters P-glycoprotein (ABCB1) and ABCG2. Drug Metab Dispos. 2009;37(2):359–65.
57. Sato H, Siddig S, Uzu M, Suzuki S, Nomura Y, Kashiba T, et al. Elacridar enhances the cytotoxic effects of sunitinib and prevents multidrug resistance in renal carcinoma cells. Eur J Pharmacol. 2015;746:258–66.
58. Kane RC, Farrell AT, Madabushi R, Booth B, Chattopadhyay S, Sridhara R, et al. Sorafenib for the treatment of unresectable hepatocellular carcinoma. Oncologist. 2009;14(1):95–100.
59. Wilhelm S, Carter C, Lynch M, Lowinger T, Dumas J, Smith RA, et al. Discovery and development of sorafenib: a multikinase inhibitor for treating cancer. Nat Rev Drug Discov. 2006;5(10):835.
60. Hu S, Chen Z, Franke R, Orwick S, Zhao M, Rudek MA, et al. Interaction of the multikinase inhibitors sorafenib and sunitinib with solute carriers and ATP-binding cassette transporters. Clin Cancer Res. 2009;15:6062–9.
61. Gupta P, Zhang Y-K, Zhang X-Y, Wang Y-J, Lu KW, Hall T, et al. Voruciclib, a potent CDK4/6 inhibitor, antagonizes ABCB1 and ABCG2-mediated multi-drug resistance in cancer cells. Cell Physiol Biochem. 2018;45(4):1515–28.
62. Sorf A, Hofman J, Kučera R, Staud F, Ceckova M. Ribociclib shows potential for pharmacokinetic drug-drug interactions being a substrate of ABCB1 and potent inhibitor of ABCB1, ABCG2 and CYP450 isoforms in vitro. Biochem Pharmacol. 2018;154:10–7.
63. Yang L, Li M, Wang F, Zhen C, Luo M, Fang X, et al. Ceritinib enhances the efficacy of substrate chemotherapeutic agent in human ABCB1-overexpressing leukemia cells in vitro, in vivo and ex-vivo. Cell Physiol Biochem. 2018;46(6):2487–99.
64. Wu C-P, Hsiao S-H, Sim H-M, Luo S-Y, Tuo W-C, Cheng H-W, et al. Human ABCB1 (P-glycoprotein) and ABCG2 mediate resistance to BI 2536, a potent and selective inhibitor of Polo-like kinase 1. Biochem Pharmacol. 2013;86(7):904–13.
65. Liu F, Xie Z H, Cai G-P, Jiang Y-Y. The effect of survivin on multidrug resistance mediated by P-glycoprotein in MCF-7 and its adriamycin resistant cells. Biol Pharm Bull. 2007;30(12):2279–83.
66. Tsubaki M, Komai M, Itoh T, Imano M, Sakamoto K, Shimaoka H, et al. By inhibiting Src, verapamil and dasatinib overcome multidrug resistance via increased expression of Bim and decreased expressions of MDR1 and survivin in human multidrug-resistant myeloma cells. Leuk Res. 2014;38(1):121–30.
67. Byrd JC, Furman RR, Coutre SE, Flinn IW, Burger JA, Blum KA, et al. Targeting BTK with ibrutinib in relapsed chronic lymphocytic leukemia. N Engl J Med. 2013;369(1):32 42.
68. Shanafelt TD, Borah BJ, Finnes HD, Chaffee KG, Ding W, Leis JF, et al. Impact of ibrutinib and idelalisib on the pharmaceutical cost of treating chronic lymphocytic leukemia at the individual and societal levels. J Oncol Pract. 2015;11(3):252–8.
69. Zhang H, Patel A, Ma SL, Li XJ, Zhang YK, Yang PQ, et al. In vitro, in vivo and ex vivo characterization of ibrutinib: a potent inhibitor of the efflux function of the transporter MRP1. Br J Pharmacol. 2014;171(24):5845–57.
70. Westover D, Li F. New trends for overcoming ABCG2/BCRP-mediated resistance to cancer therapies. J Exp Clin Cancer Res. 2015;34(1):159.
71. Li H, Krstin S, Wang S, Wink M. Capsaicin and piperine can overcome multidrug resistance in cancer cells to doxorubicin. Molecules. 2018;23(3):557.
72. Syed SB, Arya H, Fu I-H, Yeh T-K, Periyasamy L, Hsieh H-P, et al. Targeting P-glycoprotein: Investigation of piperine analogs for overcoming drug resistance in cancer. Sci Rep. 2017;7(1):7972.
73. Bar-Sela G, Epelbaum R, Schaffer M. Curcumin as an anti-cancer agent: review of the gap between basic and clinical applications. Curr Med Chem. 2010;17(3):190–7.
74. Singh S, Khar A. Biological effects of curcumin and its role in cancer chemoprevention and therapy. Anticancer Agents Med Chem. 2006;6(3):259–70.

75. Murakami M, Ohnuma S, Fukuda M, Chufan EE, Kudoh K, Kanehara K, et al. Synthetic analogs of curcumin modulate the function of multidrug resistance-linked ABC transporter ABCG2. Drug Metab Dispos. 2017;45:1166–77.
76. Limtrakul P, Chearwae W, Shukla S, Phisalphong C, Ambudkar SV. Modulation of function of three ABC drug transporters, P-glycoprotein (ABCB1), mitoxantrone resistance protein (ABCG2) and multidrug resistance protein 1 (ABCC1) by tetrahydrocurcumin, a major metabolite of curcumin. Mol Cell Biochem. 2007;296(1-2):85–95.
77. Pan Y, Shao D, Zhao Y, Zhang F, Zheng X, Tan Y, et al. Berberine reverses hypoxia-induced chemoresistance in breast cancer through the inhibition of AMPK-HIF-1α. Int J Biol Sci. 2017;13(6):794.
78. Hussain I, Waheed S, Ahmad KA, Pirog JE, Syed V. Scutellaria baicalensis targets the hypoxia-inducible factor-1α and enhances cisplatin efficacy in ovarian cancer. J Cell Biochem. 2018;119:7515–24.
79. Farabegoli F, Papi A, Bartolini G, Ostan R, Orlandi M. (-)-Epigallocatechin-3-gallate downregulates Pg-P and BCRP in a tamoxifen resistant MCF-7 cell line. Phytomedicine. 2010;17(5):356–62.
80. Bhardwaj M, Cho HJ, Paul S, Jakhar R, Khan I, Lee S-J, et al. Vitexin induces apoptosis by suppressing autophagy in multi-drug resistant colorectal cancer cells. Oncotarget. 2018;9(3):3278.
81. Cocker HA, Tiffin N, Pritchard-Jones K, Pinkerton CR, Kelland LR. In vitro prevention of the emergence of multidrug resistance in a pediatric rhabdomyosarcoma cell line. Clin Cancer Res. 2001;7(10):3193–8.
82. Kelly JX, Smilkstein MJ, Brun R, Wittlin S, Cooper RA, Lane KD, et al. Discovery of dual function acridones as a new antimalarial chemotype. Nature. 2009;459(7244):270.
83. Xia Y, Chu H, Kuang G, Jiang G, Che Y. Inhibition effects of acridone on the growth of breast cancer cells in vivo. Eur Rev Med Pharmacol Sci. 2018;22(8):2356–63.
84. Iyer VV, Priya PY, Kangeyavelu J. Effects of increased accumulation of doxorubicin due to emodin on efflux transporter and LRP1 expression in lung adenocarcinoma and colorectal carcinoma cells. Mol Cell Biochem. 2018;449:91–104.
85. Su S, Cheng X, Wink M. Natural lignans from Arctium lappa modulate P-glycoprotein efflux function in multidrug resistant cancer cells. Phytomedicine. 2015;22(2):301–7.
86. El-Readi MZ, Hamdan D, Farrag N, El-Shazly A, Wink M. Inhibition of P-glycoprotein activity by limonin and other secondary metabolites from Citrus species in human colon and leukaemia cell lines. Eur J Pharmacol. 2010;626(2-3):139–45.
87. Yoo CB, Jones PA. Epigenetic therapy of cancer: past, present and future. Nat Rev Drug Discov. 2006;5(1):37.
88. Wilson AG. Epigenetic regulation of gene expression in the inflammatory response and relevance to common diseases. J Periodontol. 2008;79(8S):1514–9.
89. Henrique R, Oliveira AI, Costa VL, Baptista T, Martins AT, Morais A, et al. Epigenetic regulation of MDR1 gene through post-translational histone modifications in prostate cancer. BMC Genomics. 2013;14(1):898.
90. Yatouji S, El-Khoury V, Trentesaux C, Trussardi-Regnier A, Benabid R, Bontems F, et al. Differential modulation of nuclear texture, histone acetylation, and MDR1 gene expression in human drug-sensitive and -resistant OV1 cell lines. Int J Oncol. 2007;30(4):1003–9.
91. Ponnusamy L, Mahalingaiah PKS, Chang Y-W, Singh KP. Reversal of epigenetic aberrations associated with the acquisition of doxorubicin resistance restores drug sensitivity in breast cancer cells. Eur J Pharm Sci. 2018;123:56–69.
92. To KK, Zhan Z, Bates SE. Aberrant promoter methylation of the ABCG2 gene in renal carcinoma. Mol Cell Biol. 2006;26(22):8572–85.
93. Martin V, Sanchez-Sanchez AM, Herrera F, Gomez-Manzano C, Fueyo J, Alvarez-Vega MA, et al. Melatonin-induced methylation of the ABCG2/BCRP promoter as a novel mechanism to overcome multidrug resistance in brain tumour stem cells. Br J Cancer. 2013;108(10):2005.

94. Wu Q, Yang Z, Xia L, Nie Y, Wu K, Shi Y, et al. Methylation of miR-129-5p CpG island modulates multi-drug resistance in gastric cancer by targeting ABC transporters. Oncotarget. 2014;5(22):11552.
95. Zhang J, da Zhang H, Chen L, Sun DW, fei Mao C, Chen W, et al. β-elemene reverses chemoresistance of breast cancer via regulating MDR-related microRNA expression. Cell Physiol Biochem. 2014;34(6):2027–37.
96. Komeili-Movahhed T, Fouladdel S, Barzegar E, Atashpour S, Ghahremani MH, Ostad SN, et al. PI3K/Akt inhibition and down-regulation of BCRP re-sensitize MCF7 breast cancer cell line to mitoxantrone chemotherapy. Iran J Basic Med Sci. 2015;18(5):472.
97. Zhang Y, Wang H, Wei L, Li G, Yu J, Gao Y, et al. Transcriptional modulation of BCRP gene to reverse multidrug resistance by toremifene in breast adenocarcinoma cells. Breast Cancer Res Treat. 2010;123(3):679–89.
98. Naik A, Al-Yahyaee A, Abdullah N, Sam J-E, Al-Zeheimi N, Yaish MW, et al. Neuropilin-1 promotes the oncogenic Tenascin-C/integrin β3 pathway and modulates chemoresistance in breast cancer cells. BMC Cancer. 2018;18(1):533.
99. Qi S-S, Sun J-H, Yu H-H, Yu S-Q. Co-delivery nanoparticles of anti-cancer drugs for improving chemotherapy efficacy. Drug Deliv. 2017;24(1):1909–26.
100. Bi Y, Hao F, Yan G, Teng L, J Lee R, Xie J. Actively targeted nanoparticles for drug delivery to tumor. Curr Drug Metab. 2016;17(8):763–82.
101. Blau R, Krivitsky A, Epshtein Y, Satchi-Fainaro R. Are nanotheranostics and nanodiagnostics-guided drug delivery stepping stones towards precision medicine? Drug Resist Updat. 2016;27:39–58. https://doi.org/10.1016/j.drup.2016.06.003.
102. Kim CK, Lim SJ. Recent progress in drug delivery systems for anticancer agents. Arch Pharm Res. 2002;25(3):229–39.
103. Markman JL, Rekechenetskiy A, Holler E, Ljubimova JY. Nanomedicine therapeutic approaches to overcome cancer drug resistance. Adv Drug Deliv Rev. 2013;65(13-14):1866–79. https://doi.org/10.1016/j.addr.2013.09.019.
104. Jin X, Zhou B, Xue L, San W. Soluplus((R)) micelles as a potential drug delivery system for reversal of resistant tumor. Biomed Pharmacother. 2015;69:388–95. https://doi.org/10.1016/j.biopha.2014.12.028.
105. Susa M, Iyer AK, Ryu K, Hornicek FJ, Mankin H, Amiji MM, et al. Doxorubicin loaded polymeric nanoparticulate delivery system to overcome drug resistance in osteosarcoma. BMC Cancer. 2009;9(1):399.
106. Eisuke Kobayashi M, Hornicek FJ, Zhenfeng DM. Lipid-functionalized dextran nanosystems to overcome multidrug resistance in cancer. Clin Orthop Relat Res. 2013;471(3):915 25.
107. Zhang X, Guo S, Fan R, Yu M, Li F, Zhu C, et al. Dual-functional liposome for tumor targeting and overcoming multidrug resistance in hepatocellular carcinoma cells. Biomaterials. 2012;33(29):7103–14.
108. Ouhtit A, Rizeq B, Saleh HA, Rahman MM, Zayed H. Novel CD44-downstream signaling pathways mediating breast tumor invasion. Int J Biol Sci. 2018;14(13):1782.
109. Wu R-L, Sedlmeier G, Kyjacova L, Schmaus A, Philipp J, Thiele W, et al. Hyaluronic acid-CD44 interactions promote BMP4/7-dependent Id1/3 expression in melanoma cells. Sci Rep. 2018;8(1):14913.
110. Song S, Qi H, Xu J, Guo P, Chen F, Li F, et al. Hyaluronan-based nanocarriers with CD44-overexpressed cancer cell targeting. Pharm Res. 2014;31(11):2988–3005.
111. Negi LM, Jaggi M, Joshi V, Ronodip K, Talegaonkar S. Hyaluronan coated liposomes as the intravenous platform for delivery of imatinib mesylate in MDR colon cancer. Int J Biol Macromol. 2015;73:222–35.
112. Gazzano E, Rolando B, Chegaev K, Salaroglio IC, Kopecka J, Pedrini I, et al. Folate-targeted liposomal nitrooxy-doxorubicin: An effective tool against P-glycoprotein-positive and folate receptor-positive tumors. J Control Release. 2018;270:37–52.

113. Bai F, Yin Y, Chen T, Chen J, Ge M, Lu Y, et al. Development of liposomal pemetrexed for enhanced therapy against multidrug resistance mediated by ABCC5 in breast cancer. Int J Nanomedicine. 2018;13:1327.
114. Wang F, Zhang D, Zhang Q, Chen Y, Zheng D, Hao L, et al. Synergistic effect of folate-mediated targeting and verapamil-mediated P-gp inhibition with paclitaxel-polymer micelles to overcome multi-drug resistance. Biomaterials. 2011;32(35):9444–56.
115. Li J, Xu R, Lu X, He J, Jin S. A simple reduction-sensitive micelles co-delivery of paclitaxel and dasatinib to overcome tumor multidrug resistance. Int J Nanomedicine. 2017;12:8043.
116. Chen T, Wang C, Liu Q, Meng Q, Sun H, Huo X, et al. Dasatinib reverses the multidrug resistance of breast cancer MCF-7 cells to doxorubicin by downregulating P-gp expression via inhibiting the activation of ERK signaling pathway. Cancer Biol Ther. 2015;16(1):106–14.
117. Bar-Zeev M, Livney YD, Assaraf YG. Targeted nanomedicine for cancer therapeutics: towards precision medicine overcoming drug resistance. Drug Resist Updat. 2017;31:15–30.
118. Tang Y, Soroush F, Tong Z, Kiani MF, Wang B. Targeted multidrug delivery system to overcome chemoresistance in breast cancer. Int J Nanomedicine. 2017;12:671.
119. Chen Y, Zhang W, Huang Y, Gao F, Sha X, Fang X. Pluronic-based functional polymeric mixed micelles for co-delivery of doxorubicin and paclitaxel to multidrug resistant tumor. Int J Pharm. 2015;488(1-2):44–58.
120. Xue H, Yu Z, Liu Y, Yuan W, Yang T, You J, et al. Delivery of miR-375 and doxorubicin hydrochloride by lipid-coated hollow mesoporous silica nanoparticles to overcome multiple drug resistance in hepatocellular carcinoma. Int J Nanomedicine. 2017;12:5271.
121. Wu M, Lin X, Tan X, Li J, Wei Z, Zhang D, et al. Photo-responsive nanovehicle for two independent wavelength light-triggered sequential release of P-gp shRNA and doxorubicin to optimize and enhance synergistic therapy of multidrug-resistant cancer. ACS Appl Mater Interfaces. 2018;10:19416–27.
122. Yu X, Yang G, Shi Y, Su C, Liu M, Feng B, et al. Intracellular targeted co-delivery of shMDR1 and gefitinib with chitosan nanoparticles for overcoming multidrug resistance. Int J Nanomedicine. 2015;10:7045.
123. Yadav S, van Vlerken LE, Little SR, Amiji MM. Evaluations of combination MDR-1 gene silencing and paclitaxel administration in biodegradable polymeric nanoparticle formulations to overcome multidrug resistance in cancer cells. Cancer Chemother Pharmacol. 2009;63(4):711–22.
124. Zheng W, Cao C, Liu Y, Yu Q, Zheng C, Sun D, et al. Multifunctional polyamidoamine-modified selenium nanoparticles dual-delivering siRNA and cisplatin to A549/DDP cells for reversal multidrug resistance. Acta Biomater. 2015;11:368–80.
125. Meng H, Mai WX, Zhang H, Xue M, Xia T, Lin S, et al. Codelivery of an optimal drug/siRNA combination using mesoporous silica nanoparticles to overcome drug resistance in breast cancer in vitro and in vivo. ACS Nano. 2013;7(2):994–1005.
126. Wang J, Ma W, Tu P. Synergistically improved anti-tumor efficacy by co-delivery doxorubicin and curcumin polymeric micelles. Macromol Biosci. 2015;15(9):1252–61.
127. Zou L, Wang D, Hu Y, Fu C, Li W, Dai L, et al. Drug resistance reversal in ovarian cancer cells of paclitaxel and borneol combination therapy mediated by PEG-PAMAM nanoparticles. Oncotarget. 2017;8(36):60453.
128. Zafar S, Negi LM, Verma AK, Kumar V, Tyagi A, Singh P, et al. Sterically stabilized polymeric nanoparticles with a combinatorial approach for multi drug resistant cancer: in vitro and in vivo investigations. Int J Pharm. 2014;477(1-2):454–68.
129. Jia X, Han Y, Pei M, Zhao X, Tian K, Zhou T, et al. Multi-functionalized hyaluronic acid nanogels crosslinked with carbon dots as dual receptor-mediated targeting tumor theranostics. Carbohydr Polym. 2016;152:391–7.
130. Ivey JW, Bonakdar M, Kanitkar A, Davalos RV, Verbridge SS. Improving cancer therapies by targeting the physical and chemical hallmarks of the tumor microenvironment. Cancer Lett. 2016;380(1):330–9.

131. Butt AM, Amin MCIM, Katas H, Abdul Murad NA, Jamal R, Kesharwani P. Doxorubicin and siRNA codelivery via chitosan-coated pH-responsive mixed micellar polyplexes for enhanced cancer therapy in multidrug-resistant tumors. Mol Pharm. 2016;13(12):4179–90.
132. Lyu L, Liu F, Wang X, Hu M, Mu J, Cheong H, et al. Stimulus-responsive short peptide nanogels for controlled intracellular drug release and for overcoming tumor resistance. Chemistry. 2017;12(7):744–52.
133. Shi Q, Zhang L, Liu M, Zhang X, Zhang X, Xu X, et al. Reversion of multidrug resistance by a pH-responsive cyclodextrin-derived nanomedicine in drug resistant cancer cells. Biomaterials. 2015;67:169–82.
134. Zhou L, Wang H, Li Y. Stimuli-responsive nanomedicines for overcoming cancer multidrug resistance. Theranostics. 2018;8(4):1059.
135. Wang Y-C, Wang F, Sun T-M, Wang J. Redox-responsive nanoparticles from the single disulfide bond-bridged block copolymer as drug carriers for overcoming multidrug resistance in cancer cells. Bioconjug Chem. 2011;22(10):1939–45.
136. Dai Z, Yao Q, Zhu L. MMP2-sensitive PEG–lipid copolymers: a new type of tumor-targeted P-glycoprotein inhibitor. ACS Appl Mater Interfaces. 2016;8(20):12661–73.
137. Li Z, Cai Y, Zhao Y, Yu H, Zhou H, Chen M. Polymeric mixed micelles loaded mitoxantrone for overcoming multidrug resistance in breast cancer via photodynamic therapy. Int J Nanomedicine. 2017;12:6595.

Chapter 6
Overcoming Resistance to PARP Inhibition

Somaira Nowsheen and Fen Xia

Abstract PARP inhibitors are one of the success stories of targeted cancer therapy. In the last few years, these drugs have been approved by the US Food and Drug Administration (FDA) for the treatment of breast and ovarian cancers. PARP inhibitors are useful in the treatment of DNA double-strand break repair deficient tumors such as those with BRCA1 or BRCA2 mutations. In this chapter, we discuss the pathophysiology of breast and ovarian cancers in association with DNA repair and genomic instability. We focus our discussion on the use of PARP inhibitors in these malignancies. We also discuss how the tumors gain resistance to these agents, including utilizing strategies such as restoration of homologous recombination-mediated DNA double-strand break repair pathway and stabilization of replication forks. We review possible approaches for overcoming resistance to PARP inhibitors including targeting protein kinases and alternate signaling pathways, exploiting cell cycle regulation, and drug pumps. We end with the benefits of novel therapies, their limitations and work that remains to be done.

Keywords DNA damage response · DNA repair · PARP inhibitor · Breast cancer · Ovarian cancer · Resistance · Radiotherapy · Targeted therapy · BRCA · p53

S. Nowsheen
Mayo Clinic Medical Scientist Training Program, Mayo Clinic Alix School of Medicine and Mayo Clinic Graduate School of Biomedical Sciences, Mayo Clinic, Rochester, MN, USA
e-mail: nowsheen.somaira@mayo.edu

F. Xia (✉)
Department of Radiation Oncology, University of Arkansas for Medical Sciences, Little Rock, AR, USA
e-mail: f.xia@uams.edu

© Springer Nature Switzerland AG 2019
M. R. Szewczuk et al. (eds.), *Current Applications for Overcoming Resistance to Targeted Therapies*, Resistance to Targeted Anti-Cancer Therapeutics 20,
https://doi.org/10.1007/978-3-030-21477-7_6

161

Abbreviations

5-FU	5-Fluorouracil
AKT	Protein kinase B
BARD1	BRCA1-associated RING domain
BET	Bromodomain and extra-terminal
BRCA1	Breast cancer gene 1
BRCA2	Breast cancer gene 2
CDK12	Cyclin-dependent kinase 12
CTIP	C-terminal binding protein interacting protein
FDA	Food and Drug Administration
HER2	Human epidermal growth factor receptor 2
HGFR	Hepatocyte growth factor receptor
HR	Homologous recombination
HSP70	Heat shock protein 70
HSP90	Heat shock protein 90
MAPK	Mitogen-activated protein kinase
MDR	Multidrug-resistant
MRN	Mre11, Rad50, NBS1
MTD	Maximally tolerated dose
NHEJ	Non-homologous end-joining
P13K	Phosphoinositide 3-kinases
PAR	Poly(ADP-ribose)
PARP	Poly(ADP-ribose) polymerase
PTIP	Pax2 transactivation domain-interacting protein
Rb	Retinoblastoma

6.1 Introduction

Our genome's fidelity is ensured by an intricate DNA damage response system that involves tumor suppressor proteins to help repair DNA damage. Two well-reported tumor suppressor genes are *BRCA1* and *BRCA2* (Breast Cancer genes 1 and 2), which encode proteins that help repair damaged DNA, specifically DNA double-strand breaks, via homologous recombination (HR). Variants or mutations in the *BRCA1* or *BRCA2* genes can lead to inadequate or absent DNA repair, which in turn, can lead to genetic mutations or trigger cell death [1]. With increasing interest and advancements in targeted therapies, it is essential to understand the cancer subtypes that will be more susceptible to specific targeted therapies. Breast cancer is the most commonly diagnosed malignancy and the second leading cause of cancer-related deaths in women in the United States [2]. As shown in Fig. 6.1, breast cancer can be broadly divided into six main molecular subtypes. It has been shown that individuals may be predisposed to breast cancer if they harbor mutations in tumor suppressor genes such as *p53*, *PALB2*, *ATM*, *BRCA1* and *BRCA2* [3–10].

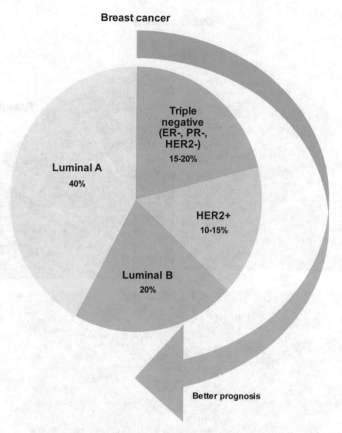

Fig. 6.1 Classification of breast cancer subtypes. Triple-negative breast cancer has the worst prognosis, while luminal A subtype confers the best prognosis

Additionally, ovarian cancer can also be classified into histological subtypes, with the most common being high-grade serous ovarian cancer (Fig. 6.2).

The non-descript symptoms of ovarian cancer lead to poor survival outcomes as women are generally diagnosed once at an advanced stage, making it one of the deadliest gynecological malignancies with a poorly understood etiology. However, similar to breast cancer, mutations in essential DNA damage response and signaling genes such as *PTEN, KRAS, BRAF, ERBB2, BRCA1* and *BRCA2* drive the development of ovarian cancer [11–16].

Current therapies for breast and ovarian cancer include chemo and radiation therapy. These systemic agents are associated with significant toxicities including fatigue, myelosuppression, rash, and gastrointestinal side effects. Thus, new targeted therapies have garnered attention.

Poly(ADP-ribose) polymerase (PARP) inhibitors are a promising option as they target cells with deficient HR-mediated DNA double-strand break repair, the same

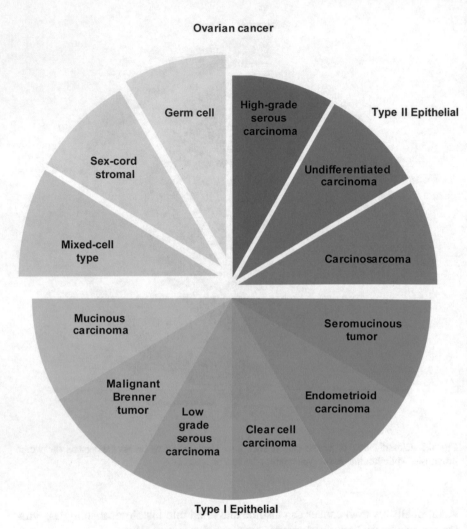

Fig. 6.2 Ovarian cancer subtypes. Ovarian cancers are divided into two main categories: Type I and Type II epithelial. Additional classifications include germ cell, sex-cord stromal and mixed-cell type

pathway that BRCA1 and BRCA2 regulate [17, 18]. PARP inhibitors have demonstrated efficacy in some patients with mutated BRCA1 and BRCA2. However, therapeutic resistance is frequently observed requiring the development of novel approaches to overcome this resistance. This chapter covers the pathophysiology of cancers treated with PARP inhibitors, with a particular focus on breast and ovarian cancers because PARP inhibitors are approved for their treatment. We also discuss mechanisms of acquired resistance to PARP inhibitors and the novel therapeutic advances and approaches to overcome this resistance.

6.2 Current Therapeutic Options for Breast and Ovarian Cancer

Patients with breast and ovarian cancer typically undergo a multimodal treatment approach (Table 6.1). More specifically, patients with high grade and large tumors or triple negative breast cancer may undergo treatment with chemotherapy that can include alkylating agents (e.g. cyclophosphamide), taxols (e.g. paclitaxel), anthracyclines (e.g. doxorubicin), and anti-metabolites (e.g. methotrexate, 5-fluorouracil and capecitabine). Furthermore, platinum-based agents such as cisplatin are often used in the metastatic setting. Specific targeted therapies are specific to a breast cancer subtype. For instance, patients with hormone receptor-positive tumors benefit from the use of endocrine therapy (aromatase inhibitors such as letrozole, anastrozole, *etc.*) while patients with human epidermal growth factor receptor 2 (HER2) positive breast cancer benefit from HER2 directed therapy such as trastuzumab.

The initial approaches to ovarian cancer treatment include debulking (surgery). Due to the risk of residual cancer cells remaining in the peritoneum and metastasizing, chemotherapy, such as paclitaxel and carboplatin, typically supplements the treatment plan [19]. The FDA recently approved PARP inhibitors (e.g., rucaparib) as an alternative therapy for women with BRCA mutations who had been treated with multiple lines of chemotherapy [20]. These tumors are typically responsive to platinum-based agents due to defects in DNA repair [21]. Other concurrent therapy options include the addition of angiogenesis inhibitor bevacizumab [22]. Despite advances in care, the overall 5-year survival for patients with ovarian cancer is around 45%, partly due to the absence of clear symptoms resulting in late detection of most ovarian cancers where survival is even more reduced (17% for stage IV disease) [2].

Table 6.1 Current therapeutic options for breast and ovarian cancer

Therapy options	Examples of therapeutic drugs and methods
Alkylating agents	Cyclophosphamide
Angiogenesis inhibitors	Bevacizumab
Anthracyclines	Doxorubicin
Antimetabolites	Methotrexate, 5-Fluorouracil, Capecitabine
CDK4/6 inhibitors	Abemaciclib
Endocrine therapy	Letrozole, Anastrozole
HER-2 Targeted therapy	Trastuzumab
Platinum-based therapy	Cisplatin, Carboplatin
Radiation therapy	
Surgery	Debulking
Taxol	Paclitaxel

6.2.1 Endocrine Therapy

Endocrine therapy has been the standard treatment option for hormone receptor-positive breast cancer. For example, anti-estrogen therapy is used in the treatment of estrogen receptor positive (ER+) cancer [23–29]. Tamoxifen is a selective estrogen receptor modulator that binds to the estrogen receptor and blocks the proliferative actions of estrogen [30]. It has been shown to substantially reduce recurrence rates of patients with ER+ disease throughout the first ten years and acts independently of progesterone receptor (PR) status (or level), age, nodal status, or use of chemotherapy, and can reduce mortality by 30%.

6.2.2 Targeted Therapy

Trastuzumab Trastuzumab is a targeted agent that has been proven to be efficacious in the treatment of patients with HER2+ breast cancers. Trastuzumab in combination with chemotherapy has significantly increased the time to disease progression and overall survival in both the metastatic and adjuvant settings when compared with chemotherapy alone [31–33]. Currently, trastuzumab is a mainstay treatment for HER2+ cancers. However, HER2-targeted therapies have been associated with a reversible decline in left ventricular ejection fraction, which is typically reversed with cessation of therapy and usage of cardiac medication such as beta-blockers [34–36].

Cyclin-Dependent Kinase 4/6 Inhibitors Cyclin-dependent kinase 4 (CDK4) and 6 (CDK6) are essential kinases that regulate the cell cycle by driving cell cycle progression into the S phase. ER-expressing breast cancer cells are highly sensitive to CDK4 and six inhibitors due to their dependence on CDK4 for proliferation [37]. Abemaciclib, a CDK4/6 inhibitor, was approved in 2017 for the treatment of patients with hormone receptor-positive, HER2-negative advanced or metastatic breast cancer that has progressed after endocrine therapy. Patients taking abemaciclib with fulvestrant, a selective estrogen receptor degrader, had a median progression-free survival (PFS) of 16.4 months compared to 9.3 months for patients taking a placebo with fulvestrant [38]. The safety and resultant efficacy of abemaciclib as a single agent showed that 19.7% of patients taking abemaciclib experienced complete or partial shrinkage of their tumors for a median of 8.6 months [39].

Inhibition of Angiogenesis Vascular endothelial growth factor (VEGF) and other cytokines activate various signaling pathways that culminate in angiogenesis, the development of aberrant vasculature. Some anti-angiogenic agents have been developed to disrupt these pathways by inhibiting extracellular growth factors and intracellular kinases [40, 41]. VEGF inhibitors, such as bevacizumab, have been efficacious in the treatment of ovarian cancer. Bevacizumab is a humanized monoclonal antibody against VEGF that binds VEGF extracellularly to prevent its interaction with the VEGF receptor (VEGFR) on the surface of endothelial cells [42, 43]. Bevacizumab, when used as maintenance therapy in ovarian cancer patients with platinum-sensitive recurrent disease, has improved PFS, but not overall survival (OS), [44]. Although bevacizumab is currently the only FDA approved antiangiogenic agent for the treatment of ovarian cancer, other antiangiogenic agents are currently being evaluated in clinical trials. For example, aflibercept is a protein that contains VEGF-binding domains from both VEGFR-1 and -2 fused to the Fc portion (tail region of the antibody that interacts with cell surface receptors) of human immunoglobulin G1 [45]. Though it is approved in colon cancer as combination therapy, it does not have significant single-agent toxicity in ovarian cancer [46].

6.2.3 Resistance to Current Therapies

Although there are a number of agents that can be used to treat cancer, cells inevitably develop resistance to these agents. For instance, secondary mutations in genes can lead to therapeutic resistance by activating alternate signaling pathways. Other factors include increased activity of drug efflux pumps and other cellular channels, activation or inactivation of signaling pathways in cells, and tumor heterogeneity. Resistance to endocrine therapy is mainly mediated by the loss of expression of the ER and reliance on other growth stimuli pathways [47]. Similarly, resistance to trastuzumab is mediated by upregulation of other HER family member proteins and alterations in the antibody binding site [48]. Loss of other cell cycle regulatory proteins such as retinoblastoma (Rb) can bestow resistance to CDK4/6 inhibitors [49] while upregulation of pro-angiogenesis gene expression can mediate resistance to anti-angiogenesis inhibitors [50].

6.3 Application of PARP Inhibitors as a Potential Option to Overcome Resistance to Targeted Therapy

Several approaches can overcome therapeutic resistance and improve survival and patient quality of life. The use of alternative targeted therapies such as poly(ADP-ribose) polymerase (PARP) inhibitors has been shown to be efficacious in early clinical trials in patients with mutated *BRCA1* and *BRCA2* and was recently approved for the treatment of advanced breast and ovarian cancer [17, 18].

6.3.1 PARP Function

PARPs are a class of enzymes that catalyze reactions in the cell by adding poly(ADP-ribose) (PAR) adducts to molecules that have various cellular roles including activation of specific signaling pathways. Perhaps the best-studied function of PARP is regarding DNA damage. PARP1 and PARP2 are activated by DNA damage, where they facilitate base excision repair as well as repair of single strand breaks. Mechanistically, PARP1 is activated upon recognizing and interacting with areas of single-strand breaks via its zinc-finger DNA-binding domain, which increases its catalytic activity. PARP uses oxidized nicotinamide adenine dinucleotide (NAD+) to create polymers of PAR and transfer it to acceptor proteins, including PARP itself. These PARylated proteins recruit other downstream factors that modulate DNA repair (Fig. 6.3) [51–53].

6.3.2 Role of PARP Inhibitors in Cancer Therapy

Maintaining a balance between DNA replication and repair is critical for cell survival. PARP inhibitors can stall replication forks, leading to an accumulation of unrepaired single-strand breaks. Some of the unrepaired breaks are converted into double-strand breaks as the cell attempts to replicate. One unrepaired double-strand break can be lethal to the cell; thus, using PARP inhibitors to prevent repair is an efficient method of killing highly proliferative cancer cells. This approach is most effective in cancers with defective HR-mediated DNA double-strand break repair. The BRCA proteins are key players in DNA double-strand break repair, specifically by the high-fidelity HR-mediated DNA repair pathway. As a result, tumors with somatic or germline mutations in BRCA1 or BRCA2 are highly sensitive to PARP inhibitors.

PARP inhibitors initially gained prominence due to their synthetic lethality in HR-deficient tumors. This concept is based on the understanding that a combination of mutations in multiple genes results in cell death, while each mutation on its own is tolerated. For instance, cells with wild-type BRCA1 or BRCA2 can repair damaged DNA via HR even when the PARP enzyme is blocked using an inhibitor. In contrast, cells with mutant BRCA1 or BRCA2 are unable to repair the DNA damage using HR. This leads to synthetic lethality in the presence of PARP inhibitors as shown in Fig. 6.4. Additionally, mutations in some genes can phenocopy mutations in BRCA1 or BRCA2. This is known as BRCAness and is characterized by an HR defect in the absence of germline BRCA1 or BRCA2 mutations. Mutations in DNA repair genes such as *BLM*, *WRN*, *NBS1*, *FANC*, *CDK12*, and *CHK2* have been associated with this phenotype [54]. PARP inhibitors are highly efficacious in these tumors.

6.3.3 Mechanism of Action of PARP Inhibitors

PARP inhibitors can be categorized based on their mechanisms of action. Some PARP inhibitors suppress PARP catalytic activity, thereby preventing the formation of PAR polymers. This blocks NAD+ from binding to the site of DNA damage,

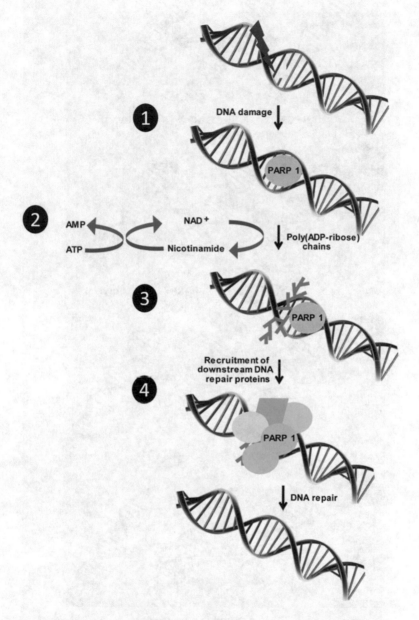

Fig. 6.3 Illustration of the catalytic function of PARP. (1) Detection of damaged DNA occurs through its DNA binding domain which activates PARP1. (2) Using ATP as its energy source and NAD+ as its substrate, (3) PARP1 generates poly(ADP-ribose) (PAR) chains on both itself and its target proteins. (4) Poly(ADP)ribosylation (PARylation) of PARP1 and other target proteins results in formation of the scaffold necessary for the accrual of various proteins that have roles in different aspects of DNA damage repair

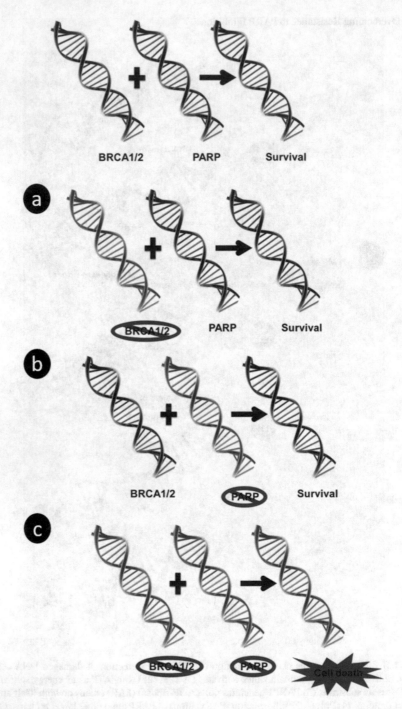

Fig. 6.4 Illustration of the concept of synthetic lethality. Loss of one gene can be tolerated (shown in **a** and **b**) while the loss of both genes leads to lethality (as shown in **d**). As shown in a and b, when PARP action is inhibited, for instance using an inhibitor, repair of single-strand breaks is inhibited. However, the single strand breaks are converted to double strand breaks during DNA replication. In cells with functional homologous recombination-mediated DNA double-strand break repair pathway, the double strand break can be efficiently repaired. (**c**) Conversely, in cells with a defect in double-strand break pathway, such as non-functional BRCA1/BRCA2, the lesions go unrepaired eventually resulting in cell death

Fig. 6.5 PARP inhibitors demonstrate a wide spectrum of PARP trapping. A list of conventional PARP inhibitors are provided here, where Talazoparib being the most trapped, compared to veliparib experiencing the least amount of PARP trapping

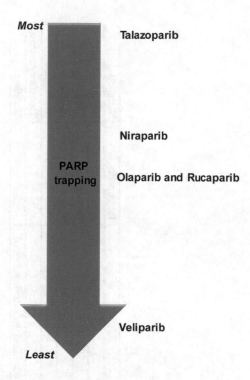

leading to a compromised DNA damage response. Some inhibitors are speculated to bind to the enzyme's NAD+ binding site, trapping PARP1 and PARP2 on the DNA. The trapped complex cannot be dissociated until the inhibitor dissociates from the active site. As a result, the complex consumes NAD+ and continues to PARylate, leading to a phenomenon known as PARP trapping, one of the critical mechanisms of action of PARP inhibitors.

Of the PARP inhibitors currently used in the clinic, the most to the least potent PARP trappers are shown in Fig. 6.5 [51, 55–58]. Over the last few years, it has become apparent that in addition to catalytic inhibition, some PARP inhibitors induce an allosteric conformational change in PARP1 and PARP2, thereby stabilizing their associations with DNA. Thus, the cytotoxicity mediated by these drugs is multifactorial.

6.3.4 Efficacy of PARP Inhibitors in Cancer Treatment

Various factors dictate the efficacy of PARP inhibitors, including NAD+ metabolism and core replication factors, DNA template switching proteins, and chromatin-remodelling proteins. Thus, these agents can hamper DNA replication. PARP inhibitors can also lead to the collapse of replication forks. However, all of the PARP inhibitors approved thus far for maintenance therapy for patients that have relapsed including, platinum-sensitive ovarian cancer, have similar efficacy but different toxicity profiles (Table 6.2).

Table 6.2 Toxicity profile of selected PARP inhibitors

Veliparib	Rucaparib	Olaparib	Talazoparib	Niraparib
Dehydration	Nausea	Leukopenia	Anemia	Nausea
Diarrhea	Anemia	Anemia	Neutropenia	Abdominal pain
Fatigue	Fatigue	Diarrhea	Thrombocytopenia	Fatigue
Febrile neutropenia	Increased liver enzymes	Fatigue		Neutropenia
Heart failure	Myelosuppression	Hypertension		Thrombocytopenia
Hyponatremia	Neutropenia	Myelosuppression (when combined with another chemo)		Vomiting
Leukopenia	Thrombocytopenia	Nausea		
Myelosuppression	Vomiting	Neutropenia		
Nausea				
Neutropenia				
Peripheral neuropathy				
Respiratory failure				
Thrombocytopenia				

PARP expression is increased in both triple negative breast cancer and cancers previously treated with chemotherapy. As a result, PARP inhibitors are efficacious in these cancers [59–61]. Although PARP inhibitors were initially studied in patients with recurrent epithelial ovarian cancer with BRCA mutations, they have also demonstrated a response in patients without mutations in BRCA1 or BRCA2. PARP inhibitors have also been used for maintenance purposes, increasing progression-free survival by at least two-fold [62]. Currently, olaparib is FDA-approved for patients with advanced ovarian cancer with deleterious or suspected deleterious germline BRCA mutations who have received ≥three lines of prior chemotherapy, or as maintenance in patients with platinum-sensitive recurrent ovarian cancer [63]. The PARP inhibitor rucaparib is approved as a monotherapy for patients with advanced disease with deleterious BRCA mutation (germline and somatic) who have been treated with ≥two kinds of chemotherapy [64, 65]. Finally, the drug niraparib is also FDA-approved as maintenance therapy in platinum-sensitive, recurrent epithelial ovarian cancer [20].

The combination of a PARP inhibitor and radiation therapy has been previously shown to be effective in preclinical models [66, 67]. This is, at least in part, due to the p53-dependent nuclear export of BRCA1 induced by radiation [68–72]. BRCA1 is localized both in the nucleus and the cytosol. Nuclear BRCA1 regulates DNA repair while cytosolic BRCA1 triggers apoptosis. BRCA1 has two nuclear localization signals that modulate its importin-mediated translocation. The BRCA1-associated Really Interesting New Gene (RING) domain protein (BARD1) has been shown to bind and mask the BRCA1 nuclear export signal. This prevents the nuclear export of BRCA1 through chromosome region maintenance 1 (CRM1). Since cytosolic BRCA1 promotes apoptosis, inhibition of this translocation leads to therapeutic resistance. Due to these modes of regulation, mutations in proteins such as p53 may confer resistance to PARP inhibitor therapy. On the other hand, cytosolic p53 and BRCA1 expression can be used as surrogate markers of response to these agents.

6.4   Development of Resistance to PARP Inhibitors and Methods of Overcoming Resistance

It is necessary to examine the development of resistance to PARP inhibitor therapy since a sustained response is rarely observed. There was an initiative to characterize differential patient response to olaparib response in an ongoing clinical trial (NCT02489058). Some of the known mechanisms of PARP resistance are depicted in Fig. 6.6.

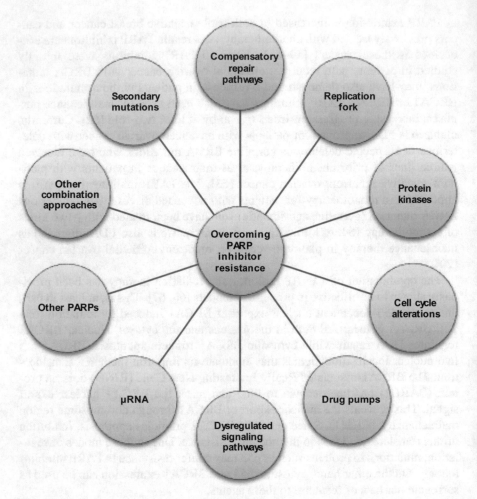

Fig. 6.6 Targets for overcoming resistance to PARP inhibitor therapy. There are several options for overcoming resistance to PARP inhibition including a combinatorial approach, targeting secondary mutations and protein kinases, to name a few

6.4.1 Secondary Mutations

The most well-known mechanism of resistance has been attributed to the restoration of the HR-mediated DNA double-strand break repair pathway. This is due to secondary mutations in genes such as BRCA1, Rad51C and Rad51D that restore the HR-mediated DNA repair capacity of the cell [73–75]. Often, truncated proteins are translated via alterations in DNA methylation that leads to restoration of the repair pathway [76, 77]. With decreasing costs of sequencing, tumor samples are sequenced more readily, and mutations are more easily identified. This knowledge can then be used to treat tumors from multiple fronts. For example, if changes in DNA methylation or acetylation status are observed, perhaps drugs that modulate histone modifications can be utilized. In this regard, bromodomain and extra-terminal motif (BET) inhibitors have been shown to increase tumor response to PARP inhibitors [78–80].

PARP inhibition is known to be a useful clinical strategy in BRCA mutant cancers; however, PARP inhibition is not effective in BRCA-proficient tumors. Multiple groups have recently shown a synergetic relationship between BET bromodomain inhibitions with PARP inhibition in BRCA-proficient cancers. This observation is multifactorial. Firstly, this is due to mitotic catastrophe secondary to impaired G2-M checkpoint and accumulation of DNA damage [79]. BET inhibitors, such as JQ1, inhibit cell cycle regulators Wee1 and TopBP1 and result in mitotic catastrophe and conclusively demonstrate the BET inhibitor mechanism of action, suppressing TopBP1and Wee1 expression. In ovarian cancer cells, JQ1 decreased the IC_{50} of Olaparib by ~50-fold, suggesting that this is a promising strategy in the treatment of repair proficient cells. The same class of drugs was also identified as being synergistic with olaparib [78]. It was found that BET inhibitors impair transcription of BRCA1 and Rad51 [78]. The most recent studies suggest that depletion of C-terminal binding protein interacting protein (CtIP) is responsible for the synergistic effect observed with BET and PARP inhibitors [80]. The authors employed PARP inhibitor resistant models to demonstrate that BET inhibitors can reverse the resistant phenotype. Mutations in genes such as KRAS and MAP 2 K1 have been suggested to confer PARP resistance [81]. Importantly, the combination of BET and PARP inhibition can reverse this resistance.

PARP has catalytic activity and binds DNA. As such, mutations both within and outside of the PARP1 DNA-binding zinc-finger domains confer resistance to PARP inhibition. These mutations also alter PARP1 trapping [82]. Interestingly, these mutations have been found in patient samples as well. However, exploiting this mechanism of resistance is challenging. One approach may involve the utilization of other PARP inhibitors since there are subtle differences in the mechanisms of action of these inhibitors. However, this approach is hypothetical thus far and is yet to be tested in clinical trials.

6.4.2 Alterations in Compensatory Repair Pathways

There are two essential DNA double-strand break repair pathways within cells: HR and non-homologous end-joining (NHEJ). Typically, there is a balance between these pathways with one inhibiting the other. BRCA1 and 53BP1 are key players in these two repair pathways. Hyper-activation of NHEJ-mediated DNA double-strand break repair pathway in HR-deficient cells can lead to PARP inhibitor resistance [83]. As proof of concept, it has been shown that loss of 53BP1 in BRCA1 null cells restores HR-mediated DNA repair. Thus, these cells gain resistance to therapy [83–85]. A recent report has shown that REV7 regulates the response to PARP inhibition by regulation end-resection [85]. REV7 is one of the members of the Shieldin complex, a 53BP1 effector complex. Others have recently shown that loss of any of the members of the Shieldin complex confers resistance to PARP inhibitors in *BRCA1*-deficient cells [86].

Also, it has been observed that HSP90 is stabilized in cells with dysfunctional BRCA1 and 53BP1 [87]. Thus, HSP90 inhibition is a promising strategy in this avenue. A clinical trial is currently in progress and is evaluating the utility of HSP90 inhibitor in combination with a PARP inhibitor (NCT02898207). More specifically, the phase I trial is evaluating the side effects and best dose of olaparib and onalespib (HSP90 inhibitor, AT13387) when given together in treating patients with solid metastatic tumors that have spread to other sites or with inoperable tumors or recurrent ovarian, fallopian tube, primary peritoneal, or triple-negative breast cancer. The primary outcome that is being measured is the maximum tolerated dose, and it is expected that by breaking up the regimen, the drugs will be better tolerated.

6.4.3 Replication Fork

Increased stabilization of replication forks also confers resistance to PARP inhibitors [88]. Replication forks are protected by the MRN (Mre11, Rad50, and NBS1) complex. Loss of the MLL3/4 complex protein and pax2 transactivation domain-interacting protein (PTIP), was shown to protect BRCA1/2-deficient cells from DNA damage and rescue the lethality of BRCA2-deficient embryonic stem cells. PTIP is an adaptor protein that has roles in end-resection and transcriptional regulation. Loss of PTIP reduces the recruitment of this complex to stalled replication forks, which protects them from degradation by Mre11 and ultimately confers resistance to PARP inhibitors. Since topoisomerases unwind DNA during replication, their inhibition leads to destabilization of the replication forks. Thus, the combination of PARP inhibition and topoisomerase inhibitors may mitigate resistance conferred through this mechanism [89, 90]. A phase I clinical trial evaluating olaparib in combination with topotecan, a topoisomerase inhibitor, in solid tumors observed a response rate of 32% (6/9 patients). Patients in four cohorts received topotecan intravenously in combination with oral olaparib for six cycles. The primary objectives were to determine safety and tolerability and to establish the maximally tolerated dose of olaparib in combination with topotecan. However, significant adverse events were observed, primarily neutropenia [91].

Currently, multiple trials are evaluating this combination therapy. A phase I dose-escalation study of oral ABT-888 (NSC #737664) plus intravenous Irinotecan (CPT-11, NSC#616348) administered in patients with advanced solid tumors (NCT00576654) has stopped recruitment. Patients received irinotecan hydrochloride and veliparib. It is expected that veliparib will potentiate the effect of irinotecan.

A similar phase I study is evaluating the utility of liposomal irinotecan and veliparib in treating patients with solid tumors (NCT02631733). In this study, patients receive liposomal irinotecan and veliparib. Courses repeat every 28 days in the absence of disease progression or unacceptable toxicity. Within 2–6 days before beginning liposomal irinotecan treatment, patients may optionally receive Ferumoxytol (an iron preparation) and undergo MRI at baseline and 24 h after Ferumoxytol infusion. After completion of study treatment, patients are followed up for four weeks.

Another trial underway is a phase I/II study evaluating the side effects and optimal dose of veliparib and topotecan hydrochloride to see how well they work in treating patients with solid tumors, recurrent ovarian cancer, ovarian cancer that does not respond to treatment, or primary peritoneal cancer (NCT01012817). Patients receive veliparib, and topotecan hydrochloride and courses repeat every 28 days in the absence of disease progression or unacceptable toxicity. After completion of study treatment, patients are followed up at three months (phase I) or every 3 or 6 months for five years (phase II). In all of these trials, it is expected that veliparib will potentiate the effect of the DNA damaging agents.

As discussed, there is currently much effort being put into utilizing this approach in overcoming resistance to PARP inhibitors.

6.4.4   Protein Kinases in the DNA Damage Response Pathway

The apical kinases in the DNA damage response pathway, ataxia-telangiectasia mutated (ATM) and ataxia telangiectasia and Rad3-related protein (ATR), activate various downstream proteins by phosphorylating them. This triggers a cascade of events that mobilize repair complexes. Since proficient DNA repair can lead to a therapeutic response, targeting these kinases has been considered as an approach to overcome resistance to PARP inhibitors. To this end, a clinical trial is underway evaluating the efficacy of Veliparib (ABT-888), an oral PARP inhibitor, and VX-970, an ATR inhibitor, in combination with cisplatin in patients with refractory solid tumors (NCT02723864). It is expected that this regimen will demonstrate significant toxicity, primarily due to non-specificity.

6.4.5   Cell Cycle Alterations

The HR-mediated DNA double-strand break repair pathway is dependent on the cell cycle process because it requires the sister chromatid as a template for faithful repair of damaged DNA. Thus, alterations in cell cycle regulators such as cyclin-dependent kinase 12 (CDK12) and Wee1 lead to resistance to PARP inhibitors [92]. Since knockdown of CDK12 leads to concomitant downregulation of DNA repair proteins (such as BRCA1, FANC1, and ATR) and a subsequent "BRCAness" phenotype, the reverse process leads to resistance. Similarly, increased expression of cell cycle regulator Wee1 that promotes reversible cell cycle arrest to allow for DNA repair to occur, leading to therapeutic resistance [93]. As a result, targeting the cell cycle has been considered as an approach to overcome PARP inhibitor resistance. There are multiple clinical trials underway evaluating cell cycle modifiers. A phase I trial is evaluating the side effects and the best dose of veliparib and dinaciclib (CDK12 inhibitor, SCH727965) in treating patients with solid metastatic tumors that cannot be cured or controlled with treatment (NCT01434316). It is expected that this regimen will be tolerable and that veliparib and dinaciclib may stop the growth of tumor cells by blocking some of the enzymes needed for cell growth.

Another suspended clinical trial, currently undergoing interim monitoring, evaluated the efficacy of Wee1 inhibitor in combination with a PARP inhibitor (NCT01827384). This randomized pilot phase II trial assessed molecular profiling-based targeted therapy in treating patients with solid metastatic tumors that usually cannot be cured or controlled with treatment. The Wee1 inhibitor AZD1775, everolimus, and trametinib are drugs that each target a specific variation in tumors by blocking different proteins needed for cell growth.

6.4.6   Drug Efflux Pumps

Drug efflux is another dominant mode of resistance [94]. Upregulation of some p-glycoproteins has been associated with resistance to therapy. The p-glycoproteins (multidrug resistance; MDR proteins) are upregulated in response to both treatment and maintenance dosing of olaparib while inhibiting the p-glycoproteins with the tariquidar in recurrent tumors re-sensitized the tumors to PARP inhibitor. Several nanomedicine-based strategies have been evaluated to overcome resistance at the cellular level including exploitation of endocytosis, usage of Pluronic nanocarriers, co-delivery of MDR modulators together with chemotherapeutic drugs, and co-delivery of anti-MDR siRNA together with chemotherapeutic drugs [95–99]. Trials targeting MDR have failed in the past, though they were not in the context of PARP inhibition [100]. Further research is warranted to test this approach.

6.4.7   Dysregulated Signaling Pathways

Signaling pathways such as the phosphoinositide 3-kinases (PI3K) pathway are required for cell survival. As a result, aberrant MET/HGFR and PI3K/AKT signaling pathways contribute to tumorigenesis and resistance [101]. In an integrated genome analysis of ovarian carcinoma, the receptor tyrosine kinase MET/HGFR was reported to be amplified or upregulated in 10% of samples [102]. Since MET directly phosphorylates PARP1 to increase PARP activity and reduces the binding activity of PARP inhibitor, upregulation or amplification of MET leads to resistance to therapy. Also, as a compensatory mechanism, PARP inhibitors can upregulate the PI3K/AKT pathway. Preexisting or acquired KRAS mutations or elevated RAS/MAPK activity mediates PARP inhibitor resistance.

A phase II signal-searching study is underway (NCT02576444) in a range of tumor types with the potential to identify novel tumor indications for combination therapy with olaparib that can subsequently be explored in dedicated studies. Patients are enrolled in this study based on molecular markers from genetic profiling performed on their tumors before study entry (outside of protocol). The trial will also identify genetic determinants of response and resistance. Patients with tumors harboring mutations in DNA damage repair genes will be treated with olaparib while those with tumors harboring either *TP53* or *KRAS* mutations or mutations in *KRAS* and *TP53* will be treated with AZD1775 plus olaparib. Patients with tumors harboring *PIK3CA*, *AKT*, or *ARID1A* mutations or other molecular aberrations leading to dysregulation of the PI3K/AKT pathway will be treated with AZD5363 plus olaparib. Finally, in patients with tumors harboring mutations in *TORC1/2*, *TSC1/2*, or *LKB1*, or tumors that are PTEN-deficient (determined either by genetic mutation or by immunohistochemistry) will be treated with AZD2014 plus olaparib. The primary aim of this trial is to assess the overall response rate. It is expected that significant response will be observed with this treatment regimen, but it is also highly likely to present with significant toxicity.

Trials evaluating VEGF inhibitors in combination with PARP inhibitors are also underway. One of these trials, NCT02354131, is phase Ia trial evaluating the safety and tolerability of the bevacizumab-niraparib combination. Here, the goal is to determine whether niraparib combined with bevacizumab is superior to niraparib. The subjects are patients with platinum-sensitive epithelial ovarian, fallopian tube, or primary peritoneal cancer. Disease control rate and progression-free survival rate will be assessed.

Another trial (NCT02208375) is determining the highest tolerable doses and combinations of the drugs Lynparza™ (olaparib), AZD2014, and AZD5363 that can be given to patients with recurrent endometrial, triple negative breast, ovarian, primary peritoneal, or fallopian tube cancer. The safety of these drugs and drug combinations is also being studied.

6.4.8   MicroRNA

Other causes of PARP inhibitor resistance include alterations in microRNA profiles that downregulate critical DNA repair genes [103]. For instance, miR-622 selectively blocks non-homologous end joining (NHEJ)-mediated DNA double-strand break repair upon DNA damage. High expression of miR-622 has been correlated with worse prognosis [103]. In contrast, miRNA-182 increases sensitivity to PARP inhibitors via downregulation of BRCA1 [104]. Thus, miRNAs modulate response to therapy. While targeting microRNAs for therapy sounds promising, so far, they are not clinically targetable. Perhaps with the advent of better technology, this approach can be evaluated in the future.

6.4.9   Other PARPs

Not all of the 17 identified PARPs, which have varying levels of activity, are targeted by the current PARP inhibitors. Though PARP1, PARP2 and PARP3 are involved directly in the repair of single strand breaks in the DNA, the inhibitors developed are more selective for PARP1 and PARP2. Thus, upregulation of the expression of other PARPs can compensate for the enzymes that are targeted, and decreased dependence on the specific PARPs that are targeted by these drugs render cancer cells resistant to maximal effects of PARP inhibition [105, 106]. As a result, one approach may be to switch inhibitors during therapy to target a more large number of PARPs. For instance, inhibitors for other PARPs such as PARP3 can be developed. Also, drugs that target PARP and augment cell death can be developed' however, this approach has not been evaluated as of yet.

6.4.10   Other Approaches

Aside from the avenues discussed above, immune modulators are being evaluated in combination with PARP inhibitors. PD-1 is a checkpoint protein on T-cells that has recently been heavily exploited for therapy. Recently developed monoclonal antibodies target the interaction between PD1 and its ligand PD-L1, boosting the immune response against cancer cells. One such clinical trial with PD1 inhibitor (NCT02657889), is a phase I/II study evaluating the safety and efficacy of combination treatment with niraparib and pembrolizumab (MK-3475) in patients with advanced or metastatic triple-negative breast cancer or recurrent ovarian cancer. Parameters being evaluated include overall response rate, dose-limiting toxicities, safety and tolerability, duration of response, disease control rate, progression-free survival, overall survival, clearance after oral administration, the volume of distribution, *etc.* The approach of targeting PD-1 and PD-L1 has garnered significant interest, especially in the last few years. It is hoped that this approach will be efficacious but may present with significant toxicity.

Another phase Ib, open-label, non-randomized study in patients with previously treated advanced ovarian or endometrial cancer (Part 1) and platinum-sensitive ovarian cancer or triple-negative breast cancer (Part 2) is investigating the dose, safety, pharmacokinetics, and preliminary efficacy of rucaparib in combination with atezolizumab. Approximately 6–18 participants with advanced gynecological cancers will receive different doses of rucaparib with a fixed dose of atezolizumab. While it is hoped that this trial will yield positive results, treatment of any advanced, recurrent malignancy poses a significant challenge and thus warrants cautious optimism.

Finally, the combination of a PARP inhibitor and radiation therapy has previously been shown to be effective in preclinical models [66, 67]. This is, at least in part, due to the nuclear export of BRCA1 induced by radiation. Completion of trials underway will help us evaluate this approach is greater detail (Table 6.3).

Table 6.3 Clinical trials evaluating the efficacy of PARP inhibitor and radiation therapy

Clinical trial title	Phase	Primary outcome
Olaparib and radiotherapy in inoperable breast cancer	I	Determination of the maximally tolerated dose of Olaparib administered with concurrent loco regional radiotherapy
A clinical study conducted in multiple centers evaluating escalating doses of Veliparib in combination with capecitabine and radiation in patients with locally advanced rectal cancer	I	Determine the maximum tolerated dose and/or establish the recommended phase II dose
Phase I/IIa study of concomitant radiotherapy with Olaparib and temozolomide in unresectable high-grade glioma patients	I/II	I: Recommended phase II dose II: Overall survival
Olaparib & radiation therapy for patients with triple negative breast cancer	I	Determination of the maximally tolerated dose of Olaparib administered with concurrent loco regional radiotherapy
Study of the poly (ADP-ribose) polymerase-1 (PARP-1) inhibitor BSI-201 in patients with newly diagnosed glioma	I/II	Determine the maximum tolerated dose of BSI-201 administered as an IV infusion in patients with newly diagnosed malignant glioma when given temozolomide after the completion of standard radiation therapy and concomitant temozolomide
Olaparib and radiotherapy in head and neck cancer	I	Incidence of dose-limiting toxicities
Veliparib with radiation therapy in patients with inflammatory or loco-regionally recurrent breast cancer	I	To determine the maximum tolerated dose of veliparib that can be administered concurrently with standard doses of radiotherapy to the chest wall and regional nodes
A trial evaluating concurrent whole brain radiotherapy and Iniparib in multiple nonoperable brain metastases	I	To determine the maximum tolerated dose
Veliparib, radiation therapy, and temozolomide in treating younger patients with newly diagnosed diffuse pontine gliomas	I/II	I: Recommended phase II dose II: Overall survival
Veliparib with radiation therapy in treating patients with advanced solid malignancies with peritoneal carcinomatosis, epithelial ovarian, fallopian, or primary peritoneal cancer	I	Determine the maximal tolerated dose of veliparib in combination with low-dose fractionated whole abdominal radiation therapy (LDFWAR) in patients with peritoneal carcinomatosis from advanced solid malignancies Determine the safety and toxicity of the combination of veliparib in conjunction with LDFWAR in patients
A phase I study of ABT-888 in combination with conventional whole brain radiation therapy in cancer patients with brain metastases	I	Determine the maximum tolerated dose of ABT-888 in combination with whole brain radiation therapy

(continued)

Table 6.3 (continued)

Clinical trial title	Phase	Primary outcome
Veliparib with or without radiation therapy, carboplatin, and paclitaxel in patients with stage III non-small cell lung cancer that cannot be removed by surgery	I/II	I: Maximum tolerated dose of veliparib when given concurrently with standard carboplatin/paclitaxel and radiotherapy
		II: Progression free survival of patients treated with chemoradiotherapy plus veliparib assessed by Response Evaluation Criteria in Solid Tumors
Olaparib dose-escalating trial + concurrent radiation therapy with or without cisplatin in locally advanced non-small cell lung cancer	I	The incidence of dose limiting toxicities
A study evaluating the efficacy and tolerability of Veliparib in combination with paclitaxel/carboplatin-based chemoradiotherapy followed by Veliparib and paclitaxel/carboplatin consolidation in subjects with stage III non-small cell lung cancer	I/II	I: Recommended phase II dose of veliparib in combination with radiotherapy, paclitaxel and carboplatin
		II: Progression-free survival
Phase I study of Olaparib combined with cisplatin-based chemo-radiotherapy to treat locally advanced head and neck cancer	I	Occurrence of dose-limiting toxicity

One of the benefits of the novel treatment options suggested above is that they target the tumors from a different perspective. It is anticipated that at least some of the malignant cells will respond to this therapy. Due to tumors heterogeneity, attacking the malignancy from multiple fronts may be beneficial, as often, the microenvironment is not taken into consideration when treating cancer. Thus, it is anticipated that the new therapeutic approaches will mitigate this issue of the milieu fostering therapeutic resistance.

6.5 Limitations and Future Directions

Similar to any therapy being developed, there are some considerations for developing a new treatment approach. Chemotherapy is toxic, often affecting both normal and cancer cells. Also, frequently, the patients are quite sick from the battery of treatments that they undergo. As a result, the drug side effect profile should be considered. Immunosuppression/myelosuppression, nausea and vomiting, and other adverse reactions should be taken into account when developing a new therapy.

Tumors evolve at a fast rate and are heterogeneous. Thus, we have to remain a step ahead in order to achieve better results. Knowledge of the DNA damage response pathway, as well as mutational profiles of therapy-resistant tumors, will help improve outcomes. Recently, there has been an increased effort in this respect [107, 108], with invaluable benefit in developing new strategies to treat treatment-resistant tumors.

Also, identifying patients who will benefit the most from PARP inhibitor therapy is a priority. As mentioned above, perhaps immunohistochemistry for BRCA1 and p53 can be used as surrogate markers to predict resistance and response [66, 69, 70, 71]. Further work is warranted to explore this avenue. Data from ongoing clinical trials will inform us what the best biomarkers are for predicting response to PARP inhibitors.

6.6   Conclusion

In conclusion, breast and ovarian cancer therapies have improved significantly over the last few decades. Cancer continues to affect millions of people every year, claiming lives and decreasing the quality of life of survivors. One of the causes for this is that the tumors eventually escape the treatment that they are subjected to. As a result, it is imperative that new strategies are developed to treat treatment-resistant diseases.

To date, there has been limited success in treating cancers with targeted agents such as PARP inhibitors. This is primarily because PARP inhibitors are not frequently used as frontline therapy. When cancers are treated with these drugs, mutations have been acquired that make them resistant to PARP inhibitors. Perhaps, tailoring treatment to each patient, i.e. personalized therapy, is the approach that needs to be taken. However, this poses additional challenges, particularly in the marketing and commercialization of drugs. In order to become better established in the clinic, PARP inhibitors will need to find their niche and area of unmet need. Other strategies include combining PARP inhibitors with inhibition of angiogenic, immune checkpoint, PI3K/AKT, Wee1 and ATR pathways. Perhaps, this multi-front approach will mitigate the issue of PARP inhibitor resistance.

Conflict of Interest   No potential conflicts of interest were disclosed.

References

1. Roy R, Chun J, Powell SN. BRCA1 and BRCA2: different roles in a common pathway of genome protection. Nat Rev Cancer. 2011;12:68. https://doi.org/10.1038/nrc3181.
2. Rebecca SL, Kimberly MD, Ahmedin J. Cancer statistics, 2018. CA Cancer J Clin. 2018;68(1):7–30. https://doi.org/10.3322/caac.21442.
3. Antoniou AC, Casadei S, Heikkinen T, Barrowdale D, Pylkäs K, Roberts J, et al. Breast-cancer risk in families with mutations in PALB2. N Engl J Med. 2014;371(6):497–506.
4. Meijers-Heijboer H, van Geel B, van Putten WL, Henzen-Logmans SC, Seynaeve C, Menke-Pluymers MB, et al. Breast cancer after prophylactic bilateral mastectomy in women with a BRCA1 or BRCA2 mutation. N Engl J Med. 2001;345(3):159–64.
5. Hollstein M, Sidransky D, Vogelstein B, Harris CC. p53 mutations in human cancers. Science. 1991;253(5015):49–53.

6. Lakhani SR, Van De Vijver MJ, Jacquemier J, Anderson TJ, Osin PP, McGuffog L, et al. The pathology of familial breast cancer: predictive value of immunohistochemical markers estrogen receptor, progesterone receptor, HER-2, and p53 in patients with mutations in BRCA1 and BRCA2. J Clin Oncol. 2002;20(9):2310–8.
7. Malkin D, Li FP, Strong LC, Fraumeni JF, Nelson CE, Kim DH, et al. Germ line p53 mutations in a familial syndrome of breast cancer, sarcomas, and other neoplasms. Science. 1990;250(4985):1233–8.
8. Renwick A, Thompson D, Seal S, Kelly P, Chagtai T, Ahmed M, et al. ATM mutations that cause ataxia-telangiectasia are breast cancer susceptibility alleles. Nat Genet. 2006;38(8):873.
9. Nik-Zainal S, Davies H, Staaf J, Ramakrishna M, Glodzik D, Zou X, et al. Landscape of somatic mutations in 560 breast cancer whole-genome sequences. Nature. 2016;534(7605):47.
10. Couch FJ, Hart SN, Sharma P, Toland AE, Wang X, Miron P, et al. Inherited mutations in 17 breast cancer susceptibility genes among a large triple-negative breast cancer cohort unselected for family history of breast cancer. J Clin Oncol. 2015;33(4):304.
11. Patch A-M, Christie EL, Etemadmoghadam D, Garsed DW, George J, Fereday S, et al. Whole–genome characterization of chemoresistant ovarian cancer. Nature. 2015;521(7553):489.
12. Song H, Dicks SJR, Tyrer JP, Intermaggio MP, Hayward J, Edlund CK, et al. Contribution of germline mutations in the RAD51B, RAD51C, and RAD51D genes to ovarian cancer in the population. J Clin Oncol. 2015;33(26):2901.
13. Ramus SJ, Song H, Dicks E, Tyrer JP, Rosenthal AN, Intermaggio MP, et al. Germline mutations in the BRIP1, BARD1, PALB2, and NBN genes in women with ovarian cancer. J Natl Cancer Inst. 2015;107(11).
14. Jayson GC, Kohn EC, Kitchener HC, Ledermann JA. Ovarian cancer. Lancet. 2014;384(9951):1376–88.
15. Daly MB, Pilarski R, Axilbund JE, Berry M, Buys SS, Crawford B, et al. Genetic/familial high-risk assessment: breast and ovarian, version 2.2015. J Natl Compr Cancer Netw. 2016;14(2):153–62.
16. McConechy MK, Ding J, Senz J, Yang W, Melnyk N, Tone AA, et al. Ovarian and endometrial endometrioid carcinomas have distinct CTNNB1 and PTEN mutation profiles. Mod Pathol. 2014;27(1):128.
17. Robson M, Im S-A, Senkus E, Xu B, Domchek SM, Masuda N, et al. Olaparib for metastatic breast cancer in patients with a germline BRCA mutation. N Engl J Med. 2017;377(6):523–33.
18. Livraghi L, Garber JE. PARP inhibitors in the management of breast cancer: current data and future prospects. BMC Med. 2015;13(1):188. https://doi.org/10.1186/s12916-015-0425-1.
19. Cortez AJ, Tudrej P, Kujawa KA, Lisowska KM. Advances in ovarian cancer therapy. Cancer Chemother Pharmacol. 2018;81(1):17–38. https://doi.org/10.1007/s00280-017-3501-8.
20. Mirza MR, Monk BJ, Herrstedt J, Oza AM, Mahner S, Redondo A, et al. Niraparib maintenance therapy in platinum-sensitive, recurrent ovarian cancer. N Engl J Med. 2016;375(22):2154–64. https://doi.org/10.1056/NEJMoa1611310.
21. Armstrong DK, Bundy B, Wenzel L, Huang HQ, Baergen R, Lele S, et al. Intraperitoneal cisplatin and paclitaxel in ovarian cancer. N Engl J Med. 2006;354(1):34–43. https://doi.org/10.1056/NEJMoa052985.
22. Burger RA, Brady MF, Bookman MA, Fleming GF, Monk BJ, Huang H, et al. Incorporation of bevacizumab in the primary treatment of ovarian cancer. N Engl J Med. 2011;365(26):2473–83. https://doi.org/10.1056/NEJMoa1104390.
23. Miller WR. Aromatase inhibitors: mechanism of action and role in the treatment of breast cancer. Semin Oncol. 2003;30:3–11.
24. Padmanabhan N, Howell A, Rubens R. Mechanism of action of adjuvant chemotherapy in early breast cancer. Lancet. 1986;328(8504):411–4.
25. Bryant HU. Mechanism of action and preclinical profile of raloxifene, a selective estrogen receptor modulator. Rev Endocr Metab Disord. 2001;2(1):129–38.
26. Lewis JS, Jordan VC. Selective estrogen receptor modulators (SERMs): mechanisms of anticarcinogenesis and drug resistance. Mutat Res. 2005;591(1):247–63.

27. Jordan V, Dix C, Rowsby L, Prestwich G. Studies on the mechanism of action of the nonsteroidal antioestrogen tamoxifen (ICI 46,474) in the rat. Mol Cell Endocrinol. 1977;7(2):177–92.
28. Sawka CA, Pritchard KI, Paterson AH, Sutherland DJ, Thomson DB, Shelley WE, et al. Role and mechanism of action of tamoxifen in premenopausal women with metastatic breast carcinoma. Cancer Res. 1986;46(6):3152–6.
29. Osborne C, Wakeling A, Nicholson R. Fulvestrant: an oestrogen receptor antagonist with a novel mechanism of action. Br J Cancer. 2004;90(S1):S2.
30. Davies C, Godwin J, Gray R, Clarke M, Cutter D, Darby S, et al. Relevance of breast cancer hormone receptors and other factors to the efficacy of adjuvant tamoxifen: patient-level meta-analysis of randomised trials. Lancet. 2011;378(9793):771–84. https://doi.org/10.1016/s0140-6736(11)60993-8.
31. Vogel CL, Cobleigh MA, Tripathy D, Gutheil JC, Harris LN, Fehrenbacher L, et al. Efficacy and safety of trastuzumab as a single agent in first-line treatment of HER2-overexpressing metastatic breast cancer. J Clin Oncol. 2002;20(3):719–26.
32. Romond EH, Perez EA, Bryant J, Suman VJ, Geyer CE Jr, Davidson NE, et al. Trastuzumab plus adjuvant chemotherapy for operable HER2-positive breast cancer. N Engl J Med. 2005;353(16):1673–84.
33. Piccart-Gebhart MJ, Procter M, Leyland-Jones B, Goldhirsch A, Untch M, Smith I, et al. Trastuzumab after adjuvant chemotherapy in HER2-positive breast cancer. N Engl J Med. 2005;353(16):1659–72.
34. O'Sullivan CC, Ruddy KJ. Management of potential long-term toxicities in breast cancer patients. Curr Breast Cancer Rep. 2016;8(4):183–92. https://doi.org/10.1007/s12609-016-0229-0.
35. Nowsheen S, Viscuse PV, O'Sullivan CC, Sandhu NP, Haddad TC, Blaes A, et al. Incidence, diagnosis, and treatment of cardiac toxicity from trastuzumab in patients with breast cancer. Curr Breast Cancer Rep. 2017;9(3):173–82. https://doi.org/10.1007/s12609-017-0249-4.
36. Nowsheen S, Duma N, Ruddy KJ. Preventing today's survivors of breast cancer from becoming tomorrow's cardiac patients. J Oncol Pract. 2018;14(4):213–4. https://doi.org/10.1200/JOP.18.00130.
37. Yu Q, Sicinska E, Geng Y, Ahnström M, Zagozdzon A, Kong Y, et al. Requirement for CDK4 kinase function in breast cancer. Cancer Cell. 2006;9(1):23–32.
38. Sledge GW Jr, Toi M, Neven P, Sohn J, Inoue K, Pivot X, et al. MONARCH 2: abemaciclib in combination with fulvestrant in women with HR+/HER2− advanced breast cancer who had progressed while receiving endocrine therapy. J Clin Oncol. 2017;35(25):2875–84.
39. Dickler MN, Tolaney SM, Rugo HS, Cortés J, Diéras V, Patt D, et al. MONARCH 1, a phase II study of Abemaciclib, a CDK4 and CDK6 inhibitor, as a single agent, in patients with refractory HR+/HER2− metastatic breast cancer. Clin Cancer Res. 2017;23(17):5218–24. https://doi.org/10.1158/1078-0432.ccr-17-0754.
40. Homsi J, Daud AI. Spectrum of activity and mechanism of action of VEGF/PDGF inhibitors. Cancer Control. 2007;14(3):285–94.
41. Gotink KJ, Verheul HM. Anti-angiogenic tyrosine kinase inhibitors: what is their mechanism of action? Angiogenesis. 2010;13(1):1–14.
42. Ellis LM. Mechanisms of action of bevacizumab as a component of therapy for metastatic colorectal cancer. Semin Oncol. 2006;33:S1–7.
43. Kazazi-Hyseni F, Beijnen JH, Schellens JHM. Bevacizumab. Oncologist. 2010;15(8):819–25. https://doi.org/10.1634/theoncologist.2009-0317.
44. Oza AM, Cook AD, Pfisterer J, Embleton A, Ledermann JA, Pujade-Lauraine E, et al. Standard chemotherapy with or without bevacizumab for women with newly diagnosed ovarian cancer (ICON7): overall survival results of a phase 3 randomised trial. Lancet Oncol. 2015;16(8):928–36.
45. Ciombor KK, Berlin J. Aflibercept—a decoy VEGF receptor. Curr Oncol Rep. 2014;16(2):368.
46. Benson AB, Bekaii-Saab T, Chan E, Chen Y-J, Choti MA, Cooper HS, et al. Metastatic colon cancer, version 3.2013 featured updates to the NCCN guidelines. J Natl Compr Cancer Netw. 2013;11(2):141–52.

47. Fan W, Chang J, Fu P. Endocrine therapy resistance in breast cancer: current status, possible mechanisms and overcoming strategies. Future Med Chem. 2015;7(12):1511–9. https://doi.org/10.4155/fmc.15.93.
48. Luque-Cabal M, García-Teijido P, Fernández-Pérez Y, Sánchez-Lorenzo L, Palacio-Vázquez I. Mechanisms behind the resistance to Trastuzumab in HER2-amplified breast cancer and strategies to overcome it. Clin Med Insights Oncol. 2016;10(Suppl 1):21–30. https://doi.org/10.4137/CMO.S34537.
49. Knudsen ES, Witkiewicz AK. The strange case of CDK4/6 inhibitors: mechanisms, resistance, and combination strategies. Trends Cancer. 2017;3(1):39–55. https://doi.org/10.1016/j.trecan.2016.11.006.
50. Loges S, Schmidt T, Carmeliet P. Mechanisms of resistance to anti-angiogenic therapy and development of third-generation anti-angiogenic drug candidates. Genes Cancer. 2010;1(1):12–25. https://doi.org/10.1177/1947601909356574.
51. Rouleau M, Patel A, Hendzel MJ, Kaufmann SH, Poirier GG. PARP inhibition: PARP1 and beyond. Nat Rev Cancer. 2010;10(4):293.
52. Underhill C, Toulmonde M, Bonnefoi H. A review of PARP inhibitors: from bench to bedside. Ann Oncol. 2010;22(2):268–79.
53. Curtin NJ. PARP inhibitors for cancer therapy. Expert Rev Mol Med. 2005;7(4):1–20.
54. Lord CJ, Ashworth A. BRCAness revisited. Nat Rev Cancer. 2016;16:110. https://doi.org/10.1038/nrc.2015.21.
55. Murai J, Shar-yin NH, Das BB, Renaud A, Zhang Y, Doroshow JH, et al. Trapping of PARP1 and PARP2 by clinical PARP inhibitors. Cancer Res. 2012;72(21):5588–99.
56. Brown JS, Kaye SB, Yap TA. PARP inhibitors: the race is on. Br J Cancer. 2016;114:713–5.
57. Yap TA, Sandhu SK, Carden CP, de Bono JS. Poly (ADP-Ribose) polymerase (PARP) inhibitors: exploiting a synthetic lethal strategy in the clinic. CA Cancer J Clin. 2011;61(1):31–49.
58. Brown JS, O'Carrigan B, Jackson SP, Yap TA. Targeting DNA repair in cancer: beyond PARP inhibitors. Cancer Discov. 2017;7(1):20–37.
59. Ibrahim YH, García-García C, Serra V, He L, Torres-Lockhart K, Prat A, et al. PI3K inhibition impairs BRCA1/2 expression and sensitizes BRCA-proficient triple-negative breast cancer to PARP inhibition. Cancer Discov. 2012;2(11):1036–47.
60. O'Shaughnessy J, Osborne C, Pippen J, Yoffe M, Patt D, Monaghan G, et al. Efficacy of BSI-201, a poly (ADP-ribose) polymerase-1 (PARP1) inhibitor, in combination with gemcitabine/carboplatin (G/C) in patients with metastatic triple-negative breast cancer (TNBC): results of a randomized phase II trial. J Clin Oncol. 2009;27(18S):3.
61. Ossovskaya V, Koo IC, Kaldjian EP, Alvares C, Sherman BM. Upregulation of poly (ADP-ribose) polymerase-1 (PARP1) in triple-negative breast cancer and other primary human tumor types. Genes Cancer. 2010;1(8):812–21.
62. Ledermann J, Harter P, Gourley C, Friedlander M, Vergote I, Rustin G, et al. Olaparib maintenance therapy in platinum-sensitive relapsed ovarian cancer. N Engl J Med. 2012;366(15):1382–92.
63. Pujade-Lauraine E, Ledermann JA, Selle F, Gebski V, Penson RT, Oza AM, et al. Olaparib tablets as maintenance therapy in patients with platinum-sensitive, relapsed ovarian cancer and a BRCA1/2 mutation (SOLO2/ENGOT-Ov21): a double-blind, randomised, placebo-controlled, phase 3 trial. Lancet Oncol. 2017;18(9):1274–84.
64. Coleman RL, Oza AM, Lorusso D, Aghajanian C, Oaknin A, Dean A, et al. Rucaparib maintenance treatment for recurrent ovarian carcinoma after response to platinum therapy (ARIEL3): a randomised, double-blind, placebo-controlled, phase 3 trial. Lancet. 2017;390(10106):1949–61.
65. Swisher EM, Lin KK, Oza AM, Scott CL, Giordano H, Sun J, et al. Rucaparib in relapsed, platinum-sensitive high-grade ovarian carcinoma (ARIEL2 Part 1): an international, multicentre, open-label, phase 2 trial. Lancet Oncol. 2017;18(1):75–87.
66. Sizemore ST, Mohammed R, Sizemore GM, Nowsheen S, Yu H, Ostrowski MC, et al. Synthetic lethality of PARP inhibition and ionizing radiation is p53-dependent. Mol Cancer Res. 2018;16:1092–102. https://doi.org/10.1158/1541-7786.MCR-18-0106.

67. Wiltshire TD, Lovejoy CA, Wang T, Xia F, O'Connor MJ, Cortez D. Sensitivity to poly(ADP-ribose) polymerase (PARP) inhibition identifies ubiquitin-specific peptidase 11 (USP11) as a regulator of DNA double-strand break repair. J Biol Chem. 2010;285(19):14565–71. https://doi.org/10.1074/jbc.M110.104745.

68. Wang H, Yang ES, Jiang J, Nowsheen S, Xia F. DNA damage-induced cytotoxicity is dissociated from BRCA1's DNA repair function but is dependent on its cytosolic accumulation. Cancer Res. 2010;70(15):6258–67. https://doi.org/10.1158/0008-5472.can-09-4713.

69. Jiang J, Yang ES, Jiang G, Nowsheen S, Wang H, Wang T, et al. p53-dependent BRCA1 nuclear export controls cellular susceptibility to DNA damage. Cancer Res. 2011;71(16):5546–57. https://doi.org/10.1158/0008-5472.can-10-3423.

70. Yang ES, Nowsheen S, Rahman MA, Cook RS, Xia F. Targeting BRCA1 localization to augment breast tumor sensitivity to poly(ADP-Ribose) polymerase inhibition. Cancer Res. 2012;72(21):5547–55. https://doi.org/10.1158/0008-5472.can-12-0934.

71. Feng Z, Kachnic L, Zhang J, Powell SN, Xia F. DNA damage induces p53-dependent BRCA1 nuclear export. J Biol Chem. 2004;279(27):28574–84. https://doi.org/10.1074/jbc.M404137200.

72. Xia F, Powell SN. The molecular basis of radiosensitivity and chemosensitivity in the treatment of breast cancer. Semin Radiat Oncol. 2002;12(4):296–304. https://doi.org/10.1053/srao.2002.35250.

73. Barber LJ, Sandhu S, Chen L, Campbell J, Kozarewa I, Fenwick K, et al. Secondary mutations in BRCA2 associated with clinical resistance to a PARP inhibitor. J Pathol. 2013;229(3):422–9. https://doi.org/10.1002/path.4140.

74. Norquist B, Wurz KA, Pennil CC, Garcia R, Gross J, Sakai W, et al. Secondary somatic mutations restoring BRCA1/2 predict chemotherapy resistance in hereditary ovarian carcinomas. J Clin Oncol. 2011;29(22):3008–15. https://doi.org/10.1200/JCO.2010.34.2980.

75. Kondrashova O, Nguyen M, Shield-Artin K, Tinker AV, Teng NNH, Harrell MI, et al. Secondary somatic mutations restoring RAD51C and RAD51D associated with acquired resistance to the PARP inhibitor Rucaparib in high-grade ovarian carcinoma. Cancer Discov. 2017;7(9):984–98. https://doi.org/10.1158/2159-8290.CD-17-0419.

76. Island BC. BRCA1 CpG island hypermethylation predicts sensitivity to poly (adenosine diphosphate)-ribose polymerase inhibitors. J Clin Oncol. 2010;28(29):e563–e4.

77. Jacot W, Thezenas S, Senal R, Viglianti C, Laberenne A-C, Lopez-Crapez E, et al. BRCA1 promoter hypermethylation, 53BP1 protein expression and PARP-1 activity as biomarkers of DNA repair deficit in breast cancer. BMC Cancer. 2013;13(1):523.

78. Yang L, Zhang Y, Shan W, Hu Z, Yuan J, Pi J, et al. Repression of BET activity sensitizes homologous recombination–proficient cancers to PARP inhibition. Sci Transl Med. 2017;9(400):eaal1645.

79. Karakashev S, Zhu H, Yokoyama Y, Zhao B, Fatkhutdinov N, Kossenkov AV, et al. BET bromodomain inhibition synergizes with PARP inhibitor in epithelial ovarian cancer. Cell Rep. 2017;21(12):3398–405. https://doi.org/10.1016/j.celrep.2017.11.095.

80. Sun C, Yin J, Fang Y, Chen J, Jeong KJ, Chen X, et al. BRD4 inhibition is synthetic lethal with PARP inhibitors through the induction of homologous recombination deficiency. Cancer Cell. 2018;33(3):401–16.e8. https://doi.org/10.1016/j.ccell.2018.01.019.

81. Sun C, Fang Y, Yin J, Chen J, Ju Z, Zhang D, et al. Rational combination therapy with PARP and MEK inhibitors capitalizes on therapeutic liabilities in RAS mutant cancers. Sci Transl Med. 2017;9.

82. Pettitt SJ, Krastev DB, Brandsma I, Dréan A, Song F, Aleksandrov R, et al. Genome-wide and high-density CRISPR-Cas9 screens identify point mutations in PARP1 causing PARP inhibitor resistance. Nat Commun. 2018;9(1):1849. https://doi.org/10.1038/s41467-018-03917-2.

83. Bunting SF, Callen E, Wong N, Chen HT, Polato F, Gunn A, et al. 53BP1 inhibits homologous recombination in Brca1-deficient cells by blocking resection of DNA breaks. Cell. 2010;141(2):243–54. https://doi.org/10.1016/j.cell.2010.03.012.

84. Jaspers JE, Kersbergen A, Boon U, Sol W, van Deemter L, Zander SA, et al. Loss of 53BP1 causes PARP inhibitor resistance in Brca1-mutated mouse mammary tumors. Cancer Discov. 2013;3(1):68–81. https://doi.org/10.1158/2159-8290.CD-12-0049.

85. Xu G, Chapman JR, Brandsma I, Yuan J, Mistrik M, Bouwman P, et al. REV7 counteracts DNA double-strand break resection and affects PARP inhibition. Nature. 2015;521(7553):541–4. https://doi.org/10.1038/nature14328.

86. Gupta R, Somyajit K, Narita T, Maskey E, Stanlie A, Kremer M, et al. DNA repair network analysis reveals Shieldin as a key regulator of NHEJ and PARP inhibitor sensitivity. Cell. 2018;173(4):972–88.e23. https://doi.org/10.1016/j.cell.2018.03.050.

87. Johnson N, Johnson SF, Yao W, Li YC, Choi YE, Bernhardy AJ, et al. Stabilization of mutant BRCA1 protein confers PARP inhibitor and platinum resistance. Proc Natl Acad Sci U S A. 2013;110(42):17041–6. https://doi.org/10.1073/pnas.1305170110.

88. Ray Chaudhuri A, Callen E, Ding X, Gogola E, Duarte AA, Lee JE, et al. Replication fork stability confers chemoresistance in BRCA-deficient cells. Nature. 2016;535(7612):382–7. https://doi.org/10.1038/nature18325.

89. Patel AG, Flatten KS, Schneider PA, Dai NT, McDonald JS, Poirier GG, et al. Enhanced killing of cancer cells by poly (ADP-ribose) polymerase inhibitors and topoisomerase I inhibitors reflects poisoning of both enzymes. J Biol Chem. 2012;287(6):4198–210.

90. Znojek P, Willmore E, Curtin NJ. Preferential potentiation of topoisomerase I poison cytotoxicity by PARP inhibition in S phase. Br J Cancer. 2014;111(7):1319–26. https://doi.org/10.1038/bjc.2014.378.

91. Samol J, Ranson M, Scott E, Macpherson E, Carmichael J, Thomas A, et al. Safety and tolerability of the poly(ADP-ribose) polymerase (PARP) inhibitor, olaparib (AZD2281) in combination with topotecan for the treatment of patients with advanced solid tumors: a phase I study. Investig New Drugs. 2012;30(4):1493–500. https://doi.org/10.1007/s10637-011-9682-9.

92. Johnson SF, Cruz C, Greifenberg AK, Dust S, Stover DG, Chi D, et al. CDK12 inhibition reverses de novo and acquired PARP inhibitor resistance in BRCA wild-type and mutated models of triple-negative breast cancer. Cell Rep. 2016;17(9):2367–81. https://doi.org/10.1016/j.celrep.2016.10.077.

93. Garcia TB, Snedeker JC, Baturin D, Gardner L, Fosmire SP, Zhou C, et al. A small-molecule inhibitor of WEE1, AZD1775, synergizes with Olaparib by impairing homologous recombination and enhancing DNA damage and apoptosis in acute leukemia. Mol Cancer Ther. 2017;16(10):2058–68. https://doi.org/10.1158/1535-7163.MCT-16-0660.

94. Rottenberg S, Jaspers JE, Kersbergen A, van der Burg E, Nygren AO, Zander SA, et al. High sensitivity of BRCA1-deficient mammary tumors to the PARP inhibitor AZD2281 alone and in combination with platinum drugs. Proc Natl Acad Sci U S A. 2008;105(44):17079–84. https://doi.org/10.1073/pnas.0806092105.

95. Kievit FM, Wang FY, Fang C, Mok H, Wang K, Silber JR, et al. Doxorubicin loaded iron oxide nanoparticles overcome multidrug resistance in cancer in vitro. J Control Release. 2011;152(1):76–83. https://doi.org/10.1016/j.jconrel.2011.01.024.

96. Batrakova EV, Kabanov AV. Pluronic block copolymers: evolution of drug delivery concept from inert nanocarriers to biological response modifiers. J Control Release. 2008;130(2):98–106. https://doi.org/10.1016/j.jconrel.2008.04.013.

97. Chen Y, Zhang W, Gu J, Ren Q, Fan Z, Zhong W, et al. Enhanced antitumor efficacy by methotrexate conjugated pluronic mixed micelles against KBv multidrug resistant cancer. Int J Pharm. 2013;452(1–2):421–33. https://doi.org/10.1016/j.ijpharm.2013.05.015.

98. Patel NR, Rathi A, Mongayt D, Torchilin VP. Reversal of multidrug resistance by co-delivery of tariquidar (XR9576) and paclitaxel using long-circulating liposomes. Int J Pharm. 2011;416(1):296–9. https://doi.org/10.1016/j.ijpharm.2011.05.082.

99. Meng H, Mai WX, Zhang H, Xue M, Xia T, Lin S, et al. Codelivery of an optimal drug/siRNA combination using mesoporous silica nanoparticles to overcome drug resistance in breast cancer in vitro and in vivo. ACS Nano. 2013;7(2):994–1005. https://doi.org/10.1021/nn3044066.

100. Amiri-Kordestani L, Basseville A, Kurdziel K, Fojo AT, Bates SE. Targeting MDR in breast and lung cancer: discriminating its potential importance from the failure of drug resistance reversal studies. Drug Resist Updat. 2012;15(1–2):50–61. https://doi.org/10.1016/j.drup.2012.02.002.

101. Du Y, Yamaguchi H, Wei Y, Hsu JL, Wang HL, Hsu YH, et al. Blocking c-Met-mediated PARP1 phosphorylation enhances anti-tumor effects of PARP inhibitors. Nat Med. 2016;22(2):194–201. https://doi.org/10.1038/nm.4032.
102. Cancer Genome Atlas Research Network. Integrated genomic analyses of ovarian carcinoma. Nature. 2011;474(7353):609–15. https://doi.org/10.1038/nature10166.
103. Choi YE, Meghani K, Brault M-E, Leclerc L, He YJ, Day TA, et al. Platinum and PARP inhibitor resistance due to overexpression of microRNA-622 in BRCA1-mutant ovarian cancer. Cell Rep. 2016;14(3):429–39.
104. Moskwa P, Buffa FM, Pan Y, Panchakshari R, Gottipati P, Muschel RJ, et al. miR-182-mediated downregulation of BRCA1 impacts DNA repair and sensitivity to PARP inhibitors. Mol Cell. 2011;41(2):210–20.
105. Byers LA, Wang J, Nilsson MB, Fujimoto J, Saintigny P, Yordy J, et al. Proteomic profiling identifies dysregulated pathways in small cell lung cancer and novel therapeutic targets including PARP1. Cancer Discov. 2012;2(9):798–811. https://doi.org/10.1158/2159-8290. CD-12-0112.
106. Murai J, Huang SY, Das BB, Renaud A, Zhang Y, Doroshow JH, et al. Trapping of PARP1 and PARP2 by clinical PARP inhibitors. Cancer Res. 2012;72(21):5588–99. https://doi. org/10.1158/0008-5472.CAN-12-2753.
107. Zehir A, Benayed R, Shah RH, Syed A, Middha S, Kim HR, et al. Mutational landscape of metastatic cancer revealed from prospective clinical sequencing of 10,000 patients. Nat Med. 2017;23:703. https://doi.org/10.1038/nm.4333.
108. Yates LR, Knappskog S, Wedge D, Farmery JH, Gonzalez S, Martincorena I, et al. Genomic evolution of breast cancer metastasis and relapse. Cancer Cell. 2017;32(2):169–84.e7.

Chapter 7
Novel Therapies to Overcome HER2 Therapy Resistance in Breast Cancer

Rita Nahta

Abstract Human epidermal growth factor receptor 2 (HER2) is a receptor tyrosine kinase that is overexpressed in approximately 15–20% of breast cancers. Trastuzumab was the first HER2-targeted therapy to be approved for clinical use against HER2-overexpressing metastatic breast cancer. However, some patients fail to respond, and many eventually develop progressive disease despite receiving treatment, which may be attributed to the development of a resistant phenotype. New therapies have been developed and approved in combination with trastuzumab for newly diagnosed disease. However, this combinatory regimen also fails and leads to treatment resistance. In this chapter, we review currently used HER2-targeted therapies for breast cancer, available therapies for HER2 antibody therapy-resistant breast cancer, and molecular mechanisms that contribute to the development of resistance. The primary focus is on novel approaches to overcome HER2 therapy resistance in the treatment of breast cancer. We discuss approaches to target HER2 with antibodies, tyrosine kinase inhibitors, or antibody-drug conjugates, as well as targeting downstream signaling, immune pathways, cell cycle regulators, and estrogen receptor signaling. Ultimately, this chapter will provide a detailed overview of the mechanisms of resistance in HER2-positive breast cancers and therapeutic strategies for patients who have developed progressive disease while being treated with HER2 antibody therapy.

Keywords Breast cancer · Herceptin · HER2 · Lapatinib · Pertuzumab · Receptor tyrosine kinase · Resistance · Trastuzumab

R. Nahta (✉)
Department of Pharmacology, Emory University School of Medicine, Atlanta, GA, USA

Department of Hematology and Medical Oncology, Emory University School of Medicine, Atlanta, GA, USA

Winship Cancer Institute, Emory University, Atlanta, GA, USA

Molecular and Systems Pharmacology Program, Graduate Division of Biological and Biomedical Sciences, Emory University, Atlanta, GA, USA
e-mail: Rnahta@emory.edu

© Springer Nature Switzerland AG 2019
M. R. Szewczuk et al. (eds.), *Current Applications for Overcoming Resistance to Targeted Therapies*, Resistance to Targeted Anti-Cancer Therapeutics 20,
https://doi.org/10.1007/978-3-030-21477-7_7

Abbreviations

ADCC	Antibody-dependent cellular cytotoxicity
CDK	Cyclin-dependent kinase
CNS	Central nervous system
CTLA-4	Cytotoxic T lymphocyte-associated protein-4
EMT	Epithelial-mesenchymal transition
ER	Estrogen receptor
FAK	Focal adhesion kinase
FDA	Food and Drug Administration
FoxM1	Forkhead box M1
GDF15	Growth differentiation factor 15
HER2	Human epidermal growth factor receptor 2
HGF	Hepatocyte growth factor
HR	Hormone receptor
Hsp90	Heat shock protein 90
IGF-1R	Insulin-like growth factor-1 receptor
MAPK	Mitogen-activated protein kinase
mTOR	Mammalian target of rapamycin
MUC-4	Mucin 4
NK	Natural killer
OS	Overall survival
pCR	Pathological complete response
PD-L1	Programmed death-ligand 1
PFS	Progression-free survival
PI3K	Phosphatidylinositol-3-kinase
PTEN	Phosphatase and tensin homolog
RTK	Receptor tyrosine kinase
T-DM1	Trastuzumab emtansine
TIL	Tumor-infiltrating lymphocyte
TKI	Tyrosine kinase inhibitor

7.1 Introduction

Breast cancer is the most commonly diagnosed cancer, accounting for approximately 30% of new cancer diagnoses and 15% of cancer-related deaths among female patients [1]. At the time of diagnosis, most breast cancers are localized and have a favourable prognosis with a 5-year relative survival rate of 80% or higher depending on the stage. However, up to 6% of breast cancers have metastasized at the time of diagnosis [1], with another 30% of localized or regional disease ultimately developing into metastatic disease [2]. Breast cancer is a heterogeneous disease consisting of multiple intrinsic molecular subgroups defined by a unique gene expression profile and hormone receptor or human epidermal growth factor receptor

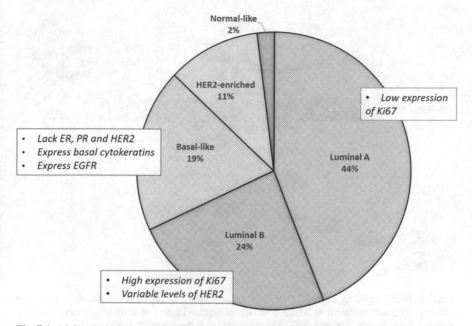

Fig. 7.1 Molecular subgroups of breast cancer. Approximately 75% of breast cancers are luminal, defined as positive for estrogen and progesterone receptors (ER and PR) [3]. Luminal A are low-grade, Ki67-low, HER2-negative tumors, whereas luminal B breast tumors are higher grade, express high levels of Ki67 and variable levels of HER2, with a worse prognosis compared to luminal A [3]. About 10–15% of luminal B tumors overexpress HER2, and another 10% of ER-negative breast cancers overexpress HER2, defined as IHC 3+ or fluorescent in situ hybridization ≥2.0 [3]. Basal breast cancers account for 10–15% of breast tumors, lack ER, PR, and HER2 expression, and may express high levels of basal cytokeratin markers or epidermal growth factor (EGFR) [3]. TNBCs as a group are heterogeneous, with six distinct subtypes, two basal-like, an immunomodulatory, mesenchymal, mesenchymal stem-like, and luminal androgen receptor subtype [9]

2 (HER2) expression status (Fig. 7.1). The stratification into molecular subgroups allows for increasingly accurate prognosis and treatment decisions [3].

HER2/erbB2 is a member of the epidermal growth factor receptor (EGFR also called HER1) family of receptor tyrosine kinases (RTKs), which also consists of HER3/erbB3 and HER4/erbB4. Ligand binding results in kinase activation, which promotes autophosphorylation and subsequent downstream signaling through several pathways, including the phosphatidylinositol-3-kinase (PI3K)/mammalian target of rapamycin (mTOR) and mitogen-activated protein kinase (MAPK) cascades (Fig. 7.2). Different downstream pathways are activated depending on the homo- or heterodimers formed. Interestingly, a specific ligand has not been identified for HER2; rather, HER2 can exist at the cell surface in an open conformation in the absence of ligand, facilitating dimerization and signaling. Thus, HER2 is the preferred partner for heterodimers when a ligand binds to EGFR, HER3, or HER4 due to its increased ligand-binding affinity and catalytic activity relative to other HER family heterodimer complexes [4]. Overexpression of HER2 results in constitutive

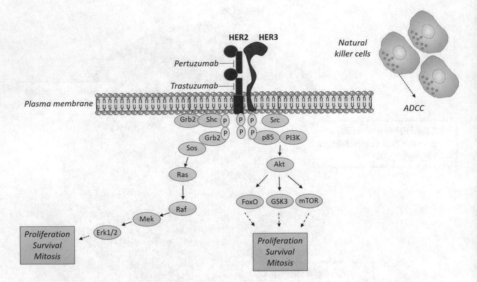

Fig. 7.2 HER2 signaling and HER2 antibody therapy. HER2 homo- or heterodimerizes with other HER family members, such as HER3, inducing phosphorylation and activating downstream signaling through Ras-MAPK and PI3K-Akt. Sustained signaling through HER2 results in numerous biological hallmarks of cancer, including proliferation and cell survival. HER2 dual antibody therapy trastuzumab and pertuzumab reduce HER2 signaling and downstream biological effects. Immune cells, such as natural killer cells, are also activated upon interaction with antibody therapy, resulting in antibody-dependent cellular cytotoxicity (ADCC)

dimerization and activation, with subsequent constitutive signaling through MAPK for homodimers or MAPK and PI3K for heterodimers, propagating many of the hallmark processes of cancer progression, including proliferation, mitosis, angiogenesis, invasion, and metastasis [5, 6]. Thus, it is not surprising that a 2- to 20-fold increase in *HER2* copy number occurs in a subset of breast tumors and is associated with aggressive disease, increased metastatic potential, and reduced survival relative to other breast cancer subtypes [7–9].

The discovery that abnormal HER2 signaling is associated with poor prognosis led to the search for therapeutic approaches to target this oncogene in breast cancer. Trastuzumab (Herceptin™; Genentech, San Francisco, California) was the first HER2-targeted therapy approved for HER2-overexpressing metastatic breast cancers. The approval of trastuzumab revolutionized treatment and survival outcomes for patients within this molecular subgroup. However, clinical experience demonstrated that not all patients were responsive to treatment. The original trial that led to approval of single-agent trastuzumab showed an objective response rate of 15% and median duration of response of only 9 months [10], indicating that a large number of patients harbour resistance, and responses are short-lived. Response rates improve when trastuzumab is combined with conventional chemotherapeutics, but intrinsic resistance remains in a subset of patients, with median time to progression of less than 1 year, indicating that acquired resistance is a significant problem impacting treatment [11].

This chapter discusses currently used HER2-targeted therapies for breast cancer and explores mechanisms of acquired resistance to these therapies. The primary focus will be novel approaches to overcome HER2 therapy resistance in the treatment of breast cancer.

7.2   HER2-Targeted Therapies for Breast Cancer

7.2.1   Trastuzumab

Trastuzumab, a recombinant humanized monoclonal antibody against a juxtamembrane region of the extracellular domain of HER2, was the first HER2-targeted therapy to be approved by the Food and Drug Administration (FDA) for metastatic HER2-overexpressing breast cancer [12]. Initial clinical trials of single-agent trastuzumab in HER2-overexpressing metastatic breast cancer demonstrated a 12–34% response rate for a median duration of 9 months [10, 13, 14]. Phase III trials of trastuzumab in combination with a taxane (paclitaxel or docetaxel) demonstrated increased response rates, time to disease progression (7.4 months), and overall survival (OS) compared to single-agent chemotherapy (4.9 months) [11, 15, 16].

Trastuzumab's anti-cancer activity is the result of a number of mechanisms of action [5, 17–21]. Trastuzumab-treated cell lines show downregulation of HER2 cell surface levels with reduced downstream PI3K and MAPK signaling [22, 23]. Trastuzumab may selectively inhibit HER2-HER3 heterodimerization, diminishing HER3-associated PI3K signaling [23, 24]. In some breast tumors, the extracellular domain of HER2 is proteolytically cleaved, yielding a truncated, membrane-bound 95-kiloDalton HER2 protein with constitutively active tyrosine kinase (p95 HER2). Trastuzumab can prevent the cleavage of the extracellular domain [23, 25]. The ability of trastuzumab to inhibit growth is also due to increased expression of cyclin-dependent kinase (CDK) inhibitor p27kip1 and subsequent inhibition of CDK2 activity [26, 27].

Another important biological action of trastuzumab includes inhibition of angiogenesis, which is related to reduced PI3K signaling, resulting in lower levels of vascular endothelial growth factor, reduced endothelial cell migration and vascular permeability [28, 29]. Normalization of tumor vasculature may improve responses to chemotherapeutic agents by increasing the efficiency by which agents are delivered. In addition to effects on the vasculature, immune system effects contribute to trastuzumab's mechanism of action. Trastuzumab-bound cells are recognized by immune cells, resulting in antibody-dependent cellular cytotoxicity (ADCC) and tumor cell lysis [30, 31]. An intact immune response is likely a critical factor for optimal response to trastuzumab. It is therefore not surprising that mice lacking Fc gamma receptors, which are generally present on immune natural killer cells and macrophages and bind to the Fc gamma regions of an antibody, fail to demonstrate tumor regression following trastuzumab treatment [31].

Currently, trastuzumab is approved as a first-line treatment for HER2-overexpressing metastatic breast cancer delivered in combination with paclitaxel or as a single agent following progression on one or more chemotherapeutic agents [32]. Additional approvals for trastuzumab include as an adjuvant for HER2-overexpressing, node-positive breast cancer or HER2-overexpressing, node-negative, ER/PR-negative/high-risk early-stage breast cancer [32]. Cardiac dysfunction is a rare but serious adverse event associated with trastuzumab that increases in frequency if an anthracycline is also administered (25% vs. <10% treated with anthracycline and cyclophosphamide alone) [15, 16]. Cardiac dysfunction occurred in 13% of patients treated with paclitaxel and trastuzumab vs. 1% treated with paclitaxel alone [16].

Despite being a highly effective therapy, there are a significant number of patients who show partial or complete resistance to trastuzumab-based therapy. Among those who do respond, the median time to acquire partial or complete resistance and demonstrate disease progression is less than 1 year. In the following sections, we review the proposed mechanisms of resistance and therapeutic strategies for resistant disease. One suggested mechanism of trastuzumab resistance observed in preclinical studies is epitope masking, where trastuzumab cannot recognize or physically interact with HER2. Although a therapeutic strategy has not resulted from this finding, this discovery may provide a useful biomarker to predict response to therapy. In these studies, a membrane protein, such as the transmembrane glycoprotein mucin 4 (MUC4), interacts with HER2, sterically hindering drug-antigen interaction. MUC4 has been shown to interact with and activate HER2 [33], with anti-MUC4 antibodies disrupting trastuzumab-HER2 interactions. A model of primary trastuzumab resistance showed MUC4-mediated epitope masking as a potential mechanism of resistance [34]. If molecules such as MUC4 are overexpressed in breast tumors, they may serve as biomarkers, indicating that HER2-directed therapies that bind to epitopes different from trastuzumab may be more beneficial. MUC4 knockdown improved HER2-trastuzumab interactions in preclinical studies, suggesting a potential therapeutic strategy that may be developed in the future.

As a result of understanding mechanisms of resistance, new HER2-targeted therapies have been developed and evaluated as first-line or later-line agents, with several of these treatments now approved for clinical use, either in combination with trastuzumab or for the treatment of resistant disease.

7.2.2   Pertuzumab

Pertuzumab (Perjeta®; Genentech), another humanized anti-HER2 monoclonal antibody, binds to an extracellular epitope distinct from the trastuzumab-binding site and disrupts heterodimerization between HER2-EGFR and HER2-HER3 [35]. The phase III CLEOPATRA trial established a significantly improved median OS of 56.5 months with pertuzumab, trastuzumab, and docetaxel vs. 40.8 months with placebo, trastuzumab, and docetaxel as first-line treatment of HER2-positive metastatic breast cancer [36]. Median progression-free survival (PFS) and duration of response were also improved by approximately 6 and 8 months, respectively [36].

There are potential mechanisms of synergy between trastuzumab and pertuzumab, such as increased ADCC and reduced HER2 extracellular domain cleavage. Pertuzumab is approved for use in combination with trastuzumab plus docetaxel as a first-line treatment for HER2-positive metastatic breast cancer or as a neoadjuvant treatment for HER2-positive, locally advanced, inflammatory, or early-stage breast cancer.

Thus, the current standard of care for first-line treatment of patients with HER2-positive metastatic breast cancer is the combination of HER2-targeted antibodies pertuzumab and trastuzumab plus docetaxel chemotherapy. However, the median duration of response to combination therapy reported in the initial trial was less than 2 years compared with approximately 1 year for trastuzumab treatment, suggesting that acquisition of resistance remains a clinical concern even with dual HER2-targeted antibody therapy [36].

7.3 Therapies to Overcome HER2 Antibody-Resistant Disease

Multiple biological and molecular mechanisms have been implicated in the acquisition of resistance to HER2-targeted antibody therapies. Identification of the molecular underpinnings of cancer therapy resistance is essential for developing new treatment regimens. As a result of decades of research investigating resistance to trastuzumab, several new targeted approaches have been clinically tested or approved for practice. In the following section, we discuss these approaches and review established mechanisms of resistance.

7.3.1 Antibody-Drug Conjugate

Antibody-drug conjugates consist of an antibody targeting a cancer-related antigen, such as HER2, conjugated with another molecule, such as a cytotoxic agent. Trastuzumab emtansine (T-DM1) is an antibody-drug conjugate of trastuzumab covalently linked with emtansine (DM1), a microtubule-inhibiting cytotoxic chemotherapeutic agent. T-DM1 allows for the selective and specific delivery of cytotoxic DM1 to HER2-overexpressing cells. The phase III EMILIA trial evaluated T-DM1 versus lapatinib and capecitabine in patients with locally advanced or metastatic HER2-positive breast cancer previously treated with trastuzumab and a taxane. This trial established significantly improved PFS (median, 9.6 vs. 6.4 months) and OS (median, 30.9 vs. 25.1 months) in the T-DM1 vs. control arm [37]. Based on these results, T-DM1 is approved as a second-line treatment for HER2-positive metastatic breast cancer that has progressed after prior treatment with trastuzumab and a taxane. Subsequent retrospective analysis of patients in the EMILIA trial demonstrated a significantly improved OS in patients with central nervous system (CNS) metastases treated with T-DM1 vs. lapatinib plus capecitabine (median, 26.8 vs. 12.9 months) [38]. Thus, T-DM1 may prove to be an essential therapy for the subset of patients with HER2 antibody-resistant disease who develop CNS metastases, a subgroup for whom few effective treatments currently exist.

7.3.2 HER Tyrosine Kinase Inhibitors (TKIs) and Pan-HER Targeting

Targeting more than one HER signaling receptor through the use of multi- or pan-HER-targeting agents can have clinical benefit particularly against breast cancers that have progressed on single HER2-targeted therapy. Employing a cocktail approach integrating more than one HER kinase inhibitor is supported by current practice and supports the idea that a pan-HER antibody may also demonstrate efficacy. Antibody mixtures targeting EGFR, HER2, and HER3 reduce the expression of all three receptors with prolonged inhibition of HER2-positive breast tumor growth compared with either trastuzumab plus lapatinib, trastuzumab plus pertuzumab or T-DM1 [39]. Pan-HER inhibition blocks the growth of trastuzumab- and T-DM1-resistant tumors *in vivo*. Also, HER3 antibody blockade restored T-DM1 sensitivity in T-DM1-resistant tumors, supporting HER3 targeting as a treatment approach in T-DM1-resistant cancers. Further, trastuzumab- and T-DM1-resistant tumors showed upregulation of phosphorylated and total HER3 and increased levels of HER3 ligand neuregulin-1, which was normalized by HER3 antibody blockade. Thus, the use of pan-HER-targeting antibodies or TKIs and HER3 blockade may provide additional benefit to patients with HER2 antibody-resistant disease.

7.3.3 Lapatinib

Lapatinib is a reversible TKI of both EGFR and HER2 and is approved for use in combination with capecitabine for advanced HER2-positive breast cancer that has progressed on trastuzumab and chemotherapy, including a taxane and an anthracycline. Patients with locally advanced or metastatic HER2-overexpressing breast cancer that progressed on treatment with anthracycline, taxane, and trastuzumab showed a significantly increased time to progression in response to lapatinib plus capecitabine (8.4 months) vs. capecitabine alone (4.4 months), leading to the approval of lapatinib plus capecitabine as a later-line, post-trastuzumab treatment [40]. More recently, the phase III ALTTO trial compared trastuzumab, lapatinib, sequential trastuzumab followed by lapatinib, and the combination of the two as adjuvant therapy for 1 year [41]. At a median follow-up period of 4.5 years, a non-significant 16% reduction in disease-free survival hazard rate was found in the combination group compared to the trastuzumab group. The 4-year OS was also similar among groups, and there was no difference in CNS metastasis as the first site of relapse among groups. These results were in contrast to those anticipated from the NeoALTTO trial, which showed a significantly higher pathological complete response (pCR) rate in patients treated with neoadjuvant lapatinib plus trastuzumab compared with trastuzumab alone (51.3% vs. 29.5%) [42]. Although NeoALTTO is an example of how neoadjuvant trials provide opportunities for investigating potential therapies for disease, the differences in outcomes observed between NeoALTTO and ALTTO are a reminder that improved pCR serves as a surrogate marker but cannot always accurately predict improvements in survival endpoints.

7.3.4 Neratinib

Neratinib is an irreversible pan-HER inhibitor that is approved as extended adjuvant therapy for patients with early-stage HER2-positive breast cancer who previously received at least 1 year of post-surgical trastuzumab [43]. Neratinib covalently binds the cysteine residue in the ATP-binding sites of the EGFR, HER2, and HER4 kinase domains, blocking phosphorylation and downstream signaling. Neratinib promotes tumor regression and reduces HER2 signaling in HER2 positive breast cancer xenografts [44, 45].

Similar to lapatinib, neratinib increases p27kip1 expression, reduces cyclin D1 expression, and promotes cell cycle arrest during the G1 phase, ultimately reducing proliferation [44, 45]. Both lapatinib and neratinib suppress ligand-stimulated HER2-HER3 dimerization in breast cancer cells; however, neratinib disrupts baseline HER2-HER3 dimerization more rapidly than lapatinib [46]. Lapatinib and neratinib inhibit ligand-induced HER2 downregulation from the cell surface, increasing trastuzumab-binding and ADCC in studies examining the combination of trastuzumab with either of these TKIs [46]. In contrast to reversible EGFR TKIs gefitinib and erlotinib, which bind EGFR in both the active (i.e. open) and inactive (i.e. closed) conformations, neratinib and lapatinib bind EGFR in the inactive (i.e. closed) kinase conformation [46]. Lapatinib and neratinib each have an extra aromatic group, reducing reversion to the open position, ultimately locking receptors in an inactive conformation to prevent HER-HER dimerization. Both neratinib and lapatinib block PI3K signaling, suggesting that this pathway is a surrogate marker of drug activity [47]. The ExteNET phase III trial, in which patients with trastuzumab-resistant stage I-IIIc HER2-positive breast cancer received either neratinib or placebo for 1 year, demonstrated significantly reduced recurrence in terms of fewer invasive disease-free survival events (116 vs. 163 events) and increased invasive disease-free survival (90.2% vs. 87.7%) at a median follow-up period of 5.2 years compared to placebo [48]. The ExteNET trial outcomes ultimately resulted in neratinib approval.

7.3.5   Targeting Compensatory Signaling Pathways: Insulin-Like Growth Factor-1 Receptor (IGF-1R) Inhibition

Compensatory signaling from non-HER receptor kinases is one mechanism by which resistance to HER2-targeted therapy develops. Insulin-like growth factor-1 receptor (IGF-1R) activity is associated with reduced response to trastuzumab. For example, IGF-1R expression is elevated in some cells with acquired or intrinsic trastuzumab resistance compared to sensitive cells [49]. Further, increased IGF-1R signaling [50–52] or interaction of IGF-1R with HER2 [53, 54] promotes resistance by sustaining HER2 signaling through cross-talk, reducing expression of the endogenous cell cycle inhibitor p27kip1, and increasing cell proliferation. Several studies support increased IGF-1R signaling as a mechanism of trastuzumab resistance. Cell cycle arrest at the G1 phase and subsequent reduction in proliferation are required for trastuzumab activity [55]. HER2-overexpressing breast cancer cells that were stably transfected with an IGF-1R expression plasmid showed loss of G1 arrest in response to trastuzumab [51]. These IGF-1R/HER2-overexpressing cells retained anchorage-independent growth despite being exposed to trastuzumab, resulting in sustained proliferation and resistance. These findings are consistent with another report, which showed that the proliferation of HER2-positive, IGF-1R stable transfectants were not inhibited by a high dose of trastuzumab [56].

Additionally, HER2-overexpressing breast cancer cells with acquired resistance to trastuzumab express threefold higher levels of IGF-1R compared with parental cells [57]. Phospho-proteomics showed constitutive activation of IGF-1R in a model of intrinsic trastuzumab resistance [52]. Thus, intrinsic and acquired trastuzumab resistance may develop from heightened IGF-1R activity. Interestingly, trastuzumab-resistant cells [58, 59] that lack IGF-1R overexpression possess a novel receptor complex involving IGF-1R and HER2 [54]. Another group subsequently validated this receptor interaction and showed that HER3 is also in this complex [53]. Cross-signaling was found to occur from IGF-IR to HER2 in resistant cells, with IGF-1 inducing HER2 phosphorylation, an effect that was blocked by an IGF-1R kinase inhibitor [54]. Thus, the preclinical data support a role for IGF-1R, either overexpression or crosstalk, in trastuzumab resistance.

Although the above preclinical studies have provided evidence for the correlation between IGF-1R and trastuzumab resistance, clinical experience with IGF-1R remains controversial, with some studies supporting an association between increased IGF-1R and trastuzumab resistance [60–62], and others refuting this association [63–65]. Although no direct association was found between IGF-1R expression alone and trastuzumab response [64, 66], the combined presence of high IGF-1R expression and high mTOR signaling correlated with reduced response to trastuzumab [66]. Additionally, multivariate analysis showed that high IGF-1R expression correlated with poor prognosis in HER2-positive breast cancer patients [67] and poor response to neoadjuvant trastuzumab plus chemotherapy [61]. Taken collectively, the role of IGF-1R in trastuzumab resistance remains unclear but appears to be sufficiently supported to warrant clinical investigation of therapies targeting IGF-1R. Preclinical studies have shown benefit from combining IGF-1R-targeted therapy with HER2-directed treatments [68–71]. However, clinical trials with IGF-1R-targeted agents have been less impressive [72, 73], with many pharmaceutical companies abandoning attempts to develop IGF-1R kinase inhibitors or monoclonal antibodies for clinical use.

7.3.6   Targeting Downstream Signaling Pathways

The major signaling cascades activated by HER2 include PI3K and MAPK, both of which regulate cell proliferation, survival, and motility, among other critical biological processes [74]. Although each pathway was historically believed to signal linearly, we now know that crosstalk between components of each cascade occurs [74]. Thus, dysregulation of one molecule in a downstream pathway can result in far-reaching molecular and biological effects.

PI3K pathway hyperactivation occurs in a subset of trastuzumab-resistant breast cancers through a variety of molecular mechanisms. One mechanism is through the loss of the phosphatase and tensin homolog (PTEN), which dephosphorylates phosphoinositide substrates, including phosphatidylinositol (3,4,5)-triphosphate, resulting in the inhibition of PI3K signaling to substrate molecule Akt. Activating mutations in *PIK3CA* which result in constitutive PI3K signaling are associated with trastuzumab resistance [75, 76]. The inhibitory growth activity of trastuzumab is in part a result of PI3K inhibition, mediated by multiple mechanisms, including membrane re-localization, PTEN activation, and HER3 dephosphorylation [24, 76]. Therefore, alterations that propagate or sustain signaling through PI3K will impede trastuzumab activity.

Trastuzumab resistance in HER2-positive breast cancer cells with reduced PTEN expression and subsequently increased PI3K signaling regain trastuzumab sensitivity in response to PI3K inhibition [76]. Patients with oncogenic mutations in *PIK3CA* or low PTEN expression have inadequate responses to trastuzumab-based therapy, including reduced clinical benefit and overall response rates, and significantly shorter median progression-free survival [75, 77]. Therefore, therapeutically targeting PI3K and mTOR has clinical relevance and was tested in the BOLERO-3 phase III trial. This trial demonstrated significant improvements in PFS following the addition of mTOR inhibitor everolimus to trastuzumab plus vinorelbine in patients with HER2-positive, advanced trastuzumab-resistant breast cancer pre-treated with taxane vs. placebo (median, 7.0 vs. 5.8 months) [78]. Furthermore, the data from BOLERO-1 and BOLERO-3 demonstrated that this PFS benefit was related to PI3K hyperactivity, including *PIK3CA* activating mutations and PTEN loss [79], indicating that PI3K status may serve as a biomarker for patient stratification when considering the addition of a PI3K/mTOR inhibitor.

In contrast to trastuzumab, lapatinib sensitivity appears to be unrelated to PTEN expression status or *PIK3CA* activating mutations [80, 81]. However, an independent study suggested that PI3K hyperactivation was associated with a reduced response to lapatinib, with PI3K/mTOR inhibition restoring sensitivity [82]. Interestingly, a clinical study demonstrated that PI3K activity was associated with trastuzumab resistance and that low PTEN expression was associated with a significantly higher pCR to lapatinib [83]. The combination of mTOR inhibition with lapatinib demonstrated synergy associated with the suppression of signaling from the mTOR substrate p70 S6 kinase [84]. Further, combined treatment with PI3K inhibitor buparlisib and lapatinib achieved clinical benefit, including one complete response, in patients with trastuzumab-resistant advanced breast cancer [85]. Also, *PIK3CA* mutations were associated with shorter median PFS and OS in patients treated with capecitabine plus lapatinib, but not in patients treated with T-DM1 [86], although another study suggested that T-DM1-resistant cells may demonstrate PTEN loss, with PI3K inhibition providing a benefit [87]. A PI3K alpha-specific inhibitor, alpelisib, generated an overall response rate of 43% and clinical benefit even in those previously exposed to T-DM1 in a phase I trial (N = 14) in trastuzumab- and taxane-resistant HER2-overexpressing metastatic breast cancer [88], providing rationale for combining a PI3K inhibitor with T-DM1 in patients who have progressed on trastuzumab-containing regimens.

Elevated PI3K activity reduces the preclinical efficacy of trastuzumab [75, 76, 89, 90] and correlates with clinical resistance [75, 76, 91]. Increased PI3K signaling may occur due to downregulation of PTEN or hyperactivating *PIK3CA* mutations, as well as increased upstream growth factor signaling, such as through IGF-1R. Cells with acquired resistance to trastuzumab show increased signaling through HER2, Akt, and Erk1/2 upon stimulation with the IGF-1R ligand, IGF-1 [54]. IGF-1R tyrosine kinase inhibition or IGF-1R antibody blockade reduces HER2, Akt, and Erk1/2 phosphorylation [54]. Exogenous IGF-1 abrogates suppression of Akt and Erk1/2 phosphorylation in trastuzumab-treated cells [49]. Pharmacological inhibition of phosphoinositide-dependent kinase-1 (PDK-1) potentiates trastuzumab-mediated growth inhibition in IGF-1R-overexpressing HER2-positive cells by suppressing PDK-1/Akt signaling [56]. Downstream of IGF-1R activation, mTOR signaling is increased. Expression of mTOR was increased in almost one-fourth of tumors from patients treated with trastuzumab, and almost half showed IGF-1R overexpression [60].

Potential mechanisms through which receptors, such as IGF-1R, promote trastuzumab resistance remain unclear. One proposed mechanism of growth inhibition employed by trastuzumab, but not lapatinib, is inhibition of the non-receptor kinase Src, mediated through inhibition of Src phosphorylation on residue Y416 and disrupted interaction with HER2 [81]. Increased IGF-1R signaling drives invasion of HER2-positive breast cancers by activating Src and focal adhesion kinase (FAK) [71]. Similarly, beta 1 integrin activates Src-FAK, with beta 1 integrin knockdown or antibody blockade diminishing signaling from these pathways and inhibiting the growth of trastuzumab- and lapatinib-resistant breast cancer cells [92, 93]. Thus, in addition to IGF-1R, beta 1 integrin is a putative therapeutic target in HER2-targeted therapy-resistant breast cancer. Cells resistant to HER2-targeted and PI3K inhibition demonstrated increased expression of factors involved in extracellular matrix (ECM) integrity and cell-to-cell adhesion and increased beta 1 integrin-Src signaling [94]. Inhibition of collagen synthesis or beta 1 integrin-Src signaling inhibited tumor growth.

Further, investigators found that high collagen II expression is associated with poor response to neoadjuvant HER2 therapy. Thus, Src-FAK signaling may mediate IGF-1R-driven resistance downstream of multiple signaling pathways, not just IGF-1R. For example, activation of another receptor kinase called RET induced Src signaling and subsequent cross-talk to HER2 in trastuzumab-resistant cells [95]. Src inhibitor saracatinib improved response to trastuzumab, further supporting combination targeting of Src and HER2 in resistant tumors.

7.3.7   Cell Cycle Inhibition

Downstream signaling alters expression and activity of key cell cycle regulators. For example, stable overexpression of IGF-1R reduces expression of cyclin-dependent kinase inhibitors, including p27kip1, which we previously discussed as being critical for trastuzumab activity, and increases expression of cyclins, which promote cellular proliferation [51]. Trastuzumab-resistant cells express lower levels of p27kip1 [59] and higher levels of cyclin E than sensitive counterparts [96]. *Cyclin E* amplification and overexpression is associated with poor response to trastuzumab and reduced progression-free survival [96]. Similar to models with low p27kip1, overexpression of cyclin E increases CDK2 activity. Importantly, CDK2 inhibition limited the growth of trastuzumab-resistant tumors [96]. IGF-1R signaling induces expression of the p27kip1 ubiquitin ligase, Skp2, resulting in p27kip1 degradation [97]. This reduction in p27kip1 expression is associated with increased CDK2 activity and proliferation [59]. Proteasome inhibition restores p27kip1 expression, suggesting that CDK2 inhibition is a potential treatment strategy for resistant tumors with low p27kip1 levels. These findings support high CDK2 activity via multiple molecular mechanisms as a source of trastuzumab resistance and reveal CDK2 inhibition as a new therapeutic strategy for resistant tumors.

Other CDK inhibitors targeted against CDK4/6 are already approved for clinical use as treatments for metastatic estrogen receptor (ER)-positive breast cancer. Additionally, it has been demonstrated that cyclin D1 expression is rate-limiting for HER2-stimulated cancer, with CDK inhibition acting synergistically with trastuzumab [98–100]. For example, in mouse models of HER2-overexpressing breast tumors, recurrent tumors that developed after termination of HER2 therapy showed an increased fraction of Ki67-positive cells and changes in cell cycle regulators, including increased expression of cyclins A2, B1, B2, and D1 and CDK4 [101]. Additionally, HER2 inhibition in HER2-positive, ER-positive breast cancers can further upregulate ER signaling, driving disease progression [102]. Thus, the integration of standard ER and CDK4/6 inhibitors with HER2 therapy may yield optimal clinical benefit and may reduce the need for chemotherapy in a subset of patients. The NA-PHER2 phase II trial evaluated changes in the Ki67 proliferation marker and apoptosis from baseline to surgery among patients with untreated, invasive HER2-positive, ER-positive breast cancer treated with trastuzumab, pertu-zumab, CDK4/6 inhibitor palbociclib and fulvestrant [103]. There were significant reductions in Ki67 expression with increased apoptosis and objective clinical response in a majority of patients, with 27% achieving pCR in breast and axillary nodes. These results support the co-targeting of ER, HER2, and CDK4/6 signaling in HER2-positive, ER-positive disease, with the potential omission of chemother-apy in a subset of patients.

Given the association of cyclin D1-CDK4/6 with HER2 and ER signaling, a cocktail targeting CDK4/6, ER, and HER2 is an attractive treatment approach. As outlined above, increased cyclin D1-CDK4/6 activity is associated with resistance to trastuzumab and lapatinib, with combined HER2 and CDK4/6 inhibition reduc-ing mTOR activity, cell proliferation, and tumor growth and delaying tumor recur-rence. Thus, combination treatment with HER2 and CDK4/6 inhibitors may be beneficial in the first-line setting, reducing recurrence, as well as in disease that has progressed on prior HER2 therapy.

7.3.8   Estrogen Receptor Inhibition

ER signaling affects the response to trastuzumab. Models of acquired resistance to ER-targeted therapies demonstrate increased HER2 signaling [104–106], and acquired lapatinib resistance is associated with increased ER signaling [107]. HER2-positive breast cancer with acquired resistance to lapatinib or the combina-tion of lapatinib and trastuzumab have an increased expression of ER or ER target genes [102]. Thus, dual inhibition of ER and HER2 is a potential strategy for the treatment of HER2-positive cancers. Combined neoadjuvant treatment with lapa-tinib and trastuzumab and letrozole for ER-positive tumors in the absence of che-motherapy achieved an overall in-breast pCR of 27% [108]. Considering pCR in breast and axilla, 18% of ER-positive and 28% of ER-negative showed no residual invasive cancer; thus, ER signaling may adversely affect response to HER2-targeted therapy.

The ExteNET trial, which was previously discussed, also provided critical pre-liminary data regarding the association between ER signaling and response to HER2 TKI treatment. Patients with hormone receptor-positive, HER2-positive tumors demonstrated a higher, but not statistically significant benefit from neratinib than their hormone receptor-negative counterpart [48]. Preclinical evaluation of extended adjuvant treatment with neratinib plus ER antagonist fulvestrant was performed in mouse xenografts of HER2-positive, ER-positive tumors previously treated with chemotherapy, trastuzumab, and pertuzumab [109]. Combined fulvestrant and neratinib achieved prolonged inhibition of tumor growth compared with fulvestrant alone. Reciprocal upregulation of HER2 or ER, including cyclin D1 signaling, occurred after treatment with fulvestrant or neratinib alone, respectively, in HER2-positive, ER-positive lines. Cyclin D1 knockdown or treatment with a CDK4/6 inhibitor improved response to fulvestrant in cell lines.

The effect of pertuzumab, trastuzumab, and chemotherapy against early-stage HER2-positive breast cancer was examined in the APHINITY trial, resulting in a lower 3-year invasive disease-free survival rate in the hormone receptor-positive subgroup versus the hormone receptor-negative subgroup, although the difference did not reach statistical significance [110]. This survival rate may be due to heightened HER2 signaling, which abrogates response to endocrine agents in ER-positive breast cancer [111]. Preclinical data support this approach, as fulvestrant plus lapatinib reduced viability, possibly through inhibition of downstream MAPK signaling, in HER2-positive, ER-positive breast cancer cells [112]. Patients with HER2-positive breast cancer routinely demonstrate lower pCR to HER2 agents if tumors are hormone receptor-positive compared to patients who have hormone receptor-negative, HER2-positive breast cancer [111]. Bidirectional crosstalk resulting in increased ER or HER2 signaling upon single-agent targeting of HER2 or ER, respectively, argues for dual inhibition.

7.3.9   Immunotherapy

As previously discussed, the failure to activate ADCC is associated with trastuzumab resistance. Immune cells such as natural killer (NK) cells, monocytes, and macrophages express Fc gamma receptors. Following antibody binding to the surface of cancer cells, the Fc gamma receptors on immune cells can recognize and bind to the Fc portion of antibodies, which ultimately results in immune cell release of cytokines and cytotoxic granules that induce cancer cell death [31]. Mice lacking Fc receptors, or in which the interaction between antibodies and NK cells is lost, exhibit aberrant ADCC in HER2-positive cells in response to trastuzumab [31]. Also, complete or partial remission of patients treated with neoadjuvant trastuzumab correlates with increased immune activity in the form of immune cells infiltrating tumor tissue and higher ADCC activity [113]. NK cells and lymphocyte-associated cytotoxic granules are increased in tumor tissues from patients with HER2-positive breast cancer treated with trastuzumab plus docetaxel, with a statistically insignificant trend toward immune cell infiltration correlating with responsiveness [30]. Patients treated with trastuzumab showed an ADCC response in 15 out of 18 patients with operable disease [114]. Pathological complete response was associated with high ADCC, whereas partial responses had lower levels of ADCC. Collectively, a lack of response to trastuzumab was associated with lack of an ADCC response.

The importance of ADCC in trastuzumab response suggests that it is essential that HER2 targeted therapy is combined with immune stimulation for increased efficacy. Cytokines, such as interleukin-2 (IL-2) that stimulate the production of NK cells also promote lysis of HER2 antibody-bound breast cancer cells [115]. Among ten patients with HER2-positive breast cancer treated with trastuzumab plus IL-2, one showed a partial response, five had stable disease, and four had the progressive disease [116]. There was also an increase in NK cells and ADCC, but these did not correlate with clinical response. Additionally, minimal benefit was observed following IL-12 plus trastuzumab treatment in a small group of patients with HER2-positive breast cancer, although one complete response and two cases of stable disease lasting longer than 6 months were documented [117]. ADCC can also be stimulated using agonists that stimulate NK cell receptors, such as CD137, which is expressed on NK cells and was stimulated with an agonistic antibody to increase ADCC [118]. Such pharmacological strategies to stimulate ADCC may improve response to antibody therapies, including trastuzumab. Using a HER2 antibody cocktail is supported considering that a combination of HER2-targeted antibodies targeting distinct epitopes induces a higher level of ADCC than a single antibody treatment [119].

A recent meta-analysis demonstrated a significant association between high baseline immune cell infiltrate in breast tumors and increased pCR in patients with HER2-positive breast cancer treated with neoadjuvant trastuzumab and lapatinib and chemotherapy [120]. Retrospective analysis of the CLEOPATRA trial also supports the relevance of tumor-infiltrating lymphocytes (TILs) to treatment response in advanced HER2-positive breast cancer [121]. A higher TIL value was significantly associated with increased OS, although no association was found with PFS in patients with advanced HER2-positive breast cancer treated with docetaxel, trastuzumab, and pertuzumab. The importance of an active immune response for optimal benefit from HER2 therapy is supported by the finding that immune suppression in the form of high expression of programmed death ligand 1 (PD-L1) was associated with worse outcome among patients with HER2-positive breast cancer [122]. PD-1-positive TILs are associated with worse outcomes in patients with HER2-positive breast cancer [123, 124]. Preclinical evaluation of anti-PD-1 with HER2-directed therapy supports the use of this combination approach [125]. Further, the addition of T-DM1 with immune checkpoint inhibition targeted against cytotoxic T lymphocyte-associated protein-4 (CTLA4) and PD-1 activated a robust immune response *in vivo* and an improved response compared to immunotherapy alone [126]. An ongoing trial (PANACEA; NCT02129556) will evaluate the efficacy of PD-1-directed pembrolizumab combined with trastuzumab in trastuzumab-resistant metastatic breast cancer.

7.4 Emerging Therapeutics to Overcome HER2 Therapy Resistance

7.4.1 Trastuzumab Biosimilars

The development and approval of new HER2 therapies have improved long-term outcomes for patients with HER2-positive breast cancer. With the patent for trastuzumab soon expiring, biosimilars, which are defined as biologic products with similar bioactive components to the reference drug (in this case, trastuzumab) and no clinically meaningful differences, are now approved or are in clinical evaluation [127, 128]. Trastuzumab treatment can surpass $50,000 for a given patient, placing a financial burden on patients and their families, ultimately limiting access to many patients [129]. Access to biosimilars will allow for a more significant number of patients to be treated but will also increase the number of patients who eventually develop resistance, which in turn increases the need for new therapies. Given the complex structure and size of biologics and differences in the inactive ingredients or manufacturing procedures, biosimilars and trastuzumab cannot be considered identical products [127, 128]. Patients exposed to different biosimilars may develop resistant disease through various mechanisms, and subsequently may require different follow-up agents. Many trastuzumab biosimilars, such as compounds SB3 and CT-P6, are now approved for metastatic and neoadjuvant therapy [130]. Thus, an emerging area of research is to fully understand the mechanisms of resistance to these new agents. Further, investigations will need to identify which agents remain effective in biosimilar-resistant disease and whether these are the same new agents used for trastuzumab-resistant disease.

7.4.2 Inhibiting HER2 Degradation

Emerging mechanisms of overcoming the development of resistance to HER2 targeted therapy for HER2-positive breast cancer research relies on the identification of novel mechanisms of resistance and molecular targets. One aspect of this research is investigating mechanisms through which HER2 may be downregulated during disease progression. For example, Phase I data on the chaperone protein heat shock protein 90 (hsp90) which has multiple targets, including HER2, suggest potential clinical benefit from combination therapy with hsp90 inhibitor ganetespib with paclitaxel and trastuzumab in patients with HER2-positive metastatic breast cancer previously treated with trastuzumab, pertuzumab, and T-DM1 [131]. Sustained expression of HER2 by inhibition hsp90 is expected to increase levels of the drug target and subsequently increase response to HER2 antibody therapies.

7.4.3 Targeting Secreted Ligands That Stimulate HER2

Overexpression of secreted ligands that stimulate receptors that cross-talk with HER2 also pose a challenge to HER2-targeted therapy. For example, the Met receptor tyrosine kinase, which is overexpressed in some HER2-positive breast cancer tissues [132], increases epithelial-mesenchymal transition (EMT) and invasion of breast cancer cells through hepatocyte growth factor (HGF)-stimulated MAPK signaling, reducing epithelial protein E-cadherin and internalizing tight junction protein ZO-1 [133]. Met amplification is significantly associated with trastuzumab resistance and reduced time to progression. HGF amplification is also significantly associated with resistance, confirming a role for Met/HGF overexpression in trastuzumab resistance [134]. Co-stimulation of Met and HER2 with HGF and neuregulin-1 beta, respectively, induces Akt and Erk1/2 signaling with increased proliferation [135]. Co-inhibition of HER2 and Met using trastuzumab plus genetic knockdown or Met kinase inhibitor inhibited proliferation to a greater degree than either alone [135]. These studies provide a rationale for clinical trials using Met inhibitors against HER2-positive breast cancer pretreated with trastuzumab.

Another secreted factor, the cytokine growth differentiation factor 15 (GDF15), induces HER2 phosphorylation in HER2-positive breast cancer cells and reduces response to trastuzumab in preclinical models [136–138]. High GDF15 levels serve as a biomarker of trastuzumab resistance, with GDF15 knockdown increasing response to trastuzumab, supporting the use of GDF15 as a mediator of trastuzumab and a potential therapeutic target [136]. GDF15 binds to the glial-derived neurotrophic factor-family receptor-alpha-like (GFRAL) receptor, which activates signaling from the cell surface receptor RET kinase [139–141], activates PI3K/mTOR and MAPK signaling [136, 142–144], and promotes EMT [145, 146]. GDF15 also promotes cancer stem cell-like properties in breast cancer [143] and confers resistance to HER2-targeted therapy [136]. Increased GDF15 expression is associated with ER-negative, HER2-positive disease and high tumor grade, with knockdown inhibiting invasion in preclinical models of HER2-positive breast cancer [147].

7.4.4 Inhibiting Transcription Factors Downstream of HER2

HER2 signaling ultimately induces the expression and activity of multiple transcription factors, including the Forkhead box MI (FoxM1) protein, which is overexpressed in HER2-positive breast cancers [148]. FoxM1 overexpression is associated with poor prognosis [149] and is directly correlated with HER2 expression [150]. FoxM1 activity blocks the response to trastuzumab and lapatinib [150, 151], whereas the combined inhibition of MEK, which regulates FoxM1 activity and expression, plus lapatinib diminishes nuclear FOXM1 levels [152]. Further, MEK inhibition inhibits FoxM1 target gene expression and subsequently, mitosis [153]. FoxM1 may promote drug resistance by upregulating levels of the anti-apoptotic protein Bcl-2 and inducing EMT [154–156], possibly through increased expression of the downstream EMT target SLUG, to promote breast cancer metastasis [157, 158]. Thus, inhibition of FoxM1 activity is a therapeutic strategy currently being investigated in antibody-resistant HER2-overexpressing breast cancer.

7.4.5 Inhibiting Anti-apoptotic Regulators

Models of HER2 therapy resistance show altered expression of apoptotic regulators, including increased expression of anti-apoptotic Bcl-2 in cells with acquired trastuzumab resistance [104, 159–162]. Resistant cells are sensitive to BH3-mimetic drug ABT-737, which targets a peptide region of Bcl-2 and restores trastuzumab activity in resistant cells. Other Bcl-2 antagonists also show benefit in HER2-positive breast cancer. For example, obatoclax (GX15-070) inhibits Bcl-2, Bcl-xL, and MCL-1 and increases lapatinib-mediated cell death in breast cancer cells [163]. Lapatinib plus another Bcl-2 inhibitor, HA14-1, or obatoclax shows synergy in various breast cancer cells [164]. Knockdown of other anti-apoptotic proteins (Mcl-1 and survivin) also induces apoptosis of HER2-positive breast cancer cells, including those that are resistant to trastuzumab and lapatinib [165]. CDK inhibition reduces Mcl-1 expression [166], with combination flavopiridol plus lapatinib or trastuzumab increasing cell death in HER2-positive breast cancer cells [98, 99, 166, 167]. Further, Mcl-1 expression or Bax or Bak knockdown abrogates the apoptotic effects of combination flavopiridol plus lapatinib [167], indicating that levels of Bcl-2 family members are an important predictor of drug response. Thus, drugs that target apoptotic regulators, including those in the Bcl-2 family, are attractive, emerging therapies for antibody-resistant HER2-positive breast cancers.

7.4.6 Targeting Aberrant Forms of HER2

Targeting Truncated HER2 Earlier studies showed that trastuzumab blocks cleavage of the extracellular domain of HER2, which prevents the formation of a truncated, unusual form of HER2, which is constitutively active and referred to as p95HER2 [25]. Clinical evaluation indicates that approximately 20% of patients with HER2-positive disease may express p95HER2, with few showing responses to trastuzumab [168]. Truncated HER2 may result from matrix metalloproteinase cleavage, or alternative translation start sites [169, 170]. Trastuzumab is unable to inhibit the kinase activity of p95HER2, as this truncated receptor lacks the cell-surface binding epitope recognized by trastuzumab. Phosphorylation and dimerization of p95HER2 are stimulated by HER3 ligand heregulin, promoting interaction between p95HER2 and HER3 [171]. HER2 kinase inhibitor treatment can suppress p95HER2 signaling through PI3K and MAPK [168, 171]. Indeed, studies confirm that the HER2 TKI lapatinib, but not trastuzumab, is effective against p95HER2-positive disease [172–174].

Targeting Mutant Forms of HER2 Recent studies indicate that up to 3% of patients with breast cancer have activating mutations in HER2 without evidence of HER2 gene amplification [175]. Patients with HER2-mutant breast cancer exhibit reduced disease-free survival and resistance to HER2 antibody therapy. Further, tumors that acquire resistance to HER2 antibody treatment may develop mutations in HER2 over time. Preclinical data suggest that multi-HER TKIs, including afatinib and neratinib, retain activity in HER2-mutant breast cancers that are resistant to trastuzumab and lapatinib [176]. Clinical evaluation of HER2 mutational status may help inform treatment decisions, possibly avoiding time delay, toxicities, and costs associated with antibody therapies and improving outcomes by treating with TKIs, which may provide more significant benefit in this setting.

7.5 Conclusions

The investigational approaches discussed may improve survival outcomes for patients with metastatic HER2-positive breast cancers that have progressed on HER2 antibody therapy. As the majority of approaches involve a cocktail of agents, safety and non-specific toxicities will need to be carefully evaluated. With the number of available drugs increasing, particularly through the use of biologics, patient stratification will be more critical than ever. There is now more attention focused on establishing molecular and cellular biomarkers for predicting which patients will derive the most benefit from any given combination of agents. Importantly, as the molecular mechanisms mediating resistance are uncovered, some multi-targeted strategies, such as the ER/HER2/CDK4/6 strategy discussed above, may remove the need for chemotherapy in select patients. It is imperative that clinical trials focus on understanding when and where chemotherapy can be minimized without reducing efficacy. Ongoing trials should continue to investigate the efficacy of new agents against HER2-positive breast cancer brain metastases, a subpopulation for whom few treatment options currently exist.

References

1. Siegel RL, Miller KD, Jemal A. Cancer statistics, 2018. CA Cancer J Clin. 2018;68(1):7–30. https://doi.org/10.3322/caac.21442.
2. Redig AJ, McAllister SS. Breast cancer as a systemic disease: a view of metastasis. J Intern Med. 2013;274(2):113–26. https://doi.org/10.1111/joim.12084.
3. Dai X, Li T, Bai Z, Yang Y, Liu X, Zhan J, et al. Breast cancer intrinsic subtype classification, clinical use and future trends. Am J Cancer Res. 2015;5(10):2929–43.
4. Graus-Porta D, Beerli RR, Daly JM, Hynes NE. ErbB-2, the preferred heterodimerization partner of all ErbB receptors, is a mediator of lateral signaling. EMBO J. 1997;16(7):1647–55. https://doi.org/10.1093/emboj/16.7.1647.
5. Nahta R, Yu D, Hung MC, Hortobagyi GN, Esteva FJ. Mechanisms of disease: understanding resistance to HER2-targeted therapy in human breast cancer. Nat Clin Pract Oncol. 2006;3(5):269–80. https://doi.org/10.1038/ncponc0509.
6. Ghosh R, Narasanna A, Wang SE, Liu S, Chakrabarty A, Balko JM et al. Trastuzumab has preferential activity against breast cancers driven by HER2 homodimers. Cancer Res 2011;71(5):1871-82. https://doi.org/10.1158/0008-5472.CAN-10-1872 [pii].

7. Eccles SA. The role of c-erbB-2/HER2/neu in breast cancer progression and metastasis. J Mammary Gland Biol Neoplasia. 2001;6(4):393–406.
8. Slamon DJ, Clark GM, Wong SG, Levin WJ, Ullrich A, McGuire WL. Human breast cancer: correlation of relapse and survival with amplification of the HER-2/neu oncogene. Science. 1987;235(4785):177–82.
9. Hudziak RM, Schlessinger J, Ullrich A. Increased expression of the putative growth factor receptor p185HER2 causes transformation and tumorigenesis of NIH 3T3 cells. Proc Natl Acad Sci U S A. 1987;84(20):7159–63.
10. Cobleigh MA, Vogel CL, Tripathy D, Robert NJ, Scholl S, Fehrenbacher L, et al. Multinational study of the efficacy and safety of humanized anti-HER2 monoclonal antibody in women who have HER2-overexpressing metastatic breast cancer that has progressed after chemotherapy for metastatic disease. J Clin Oncol. 1999;17(9):2639–48.
11. Esteva FJ, Valero V, Booser D, Guerra LT, Murray JL, Pusztai L, et al. Phase II study of weekly docetaxel and trastuzumab for patients with HER-2-overexpressing metastatic breast cancer. J Clin Oncol. 2002;20(7):1800–8. https://doi.org/10.1200/JCO.2002.07.058.
12. Hudziak RM, Lewis GD, Winget M, Fendly BM, Shepard HM, Ullrich A. p185HER2 monoclonal antibody has antiproliferative effects in vitro and sensitizes human breast tumor cells to tumor necrosis factor. Mol Cell Biol. 1989;9(3):1165–72.
13. Baselga J, Tripathy D, Mendelsohn J, Baughman S, Benz CC, Dantis L, et al. Phase II study of weekly intravenous recombinant humanized anti-p185HER2 monoclonal antibody in patients with HER2/neu-overexpressing metastatic breast cancer. J Clin Oncol. 1996;14(3):737–44.
14. Vogel CL, Cobleigh MA, Tripathy D, Gutheil JC, Harris LN, Fehrenbacher L, et al. Efficacy and safety of trastuzumab as a single agent in first-line treatment of HER2-overexpressing metastatic breast cancer. J Clin Oncol. 2002;20(3):719–26.
15. Seidman AD, Fornier MN, Esteva FJ, Tan L, Kaptain S, Bach A, et al. Weekly trastuzumab and paclitaxel therapy for metastatic breast cancer with analysis of efficacy by HER2 immunophenotype and gene amplification. J Clin Oncol. 2001;19(10):2587–95 https://doi.org/10.1200/JCO.2001.19.10.2587.
16. Slamon DJ, Leyland-Jones B, Shak S, Fuchs H, Paton V, Bajamonde A, et al. Use of chemotherapy plus a monoclonal antibody against HER2 for metastatic breast cancer that overexpresses HER2. N Engl J Med. 2001;344(11):783–92. https://doi.org/10.1056/NEJM200103153441101.
17. Nahta R. Pharmacological strategies to overcome HER2 cross-talk and trastuzumab resistance. Curr Med Chem. 2012;19(7):1065–75. BSP/CMC/E-Pub/2012/086 [pii].
18. Nahta R, Esteva FJ. HER2 therapy: molecular mechanisms of trastuzumab resistance. Breast Cancer Res. 2006;8(6):215. https://doi.org/10.1186/bcr1612.
19. Nahta R, Esteva FJ. Herceptin: mechanisms of action and resistance. Cancer Lett. 2006;232(2):123–38. https://doi.org/10.1016/j.canlet.2005.01.041.
20. Nahta R, Esteva FJ. Trastuzumab: triumphs and tribulations. Oncogene. 2007;26(25):3637–43. https://doi.org/10.1038/sj.onc.1210379.
21. Nahta R, Shabaya S, Ozbay T, Rowe DL. Personalizing HER2-targeted therapy in metastatic breast cancer beyond HER2 status: what we have learned from clinical specimens. Curr Pharmacogenomics Person Med. 2009;7(4):263–74.
22. Cuello M, Ettenberg SA, Clark AS, Keane MM, Posner RH, Nau MM, et al. Down-regulation of the erbB-2 receptor by trastuzumab (herceptin) enhances tumor necrosis factor-related apoptosis-inducing ligand-mediated apoptosis in breast and ovarian cancer cell lines that overexpress erbB-2. Cancer Res. 2001;61(12):4892–900.
23. Gajria D, Chandarlapaty S. HER2-amplified breast cancer: mechanisms of trastuzumab resistance and novel targeted therapies. Expert Rev Anticancer Ther. 2011;11(2):263–75. https://doi.org/10.1586/era.10.226.
24. Junttila TT, Akita RW, Parsons K, Fields C, Lewis Phillips GD, Friedman LS, et al. Ligand-independent HER2/HER3/PI3K complex is disrupted by trastuzumab and is effectively inhibited by the PI3K inhibitor GDC-0941. Cancer Cell. 2009;15(5):429–40. https://doi.org/10.1016/j.ccr.2009.03.020.

25. Molina MA, Codony-Servat J, Albanell J, Rojo F, Arribas J, Baselga J. Trastuzumab (herceptin), a humanized anti-Her2 receptor monoclonal antibody, inhibits basal and activated Her2 ectodomain cleavage in breast cancer cells. Cancer Res. 2001;61(12):4744–9.

26. Lane HA, Motoyama AB, Beuvink I, Hynes NE. Modulation of p27/Cdk2 complex formation through 4D5-mediated inhibition of HER2 receptor signaling. Ann Oncol. 2001;12(Suppl 1):S21–2.

27. Le XF, Claret FX, Lammayot A, Tian L, Deshpande D, LaPushin R, et al. The role of cyclin-dependent kinase inhibitor p27Kip1 in anti-HER2 antibody-induced G1 cell cycle arrest and tumor growth inhibition. J Biol Chem. 2003;278(26):23441–50. https://doi.org/10.1074/jbc. M300848200. M300848200 [pii].

28. Izumi Y, Xu L, di Tomaso E, Fukumura D, Jain RK. Tumour biology: herceptin acts as an anti-angiogenic cocktail. Nature. 2002;416(6878):279–80. https://doi.org/10.1038/416279b.

29. Klos KS, Zhou X, Lee S, Zhang L, Yang W, Nagata Y, et al. Combined trastuzumab and paclitaxel treatment better inhibits ErbB-2-mediated angiogenesis in breast carcinoma through a more effective inhibition of Akt than either treatment alone. Cancer. 2003;98(7):1377–85. https://doi.org/10.1002/cncr.11656.

30. Arnould L, Gelly M, Penault-Llorca F, Benoit L, Bonnetain F, Migeon C, et al. Trastuzumab-based treatment of HER2-positive breast cancer: an antibody-dependent cellular cytotoxicity mechanism? Br J Cancer. 2006;94(2):259–67. https://doi.org/10.1038/sj.bjc.6602930. 6602930 [pii].

31. Clynes RA, Towers TL, Presta LG, Ravetch JV. Inhibitory Fc receptors modulate in vivo cytotoxicity against tumor targets. Nat Med. 2000;6(4):443–6. https://doi.org/10.1038/74704.

32. Herceptin FDA label. https://www.accessdata.fda.gov/drugsatfda_docs/label/2010/103792s5250lbl.pdf.

33. Price-Schiavi SA, Jepson S, Li P, Arango M, Rudland PS, Yee L, et al. Rat Muc4 (sialomucin complex) reduces binding of anti-ErbB2 antibodies to tumor cell surfaces, a potential mechanism for herceptin resistance. Int J Cancer. 2002;99(6):783–91. https://doi.org/10.1002/ijc.10410.

34. Nagy P, Friedlander E, Tanner M, Kapanen AI, Carraway KL, Isola J, et al. Decreased accessibility and lack of activation of ErbB2 in JIMT-1, a herceptin-resistant, MUC4-expressing breast cancer cell line. Cancer Res. 2005;65(2):473–82. 65/2/473 [pii].

35. Agus DB, Akita RW, Fox WD, Lewis GD, Higgins B, Pisacane PI, et al. Targeting ligand-activated ErbB2 signaling inhibits breast and prostate tumor growth. Cancer Cell. 2002;2(2):127–37.

36. Swain SM, Baselga J, Kim SB, Ro J, Semiglazov V, Campone M, et al. Pertuzumab, trastuzumab, and docetaxel in HER2-positive metastatic breast cancer. N Engl J Med. 2015;372(8):724–34. https://doi.org/10.1056/NEJMoa1413513.

37. Verma S, Miles D, Gianni L, Krop IE, Welslau M, Baselga J, et al. Trastuzumab emtansine for HER2-positive advanced breast cancer. N Engl J Med. 2012;367(19):1783–91. https://doi.org/10.1056/NEJMoa1209124.

38. Krop IE, Lin NU, Blackwell K, Guardino E, Huober J, Lu M, et al. Trastuzumab emtansine (T-DM1) versus lapatinib plus capecitabine in patients with HER2-positive metastatic breast cancer and central nervous system metastases: a retrospective, exploratory analysis in EMILIA. Ann Oncol. 2015;26(1):113–9. https://doi.org/10.1093/annonc/mdu486.

39. Schwarz LJ, Hutchinson KE, Rexer BN, Estrada MV, Gonzalez Ericsson PI, Sanders ME, et al. An ERBB1-3 neutralizing antibody mixture with high activity against drug-resistant HER2+ breast cancers with ERBB ligand overexpression. J Natl Cancer Inst. 2017;109(11) https://doi.org/10.1093/jnci/djx065.

40. Geyer CE, Forster J, Lindquist D, Chan S, Romieu CG, Pienkowski T, et al. Lapatinib plus capecitabine for HER2-positive advanced breast cancer. N Engl J Med. 2006;355(26):2733–43. https://doi.org/10.1056/NEJMoa064320.

41. Piccart-Gebhart M, Holmes E, Baselga J, de Azambuja E, Dueck AC, Viale G, et al. Adjuvant lapatinib and trastuzumab for early human epidermal growth factor receptor 2-positive

breast cancer: results from the randomized phase III adjuvant lapatinib and/or trastuzumab treatment optimization trial. J Clin Oncol. 2016;34(10):1034–42. https://doi.org/10.1200/JCO.2015.62.1797.

42. Baselga J, Bradbury I, Eidtmann H, Di Cosimo S, de Azambuja E, Aura C, et al. Lapatinib with trastuzumab for HER2-positive early breast cancer (NeoALTTO): a randomised, open-label, multicentre, phase 3 trial. Lancet. 2012;379(9816):633–40. https://doi.org/10.1016/S0140-6736(11)61847-3.

43. Deeks ED. Neratinib: first global approval. Drugs. 2017;77(15):1695–704. https://doi.org/10.1007/s40265-017-0811-4.

44. Rabindran SK, Discafani CM, Rosfjord EC, Baxter M, Floyd MB, Golas J, et al. Antitumor activity of HKI-272, an orally active, irreversible inhibitor of the HER-2 tyrosine kinase. Cancer Res. 2004;64(11):3958–65. https://doi.org/10.1158/0008-5472.CAN-03-2868. 64/11/3958 [pii].

45. Hegde PS, Rusnak D, Bertiaux M, Alligood K, Strum J, Gagnon R, et al. Delineation of molecular mechanisms of sensitivity to lapatinib in breast cancer cell lines using global gene expression profiles. Mol Cancer Ther. 2007;6(5):1629–40. https://doi.org/10.1158/1535-7163.MCT-05-0399. 6/5/1629 [pii].

46. Sanchez-Martin M, Pandiella A. Differential action of small molecule HER kinase inhibitors on receptor heterodimerization: therapeutic implications. Int J Cancer. 2012;131(1):244–52. https://doi.org/10.1002/ijc.26358.

47. Seyhan AA, Varadarajan U, Choe S, Liu Y, McGraw J, Woods M, et al. A genome-wide RNAi screen identifies novel targets of neratinib sensitivity leading to neratinib and pacli-taxel combination drug treatments. Mol Biosyst. 2011;7(6):1974–89. https://doi.org/10.1039/c0mb00294a.

48. Martin M, Holmes FA, Ejlertsen B, Delaloge S, Moy B, Iwata H, et al. Neratinib after trastuzumab-based adjuvant therapy in HER2-positive breast cancer (ExteNET): 5-year analysis of a randomised, double-blind, placebo-controlled, phase 3 trial. Lancet Oncol. 2017;18(12):1688–700. https://doi.org/10.1016/S1470-2045(17)30717-9.

49. Jerome L, Alami N, Belanger S, Page V, Yu Q, Paterson J, et al. Recombinant human insulin-like growth factor binding protein 3 inhibits growth of human epidermal growth factor receptor-2-overexpressing breast tumors and potentiates herceptin activity in vivo. Cancer Res. 2006;66(14):7245–52. https://doi.org/10.1158/0008-5472.CAN-05-3555.

50. Alexander PB, Chen R, Gong C, Yuan L, Jasper JS, Ding Y, et al. Distinct receptor tyro-sine kinase subsets mediate anti-HER2 drug resistance in breast cancer. J Biol Chem. 2017;292(2):748–59. https://doi.org/10.1074/jbc.M116.754960.

51. Lu Y, Zi X, Zhao Y, Mascarenhas D, Pollak M. Insulin-like growth factor-I receptor signaling and resistance to trastuzumab (Herceptin). J Natl Cancer Inst. 2001;93(24):1852–7.

52. Oliveras-Ferraros C, Vazquez-Martin A, Martin-Castillo B, Perez-Martinez MC, Cufi S, Del Barco S, et al. Pathway-focused proteomic signatures in HER2-overexpressing breast cancer with a basal-like phenotype: new insights into de novo resistance to trastuzumab (Herceptin). Int J Oncol. 2010;37(3):669–78.

53. Huang X, Gao L, Wang S, McManaman JL, Thor AD, Yang X, et al. Heterotrimerization of the growth factor receptors erbB2, erbB3, and insulin-like growth factor-i receptor in breast cancer cells resistant to herceptin. Cancer Res. 2010;70(3):1204–14. https://doi.org/10.1158/0008-5472.CAN-09-3321.

54. Nahta R, Yuan LX, Zhang B, Kobayashi R, Esteva FJ. Insulin-like growth factor-I recep-tor/human epidermal growth factor receptor 2 heterodimerization contributes to trastu-zumab resistance of breast cancer cells. Cancer Res. 2005;65(23):11118–28. https://doi.org/10.1158/0008-5472.CAN-04-3841.

55. Sliwkowski MX, Lofgren JA, Lewis GD, Hotaling TE, Fendly BM, Fox JA. Nonclinical stud-ies addressing the mechanism of action of trastuzumab (Herceptin). Semin Oncol. 1999;26(4 Suppl 12):60–70.

56. Tseng PH, Wang YC, Weng SC, Weng JR, Chen CS, Brueggemeier RW, et al. Overcoming trastuzumab resistance in HER2-overexpressing breast cancer cells by using a novel celecoxib-derived phosphoinositide-dependent kinase-1 inhibitor. Mol Pharmacol. 2006;70(5):1534–41. https://doi.org/10.1124/mol.106.023911. mol.106.023911 [pii].

57. Cornelissen B, McLarty K, Kersemans V, Reilly RM. The level of insulin growth factor-1 receptor expression is directly correlated with the tumor uptake of (111)In-IGF-1(E3R) in vivo and the clonogenic survival of breast cancer cells exposed in vitro to trastuzumab (Herceptin). Nucl Med Biol. 2008;35(6):645–53. https://doi.org/10.1016/j.nucmedbio.2008.05.010.

58. Nahta R, Esteva FJ. In vitro effects of trastuzumab and vinorelbine in trastuzumab-resistant breast cancer cells. Cancer Chemother Pharmacol. 2004;53(2):186–90. https://doi.org/10.1007/s00280-003-0728-3.

59. Nahta R, Takahashi T, Ueno NT, Hung MC, Esteva FJ. P27(kip1) down-regulation is associated with trastuzumab resistance in breast cancer cells. Cancer Res. 2004;64(11):3981–6. https://doi.org/10.1158/0008-5472.CAN-03-3900.

60. Gallardo A, Lerma E, Escuin D, Tibau A, Munoz J, Ojeda B, et al. Increased signalling of EGFR and IGF1R, and deregulation of PTEN/PI3K/Akt pathway are related with trastuzumab resistance in HER2 breast carcinomas. Br J Cancer. 2012;106(8):1367–73. https://doi.org/10.1038/bjc.2012.85.

61. Harris LN, You F, Schnitt SJ, Witkiewicz A, Lu X, Sgroi D, et al. Predictors of resistance to preoperative trastuzumab and vinorelbine for HER2-positive early breast cancer. Clin Cancer Res. 2007;13(4):1198–207. https://doi.org/10.1158/1078-0432.CCR-06-1304.

62. Sonnenblick A, Agbor-Tarh D, Bradbury I, Di Cosimo S, Azim HA Jr, Fumagalli D, et al. Impact of diabetes, insulin, and metformin use on the outcome of patients with human epidermal growth factor receptor 2-positive primary breast cancer: analysis from the ALTTO phase III randomized trial. J Clin Oncol. 2017;35(13):1421–9. https://doi.org/10.1200/JCO.2016.69.7722.

63. Browne BC, Eustace AJ, Kennedy S, O'Brien NA, Pedersen K, McDermott MS, et al. Evaluation of IGF1R and phosphorylated IGF1R as targets in HER2-positive breast cancer cell lines and tumours. Breast Cancer Res Treat. 2012;136(3):717–27. https://doi.org/10.1007/s10549-012-2260-9.

64. Kostler WJ, Hudelist G, Rabitsch W, Czerwenka K, Muller R, Singer CF, et al. Insulin-like growth factor-1 receptor (IGF-1R) expression does not predict for resistance to trastuzumab-based treatment in patients with Her-2/neu overexpressing metastatic breast cancer. J Cancer Res Clin Oncol. 2006;132(1):9–18. https://doi.org/10.1007/s00432-005-0038-8.

65. Reinholz MM, Chen B, Dueck AC, Tenner K, Ballman K, Riehle D, et al. IGF1R protein expression is not associated with differential benefit to concurrent trastuzumab in early-stage HER2(+) breast cancer from the North Central Cancer Treatment Group (Alliance) adjuvant trastuzumab trial N9831. Clin Cancer Res. 2017;23(15):4203–11. https://doi.org/10.1158/1078-0432.CCR-15-0574.

66. Smith BL, Chin D, Maltzman W, Crosby K, Hortobagyi GN, Bacus SS. The efficacy of Herceptin therapies is influenced by the expression of other erbB receptors, their ligands and the activation of downstream signalling proteins. Br J Cancer. 2004;91(6):1190–4. https://doi.org/10.1038/sj.bjc.6602090. 6602090 [pii].

67. Yerushalmi R, Gelmon KA, Leung S, Gao D, Cheang M, Pollak M, et al. Insulin-like growth factor receptor (IGF-1R) in breast cancer subtypes. Breast Cancer Res Treat. 2012;132(1):131–42. https://doi.org/10.1007/s10549-011-1529-8.

68. Browne BC, Crown J, Venkatesan N, Duffy MJ, Clynes M, Slamon D, et al. Inhibition of IGF1R activity enhances response to trastuzumab in HER-2-positive breast cancer cells. Ann Oncol. 2011;22(1):68–73. https://doi.org/10.1093/annonc/mdq349.

69. Chakraborty AK, Zerillo C, DiGiovanna MP. In vitro and in vivo studies of the combination of IGF1R inhibitor figitumumab (CP-751,871) with HER2 inhibitors trastuzumab and neratinib. Breast Cancer Res Treat. 2015;152(3):533–44. https://doi.org/10.1007/s10549-015-3504-2.

70. Esparis-Ogando A, Ocana A, Rodriguez-Barrueco R, Ferreira L, Borges J, Pandiella A. Synergic antitumoral effect of an IGF-IR inhibitor and trastuzumab on HER2-overexpressing breast cancer cells. Ann Oncol. 2008;19(11):1860–9. https://doi.org/10.1093/annonc/mdn406.

71. Sanabria-Figueroa E, Donnelly SM, Foy KC, Buss MC, Castellino RC, Paplomata E, et al. Insulin-like growth factor-1 receptor signaling increases the invasive potential of human epidermal growth factor receptor 2-overexpressing breast cancer cells via Src-focal adhesion kinase and forkhead box protein M1. Mol Pharmacol. 2015;87(2):150–61. https://doi.org/10.1124/mol.114.095380.

72. Gradishar WJ, Yardley DA, Layman R, Sparano JA, Chuang E, Northfelt DW, et al. Clinical and translational results of a phase II, randomized trial of an anti-IGF-1R (cixutumumab) in women with breast cancer that progressed on endocrine therapy. Clin Cancer Res. 2016;22(2):301–9. https://doi.org/10.1158/1078-0432.CCR-15-0588.

73. Rugo HS, Tredan O, Ro J, Morales SM, Campone M, Musolino A, et al. A randomized phase II trial of ridaforolimus, dalotuzumab, and exemestane compared with ridaforolimus and exemestane in patients with advanced breast cancer. Breast Cancer Res Treat. 2017;165(3):601–9. https://doi.org/10.1007/s10549-017-4375-5.

74. Mendoza MC, Er EE, Blenis J. The Ras-ERK and PI3K-mTOR pathways: cross-talk and compensation. Trends Biochem Sci. 2011;36(6):320–8. https://doi.org/10.1016/j.tibs.2011.03.006.

75. Berns K, Horlings HM, Hennessy BT, Madiredjo M, Hijmans EM, Beelen K, et al. A functional genetic approach identifies the PI3K pathway as a major determinant of trastuzumab resistance in breast cancer. Cancer Cell. 2007;12(4):395–402. https://doi.org/10.1016/j.ccr.2007.08.030.

76. Nagata Y, Lan KH, Zhou X, Tan M, Esteva FJ, Sahin AA, et al. PTEN activation contributes to tumor inhibition by trastuzumab, and loss of PTEN predicts trastuzumab resistance in patients. Cancer Cell. 2004;6(2):117–27. https://doi.org/10.1016/j.ccr.2004.06.022.

77. Wang L, Zhang Q, Zhang J, Sun S, Guo H, Jia Z, et al. PI3K pathway activation results in low efficacy of both trastuzumab and lapatinib. BMC Cancer. 2011;11:248. https://doi.org/10.1186/1471-2407-11-248.

78. Andre F, O'Regan R, Ozguroglu M, Toi M, Xu B, Jerusalem G, et al. Everolimus for women with trastuzumab-resistant, HER2-positive, advanced breast cancer (BOLERO-3): a randomised, double-blind, placebo-controlled phase 3 trial. Lancet Oncol. 2014;15(6):580–91. https://doi.org/10.1016/S1470-2045(14)70138-X.

79. Andre F, Hurvitz S, Fasolo A, Tseng LM, Jerusalem G, Wilks S, et al. Molecular alterations and everolimus efficacy in human epidermal growth factor receptor 2-overexpressing metastatic breast cancers: combined exploratory biomarker analysis from BOLERO-1 and BOLERO 3. J Clin Oncol. 2016;34(18):2115–24. https://doi.org/10.1200/JCO.2015.63.9161.

80. O'Brien NA, Browne BC, Chow L, Wang Y, Ginther C, Arboleda J, et al. Activated phosphoinositide 3-kinase/AKT signaling confers resistance to trastuzumab but not lapatinib. Mol Cancer Ther. 2010;9(6):1489–502. https://doi.org/10.1158/1535-7163.MCT-09-1171.

81. Xia W, Husain I, Liu L, Bacus S, Saini S, Spohn J, et al. Lapatinib antitumor activity is not dependent upon phosphatase and tensin homologue deleted on chromosome 10 in ErbB2-overexpressing breast cancers. Cancer Res. 2007;67(3):1170–5. https://doi.org/10.1158/0008-5472.CAN-06-2101.

82. Eichhorn PJ, Gili M, Scaltriti M, Serra V, Guzman M, Nijkamp W, et al. Phosphatidylinositol 3-kinase hyperactivation results in lapatinib resistance that is reversed by the mTOR/phosphatidylinositol 3-kinase inhibitor NVP-BEZ235. Cancer Res. 2008;68(22):9221–30. https://doi.org/10.1158/0008-5472.CAN-08-1740.

83. Dave B, Migliaccio I, Gutierrez MC, Wu MF, Chamness GC, Wong H, et al. Loss of phosphatase and tensin homolog or phosphoinositol-3 kinase activation and response to trastuzumab or lapatinib in human epidermal growth factor receptor 2-overexpressing locally advanced breast cancers. J Clin Oncol. 2011;29(2):166–73. https://doi.org/10.1200/JCO.2009.27.7814.

84. Vazquez-Martin A, Oliveras-Ferraros C, Colomer R, Brunet J, Menendez JA. Low-scale phos-phoproteome analyses identify the mTOR effector p70 S6 kinase 1 as a specific biomarker of the dual-HER1/HER2 tyrosine kinase inhibitor lapatinib (Tykerb) in human breast carcinoma cells. Ann Oncol. 2008;19(6):1097–109. https://doi.org/10.1093/annonc/mdm589.

85. Guerin M, Rezai K, Isambert N, Campone M, Autret A, Pakradouni J, et al. PIKHER2: a phase IB study evaluating buparlisib in combination with lapatinib in trastuzumab-resistant HER2-positive advanced breast cancer. Eur J Cancer. 2017;86:28–36. https://doi.org/10.1016/j.ejca.2017.08.025.

86. Baselga J, Lewis Phillips GD, Verma S, Ro J, Huober J, Guardino AE, et al. Relationship between tumor biomarkers and efficacy in EMILIA, a phase III study of trastuzumab emtansine in HER2-positive metastatic breast cancer. Clin Cancer Res. 2016;22(15):3755–63. https://doi.org/10.1158/1078-0432.CCR-15-2499.

87. Li G, Guo J, Shen BQ, Yadav DB, Sliwkowski MX, Crocker LM, et al. Mechanisms of acquired resistance to trastuzumab emtansine in breast cancer cells. Mol Cancer Ther. 2018;17(7):1441–53. https://doi.org/10.1158/1535-7163.MCT-17-0296.

88. Jain S, Shah AN, Santa-Maria CA, Siziopikou K, Rademaker A, Helenowski I, et al. Phase I study of alpelisib (BYL-719) and trastuzumab emtansine (T-DM1) in HER2-positive meta-static breast cancer (MBC) after trastuzumab and taxane therapy. Breast Cancer Res Treat. 2018;171(2):371–81. https://doi.org/10.1007/s10549-018-4792-0.

89. Lu CH, Wyszomierski SL, Tseng LM, Sun MH, Lan KH, Neal CL, et al. Preclinical testing of clinically applicable strategies for overcoming trastuzumab resistance caused by PTEN deficiency. Clin Cancer Res. 2007;13(19):5883–8. https://doi.org/10.1158/1078-0432.CCR-06-2837. 13/19/5883 [pii].

90. Ozbay T, Durden DL, Liu T, O'Regan RM, Nahta R. In vitro evaluation of pan-PI3-kinase inhibitor SF1126 in trastuzumab-sensitive and trastuzumab-resistant HER2-over-expressing breast cancer cells. Cancer Chemother Pharmacol. 2010;65(4):697–706. https://doi.org/10.1007/s00280-009-1075-9.

91. Esteva FJ, Guo H, Zhang S, Santa-Maria C, Stone S, Lanchbury JS, et al. PTEN, PIK3CA, p-AKT, and p-p70S6K status: association with trastuzumab response and survival in patients with HER2-positive metastatic breast cancer. Am J Pathol. 2010;177(4):1647–56. https://doi.org/10.2353/ajpath.2010.090885. S0002-9440(10)60218-0 [pii].

92. Huang C, Park CC, Hilsenbeck SG, Ward R, Rimawi MF, Wang YC, et al. beta1 integrin mediates an alternative survival pathway in breast cancer cells resistant to lapatinib. Breast Cancer Res. 2011;13(4):R84. https://doi.org/10.1186/bcr2936.

93. Park CC, Zhang H, Pallavicini M, Gray JW, Baehner F, Park CJ, et al. Beta1 integrin inhibi-tory antibody induces apoptosis of breast cancer cells, inhibits growth, and distinguishes malignant from normal phenotype in three dimensional cultures and in vivo. Cancer Res. 2006;66(3):1526–35. https://doi.org/10.1158/0008-5472.CAN-05-3071.

94. Hanker AB, Estrada MV, Bianchini G, Moore PD, Zhao J, Cheng F, et al. Extracellular matrix/integrin signaling promotes resistance to combined inhibition of HER2 and PI3K in HER2(+) breast cancer. Cancer Res. 2017;77(12):3280–92. https://doi.org/10.1158/0008-5472.CAN-16-2808.

95. Gardaneh M, Shojaei S, Kaviani A, Behnam B. GDNF induces RET-SRC-HER2-dependent growth in trastuzumab-sensitive but SRC-independent growth in resistant breast tumor cells. Breast Cancer Res Treat. 2017;162(2):231–41. https://doi.org/10.1007/s10549-016-4078-3.

96. Scaltriti M, Eichhorn PJ, Cortes J, Prudkin L, Aura C, Jimenez J, et al. Cyclin E amplification/overexpression is a mechanism of trastuzumab resistance in HER2+ breast cancer patients. Proc Natl Acad Sci U S A. 2011;108(9):3761–6. https://doi.org/10.1073/pnas.1014835108. 1014835108 [pii].

97. Lu Y, Zi X, Pollak M. Molecular mechanisms underlying IGF-I-induced attenuation of the growth-inhibitory activity of trastuzumab (Herceptin) on SKBR3 breast cancer cells. Int J Cancer. 2004;108(3):334–41. https://doi.org/10.1002/ijc.11445.

98. Nahta R, Iglehart JD, Kempkes B, Schmidt EV. Rate-limiting effects of cyclin D1 in transformation by ErbB2 predicts synergy between herceptin and flavopiridol. Cancer Res. 2002;62(8):2267–71.

99. Nahta R, Trent S, Yang C, Schmidt EV. Epidermal growth factor receptor expression is a candidate target of the synergistic combination of trastuzumab and flavopiridol in breast cancer. Cancer Res. 2003;63(13):3626–31.

100. Wu K, Wang C, D'Amico M, Lee RJ, Albanese C, Pestell RG, et al. Flavopiridol and trastuzumab synergistically inhibit proliferation of breast cancer cells: association with selective cooperative inhibition of cyclin D1-dependent kinase and Akt signaling pathways. Mol Cancer Ther. 2002;1(9):695–706.

101. Goel S, Wang Q, Watt AC, Tolaney SM, Dillon DA, Li W, et al. Overcoming therapeutic resistance in HER2-positive breast cancers with CDK4/6 inhibitors. Cancer Cell. 2016;29(3):255–69. https://doi.org/10.1016/j.ccell.2016.02.006.

102. Wang YC, Morrison G, Gillihan R, Guo J, Ward RM, Fu X, et al. Different mechanisms for resistance to trastuzumab versus lapatinib in HER2-positive breast cancers--role of estrogen receptor and HER2 reactivation. Breast Cancer Res. 2011;13(6):R121. https://doi.org/10.1186/bcr3067.

103. Gianni L, Bisagni G, Colleoni M, Del Mastro L, Zamagni C, Mansutti M, et al. Neoadjuvant treatment with trastuzumab and pertuzumab plus palbociclib and fulvestrant in HER2-positive, ER-positive breast cancer (NA-PHER2): an exploratory, open-label, phase 2 study. Lancet Oncol. 2018;19(2):249–56. https://doi.org/10.1016/S1470-2045(18)30001-9.

104. Kumar R, Mandal M, Lipton A, Harvey H, Thompson CB. Overexpression of HER2 modulates bcl-2, bcl-XL, and tamoxifen-induced apoptosis in human MCF-7 breast cancer cells. Clin Cancer Res. 1996;2(7):1215–9.

105. Kurokawa H, Lenferink AE, Simpson JF, Pisacane PI, Sliwkowski MX, Forbes JT, et al. Inhibition of HER2/neu (erbB-2) and mitogen-activated protein kinases enhances tamoxifen action against HER2-overexpressing, tamoxifen-resistant breast cancer cells. Cancer Res. 2000;60(20):5887–94.

106. Shou J, Massarweh S, Osborne CK, Wakeling AE, Ali S, Weiss H, et al. Mechanisms of tamoxifen resistance: increased estrogen receptor-HER2/neu cross-talk in ER/HER2-positive breast cancer. J Natl Cancer Inst. 2004;96(12):926–35.

107. Xia W, Bacus S, Hegde P, Husain I, Strum J, Liu L, et al. A model of acquired autoresistance to a potent ErbB2 tyrosine kinase inhibitor and a therapeutic strategy to prevent its onset in breast cancer. Proc Natl Acad Sci U S A. 2006;103(20):7795–800. https://doi.org/10.1073/pnas.0602468103.

108. Rimawi MF, Mayer IA, Forero A, Nanda R, Goetz MP, Rodriguez AA, et al. Multicenter phase II study of neoadjuvant lapatinib and trastuzumab with hormonal therapy and without chemotherapy in patients with human epidermal growth factor receptor 2-overexpressing breast cancer: TBCRC 006. J Clin Oncol. 2013;31(14):1726–31. https://doi.org/10.1200/JCO.2012.44.8027.

109. Sudhan DR, Schwarz LJ, Guerrero-Zotano A, Formisano L, Nixon MJ, Croessmann S, et al. Extended adjuvant therapy with neratinib plus fulvestrant blocks ER/HER2 crosstalk and maintains complete responses of ER+/HER2+ breast cancers: implications to the ExteNET trial. Clin Cancer Res. 2019;25(2):771–83. https://doi.org/10.1158/1078-0432.CCR-18-1131.

110. von Minckwitz G, Procter M, de Azambuja E, Zardavas D, Benyunes M, Viale G, et al. Adjuvant pertuzumab and trastuzumab in early HER2-positive breast cancer. N Engl J Med. 2017;377(2):122–31. https://doi.org/10.1056/NEJMoa1703643.

111. Paplomata E, Nahta R, O'Regan RM. Systemic therapy for early-stage HER2-positive breast cancers: time for a less-is-more approach? Cancer. 2015;121(4):517–26. https://doi.org/10.1002/cncr.29060.

112. Emde A, Mahlknecht G, Maslak K, Ribba B, Sela M, Possinger K, et al. Simultaneous inhibition of estrogen receptor and the HER2 pathway in breast cancer: Effects of HER2 abundance. Transl Oncol. 2011;4(5):293–300.

113. Gennari R, Menard S, Fagnoni F, Ponchio L, Scelsi M, Tagliabue E, et al. Pilot study of the mechanism of action of preoperative trastuzumab in patients with primary operable breast tumors overexpressing HER2. Clin Cancer Res. 2004;10(17):5650–5. https://doi.org/10.1158/1078-0432.CCR-04-0225.

114. Varchetta S, Gibelli N, Oliviero B, Nardini E, Gennari R, Gatti G, et al. Elements related to heterogeneity of antibody-dependent cell cytotoxicity in patients under trastuzumab therapy for primary operable breast cancer overexpressing Her2. Cancer Res. 2007;67(24):11991–9. https://doi.org/10.1158/0008-5472.CAN-07-2068.

115. Carson WE, Parihar R, Lindemann MJ, Personeni N, Dierksheide J, Meropol NJ, et al. Interleukin-2 enhances the natural killer cell response to Herceptin-coated Her2/neu-positive breast cancer cells. Eur J Immunol. 2001;31(10):3016–25. https://doi.org/10.1002/1521-4141(2001010)31:10<3016::AID-IMMU3016gt;3.0.CO;2-J.

116. Repka T, Chiorean EG, Gay J, Herwig KE, Kohl VK, Yee D, et al. Trastuzumab and interleukin-2 in HER2-positive metastatic breast cancer: a pilot study. Clin Cancer Res. 2003;9(7):2440–6.

117. Parihar R, Nadella P, Lewis A, Jensen R, De Hoff C, Dierksheide JE, et al. A phase I study of interleukin 12 with trastuzumab in patients with human epidermal growth factor receptor-2-overexpressing malignancies: analysis of sustained interferon gamma production in a subset of patients. Clin Cancer Res. 2004;10(15):5027–37. https://doi.org/10.1158/1078-0432.CCR-04-0265.

118. Kohrt HE, Houot R, Weiskopf K, Goldstein MJ, Scheeren F, Czerwinski D, et al. Stimulation of natural killer cells with a CD137-specific antibody enhances trastuzumab efficacy in xenotransplant models of breast cancer. J Clin Invest. 2012;122(3):1066–75. https://doi.org/10.1172/JCI61226.

119. Spiridon CI, Ghetie MA, Uhr J, Marches R, Li JL, Shen GL, et al. Targeting multiple Her-2 epitopes with monoclonal antibodies results in improved antigrowth activity of a human breast cancer cell line in vitro and in vivo. Clin Cancer Res. 2002;8(6):1720–30.

120. Solinas C, Ceppi M, Lambertini M, Scartozzi M, Buisseret L, Garaud S, et al. Tumor-infiltrating lymphocytes in patients with HER2-positive breast cancer treated with neoadjuvant chemotherapy plus trastuzumab, lapatinib or their combination: a meta-analysis of randomized controlled trials. Cancer Treat Rev. 2017;57:8–15. https://doi.org/10.1016/j.ctrv.2017.04.005.

121. Luen SJ, Salgado R, Fox S, Savas P, Eng-Wong J, Clark E, et al. Tumour-infiltrating lymphocytes in advanced HER2-positive breast cancer treated with pertuzumab or placebo in addition to trastuzumab and docetaxel: a retrospective analysis of the CLEOPATRA study. Lancet Oncol. 2017;18(1):52–62. https://doi.org/10.1016/S1470-2045(16)30631-3.

122. Tsang JY, Au WL, Lo KY, Ni YB, Hlaing T, Hu J, et al. PD-L1 expression and tumor infiltrating PD-1+ lymphocytes associated with outcome in HER2+ breast cancer patients. Breast Cancer Res Treat. 2017;162(1):19–30. https://doi.org/10.1007/s10549-016-4095-2.

123. Ghebeh H, Barhoush E, Tulbah A, Elkum N, Al-Tweigeri T, Dermime S. FOXP3+ Tregs and B7-H1+/PD-1+ T lymphocytes co-infiltrate the tumor tissues of high-risk breast cancer patients: Implication for immunotherapy. BMC Cancer. 2008;8:57. https://doi.org/10.1186/1471-2407-8-57.

124. Muenst S, Soysal SD, Gao F, Obermann EC, Oertli D, Gillanders WE. The presence of programmed death 1 (PD-1)-positive tumor-infiltrating lymphocytes is associated with poor prognosis in human breast cancer. Breast Cancer Res Treat. 2013;139(3):667–76. https://doi.org/10.1007/s10549-013-2581-3.

125. Stagg J, Loi S, Divisekera U, Ngiow SF, Duret H, Yagita H, et al. Anti-ErbB-2 mAb therapy requires type I and II interferons and synergizes with anti-PD-1 or anti-CD137 mAb therapy. Proc Natl Acad Sci U S A. 2011;108(17):7142–7. https://doi.org/10.1073/pnas.1016569108.

126. Muller P, Kreuzaler M, Khan T, Thommen DS, Martin K, Glatz K, et al. Trastuzumab emtansine (T-DM1) renders HER2+ breast cancer highly susceptible to CTLA-4/PD-1 blockade. Sci Transl Med. 2015;7(315):315ra188. https://doi.org/10.1126/scitranslmed.aac4925.

127. Blackstone EA, Joseph PF. The economics of biosimilars. Am Health Drug Benefits. 2013;6(8):469–78.
128. Macdonald JC, Hartman H, Jacobs IA. Regulatory considerations in oncologic biosimilar drug development. MAbs. 2015;7(4):653–61. https://doi.org/10.1080/19420862.2015.10409 73.
129. Nelson KM, Gallagher PC. Biosimilars lining up to compete with Herceptin--opportunity knocks. Expert Opin Ther Pat. 2014;24(11):1149–53. https://doi.org/10.1517/13543776.201 4.964683.
130. Paplomata E, Nahta R. ABP 980: promising trastuzumab biosimilar for HER2-positive breast cancer. Expert Opin Biol Ther. 2018;18(3):335–41. https://doi.org/10.1080/14712598.2018.1 430761.
131. Jhaveri K, Wang R, Teplinsky E, Chandarlapaty S, Solit D, Cadoo K, et al. A phase I trial of ganetespib in combination with paclitaxel and trastuzumab in patients with human epidermal growth factor receptor-2 (HER2)-positive metastatic breast cancer. Breast Cancer Res. 2017;19(1):89. https://doi.org/10.1186/s13058-017-0879-5.
132. Lindemann K, Resau J, Nahrig J, Kort E, Leeser B, Annecke K, et al. Differential expression of c-Met, its ligand HGF/SF and HER2/neu in DCIS and adjacent normal breast tissue. Histopathology. 2007;51(1):54–62. https://doi.org/10.1111/j.1365-2559.2007.02732.x.
133. Khoury H, Naujokas MA, Zuo D, Sangwan V, Frigault MM, Petkiewicz S, et al. HGF converts ErbB2/Neu epithelial morphogenesis to cell invasion. Mol Biol Cell. 2005;16(2):550–61. https://doi.org/10.1091/mbc.E04-07-0567.
134. Minuti G, Cappuzzo F, Duchnowska R, Jassem J, Fabi A, O'Brien T, et al. Increased MET and HGF gene copy numbers are associated with trastuzumab failure in HER2-positive metastatic breast cancer. Br J Cancer. 2012;107(5):793–9. https://doi.org/10.1038/bjc.2012.335.
135. Shattuck DL, Miller JK, Carraway KL 3rd, Sweeney C. Met receptor contributes to trastuzumab resistance of Her2-overexpressing breast cancer cells. Cancer Res. 2008;68(5):1471–7. https://doi.org/10.1158/0008-5472.CAN-07-5962. 68/5/1471 [pii].
136. Joshi JP, Brown NE, Griner SE, Nahta R. Growth differentiation factor 15 (GDF15)-mediated HER2 phosphorylation reduces trastuzumab sensitivity of HER2-overexpressing breast cancer cells. Biochem Pharmacol. 2011;82(9):1090–9. https://doi.org/10.1016/j.bcp.2011.07.082.
137. Kim KK, Lee JJ, Yang Y, You KH, Lee JH. Macrophage inhibitory cytokine-1 activates AKT and ERK-1/2 via the transactivation of ErbB2 in human breast and gastric cancer cells. Carcinogenesis. 2008;29(4):704–12. https://doi.org/10.1093/carcin/bgn031.
138. Park YJ, Lee H, Lee JH. Macrophage inhibitory cytokine-1 transactivates ErbB family receptors via the activation of Src in SK-BR-3 human breast cancer cells. BMB Rep. 2010;43(2):91–6.
139. Emmerson PJ, Wang F, Du Y, Liu Q, Pickard RT, Gonciarz MD, et al. The metabolic effects of GDF15 are mediated by the orphan receptor GFRAL. Nat Med. 2017;23(10):1215–9. https://doi.org/10.1038/nm.4393.
140. Mullican SE, Lin-Schmidt X, Chin CN, Chavez JA, Furman JL, Armstrong AA, et al. GFRAL is the receptor for GDF15 and the ligand promotes weight loss in mice and nonhuman primates. Nat Med. 2017;23(10):1150–7. https://doi.org/10.1038/nm.4392.
141. Yang L, Chang CC, Sun Z, Madsen D, Zhu H, Padkjaer SB, et al. GFRAL is the receptor for GDF15 and is required for the anti-obesity effects of the ligand. Nat Med. 2017;23(10):1158–66. https://doi.org/10.1038/nm.4394.
142. Li YL, Chang JT, Lee LY, Fan KH, Lu YC, Li YC, et al. GDF15 contributes to radioresistance and cancer stemness of head and neck cancer by regulating cellular reactive oxygen species via a SMAD-associated signaling pathway. Oncotarget. 2017;8(1):1508–28. https://doi.org/10.18632/oncotarget.13649.
143. Sasahara A, Tominaga K, Nishimura T, Yano M, Kiyokawa E, Noguchi M, et al. An autocrine/paracrine circuit of growth differentiation factor (GDF) 15 has a role for maintenance

of breast cancer stem-like cells. Oncotarget. 2017;18(5):24869–81. https://doi.org/10.18632/oncotarget.15276.

144. Xu J, Kimball TR, Lorenz JN, Brown DA, Bauskin AR, Klevitsky R, et al. GDF15/MIC-1 functions as a protective and antihypertrophic factor released from the myocardium in association with SMAD protein activation. Circ Res. 2006;98(3):342–50. https://doi.org/10.1161/01.RES.0000202804.84885.d0.

145. Griner SE, Joshi JP, Nahta R. Growth differentiation factor 15 stimulates rapamycin-sensitive ovarian cancer cell growth and invasion. Biochem Pharmacol. 2013;85(1):46–58. https://doi.org/10.1016/j.bcp.2012.10.007.

146. Li C, Wang J, Kong J, Tang J, Wu Y, Xu E, et al. GDF15 promotes EMT and metastasis in colorectal cancer. Oncotarget. 2016;7(1):860–72. https://doi.org/10.18632/oncotarget.6205.

147. Peake BF, Eze SM, Yang L, Castellino RC, Nahta R. Growth differentiation factor 15 mediates epithelial mesenchymal transition and invasion of breast cancers through IGF-1R-FoxM1 signaling. Oncotarget. 2017;8(55):94393–406. https://doi.org/10.18632/oncotarget.21765.

148. Wierstra I. The transcription factor FOXM1 (Forkhead box M1): proliferation-specific expression, transcription factor function, target genes, mouse models, and normal biological roles. Adv Cancer Res. 2013;118:97–398. https://doi.org/10.1016/B978-0-12-407173-5.00004-2.

149. Bektas N, Haaf A, Veeck J, Wild PJ, Luscher-Firzlaff J, Hartmann A, et al. Tight correlation between expression of the Forkhead transcription factor FOXM1 and HER2 in human breast cancer. BMC Cancer. 2008;8:42. https://doi.org/10.1186/1471-2407-8-42.

150. Carr JR, Park HJ, Wang Z, Kiefer MM, Raychaudhuri P. FoxM1 mediates resistance to herceptin and paclitaxel. Cancer Res. 2010;70(12):5054–63. https://doi.org/10.1158/0008-5472.CAN-10-0545.

151. Gayle SS, Castellino RC, Buss MC, Nahta R. MEK inhibition increases lapatinib sensitivity via modulation of FOXM1. Curr Med Chem. 2013;20(19):2486–99.

152. Francis RE, Myatt SS, Krol J, Hartman J, Peck B, McGovern UB, et al. FoxM1 is a downstream target and marker of HER2 overexpression in breast cancer. Int J Oncol. 2009;35(1):57–68.

153. Baselga J, Gelmon KA, Verma S, Wardley A, Conte P, Miles D, et al. Phase II trial of pertuzumab and trastuzumab in patients with human epidermal growth factor receptor 2-positive metastatic breast cancer that progressed during prior trastuzumab therapy. J Clin Oncol. 2010;28(7):1138–44. https://doi.org/10.1200/JCO.2009.24.2024. JCO.2009.24.2024 [pii].

154. Zhao F, Lam EW. Role of the forkhead transcription factor FOXO-FOXM1 axis in cancer and drug resistance. Front Med. 2012;6(4):376–80. https://doi.org/10.1007/s11684-012-0228-0.

155. Millour J, de Olano N, Horimoto Y, Monteiro LJ, Langer JK, Aligue R, et al. ATM and p53 regulate FOXM1 expression via E2F in breast cancer epirubicin treatment and resistance. Mol Cancer Ther. 2011;10(6):1046–58. https://doi.org/10.1158/1535-7163.MCT-11-0024.

156. Halasi M, Gartel AL. Suppression of FOXM1 sensitizes human cancer cells to cell death induced by DNA-damage. PLoS One. 2012;7(2):e31761. https://doi.org/10.1371/journal.pone.0031761.

157. Xue J, Lin X, Chiu WT, Chen YH, Yu G, Liu M, et al. Sustained activation of SMAD3/SMAD4 by FOXM1 promotes TGF-beta-dependent cancer metastasis. J Clin Invest. 2014;124(2):564–79. https://doi.org/10.1172/JCI71104.

158. Yang C, Chen H, Tan G, Gao W, Cheng L, Jiang X, et al. FOXM1 promotes the epithelial to mesenchymal transition by stimulating the transcription of Slug in human breast cancer. Cancer Lett. 2013;340(1):104–12. https://doi.org/10.1016/j.canlet.2013.07.004.

159. Cittelly DM, Das PM, Salvo VA, Fonseca JP, Burow ME, Jones FE. Oncogenic HER2{Delta}16 suppresses miR-15a/16 and deregulates BCL-2 to promote endocrine resistance of breast tumors. Carcinogenesis. 2010;31(12):2049–57. https://doi.org/10.1093/carcin/bgq192. bgq192 [pii].

160. Mitra D, Brumlik MJ, Okamgba SU, Zhu Y, Duplessis TT, Parvani JG, et al. An oncogenic isoform of HER2 associated with locally disseminated breast cancer and trastuzumab resistance. Mol Cancer Ther. 2009;8(8):2152–62. https://doi.org/10.1158/1535-7163.MCT-09-0295. 1535-7163.MCT-09-0295 [pii].

161. Siddiqa A, Long LM, Li L, Marciniak RA, Kazhdan I. Expression of HER-2 in MCF-7 breast cancer cells modulates anti-apoptotic proteins Survivin and Bcl-2 via the extracellular signal-related kinase (ERK) and phosphoinositide-3 kinase (PI3K) signalling pathways. BMC Cancer. 2008;8:129. https://doi.org/10.1186/1471-2407-8-129. 1471-2407-8-129 [pii].
162. Crawford A, Nahta R. Targeting Bcl-2 in herceptin-resistant breast cancer cell lines. Current Pharmacogenomics Person Med. 2011;9(3):184–90.
163. Martin AP, Mitchell C, Rahmani M, Nephew KP, Grant S, Dent P. Inhibition of MCL-1 enhances lapatinib toxicity and overcomes lapatinib resistance via BAK-dependent autophagy. Cancer Biol Ther. 2009;8(21):2084–96. 9895 [pii].
164. Witters LM, Witkoski A, Planas-Silva MD, Berger M, Viallet J, Lipton A. Synergistic inhibition of breast cancer cell lines with a dual inhibitor of EGFR-HER-2/neu and a Bcl-2 inhibitor. Oncol Rep. 2007;17(2):465–9.
165. Valabrega G, Capellero S, Cavalloni G, Zaccarello G, Petrelli A, Migliardi G, et al. HER2-positive breast cancer cells resistant to trastuzumab and lapatinib lose reliance upon HER2 and are sensitive to the multitargeted kinase inhibitor sorafenib. Breast Cancer Res Treat. 2011;130(1):29–40. https://doi.org/10.1007/s10549-010-1281-5.
166. Gojo I, Zhang B, Fenton RG. The cyclin-dependent kinase inhibitor flavopiridol induces apoptosis in multiple myeloma cells through transcriptional repression and down-regulation of Mcl-1. Clin Cancer Res. 2002;8(11):3527–38.
167. Mitchell C, Yacoub A, Hossein H, Martin AP, Bareford MD, Eulitt P, et al. Inhibition of MCL-1 in breast cancer cells promotes cell death in vitro and in vivo. Cancer Biol Ther. 2010;10(9):903–17. https://doi.org/10.4161/cbt.10.9.13273. 13273 [pii].
168. Scaltriti M, Rojo F, Ocana A, Anido J, Guzman M, Cortes J, et al. Expression of p95HER2, a truncated form of the HER2 receptor, and response to anti-HER2 therapies in breast cancer. J Natl Cancer Inst. 2007;99(8):628–38. https://doi.org/10.1093/jnci/djk134.
169. Anido J, Scaltriti M, Bech Serra JJ, Santiago Josefat B, Todo FR, Baselga J, et al. Biosynthesis of tumorigenic HER2 C-terminal fragments by alternative initiation of translation. EMBO J. 2006;25(13):3234–44. https://doi.org/10.1038/sj.emboj.7601191.
170. Pupa SM, Menard S, Morelli D, Pozzi B, De Palo G, Colnaghi MI. The extracellular domain of the c-erbB-2 oncoprotein is released from tumor cells by proteolytic cleavage. Oncogene. 1993;8(11):2917–23.
171. Xia W, Liu LH, Ho P, Spector NL. Truncated ErbB2 receptor (p95ErbB2) is regulated by heregulin through heterodimer formation with ErbB3 yet remains sensitive to the dual EGFR/ErbB2 kinase inhibitor GW572016. Oncogene. 2004;23(3):646–53. https://doi.org/10.1038/sj.onc.1207166.
172. Scaltriti M, Chandarlapaty S, Prudkin L, Aura C, Jimenez J, Angelini PD, et al. Clinical benefit of lapatinib-based therapy in patients with human epidermal growth factor receptor 2-positive breast tumors coexpressing the truncated p95HER2 receptor. Clin Cancer Res. 2010;16(9):2688–95. https://doi.org/10.1158/1078-0432.CCR-09-3407.
173. Sperinde J, Jin X, Banerjee J, Penuel E, Saha A, Diedrich G, et al. Quantitation of p95HER2 in paraffin sections by using a p95-specific antibody and correlation with outcome in a cohort of trastuzumab-treated breast cancer patients. Clin Cancer Res. 2010;16(16):4226–35. https://doi.org/10.1158/1078-0432.CCR-10-0410.
174. Vazquez-Martin A, Oliveras-Ferraros C, Cufi S, Del Barco S, Martin-Castillo B, Menendez JA. Lapatinib, a dual HER1/HER2 tyrosine kinase inhibitor, augments basal cleavage of HER2 extracellular domain (ECD) to inhibit HER2-driven cancer cell growth. J Cell Physiol. 2011;226(1):52–7. https://doi.org/10.1002/jcp.22333.
175. Wang T, Xu Y, Sheng S, Yuan H, Ouyang T, Li J, et al. HER2 somatic mutations are associated with poor survival in HER2-negative breast cancers. Cancer Sci. 2017;108(4):671–7. https://doi.org/10.1111/cas.13182.
176. Xu X, De Angelis C, Burke KA, Nardone A, Hu H, Qin L, et al. HER2 reactivation through acquisition of the HER2 L755S mutation as a mechanism of acquired resistance to HER2-targeted therapy in HER2(+) breast cancer. Clin Cancer Res. 2017;23(17):5123–34. https://doi.org/10.1158/1078-0432.CCR-16-2191.

Chapter 8
Emerging Novel Therapies in Overcoming Resistance to Targeted Therapy

Andreia V. Pinho, Jenny H. Lee, and Helen Rizos

Abstract The recent development of small molecule inhibitors and monoclonal antibodies that target cancer-specific oncogenic driver mutations has significantly improved the outcomes of patients with various tumour types including chronic myeloid leukemia, non-small cell lung cancer and melanoma. Despite high rates of response, most patients will relapse within the first year of targeted therapy due to drug resistance. Although multiple mechanisms of resistance have been defined, these often lead to the re-activation of oncogene-regulated signaling or the activation of compensatory survival cascades. This chapter focusses on emerging therapeutic strategies to overcome and circumvent resistance to targeted therapies, with an emphasis on metastatic melanoma. A variety of therapeutic salvage approaches are being explored, including novel targeted agents, new combination therapies and consideration of drug timing and sequencing. Improved clinical trial design, treatment of earlier stage cancer patients and sensitive real-time monitoring of patient responses and resistance are critical for improving the durability of cancer targeted therapies.

Keywords Targeted therapies · Melanoma · Cancer therapy resistance · Receptor tyrosine kinases · Immune checkpoint blockade therapy · Non-small cell lung cancer

A. V. Pinho · J. H. Lee · H. Rizos (✉)
Faculty of Medicine and Health Sciences, Macquarie University, Sydney, NSW, Australia

Melanoma Institute Australia, Sydney, NSW, Australia
e-mail: andreia.pinho@mq.edu.au; jenny.lee@mq.edu.au; helen.rizos@mq.edu.au

© Springer Nature Switzerland AG 2019
M. R. Szewczuk et al. (eds.), *Current Applications for Overcoming Resistance to Targeted Therapies*, Resistance to Targeted Anti-Cancer Therapeutics 20,
https://doi.org/10.1007/978-3-030-21477-7_8

223

Abbreviations

ALK	Anaplastic lymphoma kinase
CI	Confidence interval
CML	Chronic myeloid leukemia
CTLA4	Cytotoxic T-lymphocyte-associated protein 4
EGFR	Epidermal growth factor receptor
FDA	Food and drug administration
GIST	Gastrointestinal stromal tumors
HR	Hazard ratio
IGF1R	Insulin-like growth factor 1 receptor
MAPK	Mitogen-activated protein kinase
MITF	Microphthalmia-associated transcription factor
mTOR	Mammalian target of rapamycin
NF1	Neurofibromin 1
NSCLC	Non-small cell lung cancer
OS	Overall survival
PD-1	Programmed cell death protein 1
PDGFR	Platelet-derived growth factor receptor
PFS	Progression-free survival
PI3K	Phosphoinositide 3-kinase
PTEN	Phosphatase and tensin homologue
RECIST	Response evaluation criteria in solid tumors
RTK	Receptor tyrosine kinase
TK	Tyrosine kinase
TKR	Tyrosine kinase receptor

8.1 Introduction

In the past two decades, the development of molecular targeted therapies has revolutionized the treatment of cancer. These personalized therapies, which are often small molecule inhibitors or monoclonal antibodies, target cancer-specific proteins that are critical for the proliferation and survival of tumor cells [1]. The rationale behind targeted molecular therapies is the continued dependence of cancer cells on a single driver oncogene, a phenomenon known as 'oncogene addiction' [2]. This continued requirement for a single driver mutation occurs even though most common solid tumors carry an average of 33–66 protein-altering mutations and up to 200 non-synonymous mutations in highly mutated tumors such as melanoma and lung cancer [3]. Many of these additional mutations are passenger mutations that confer no selective advantage on the neoplastic process.

Molecular therapies have led to significant improvements in patient outcomes, including in tumor types with no previous effective systemic treatments. These therapies include selective inhibitors of the epidermal growth factor (EGFR) in

EGFR-mutant non-small cell lung cancer (NSCLC) [4–6] and the BRAF kinase in BRAF^{V600}-mutant metastatic melanoma [7, 8]. Despite high response rates, most patients will progress within the first year of treatment with targeted therapies. This chapter explores mechanisms of acquired resistance to molecular therapies and describes novel therapeutic approaches to overcome and circumvent resistance, with a particular focus on resistance to selective BRAF inhibitors in BRAF^{V600}-mutant melanoma.

8.2   Targeted Therapies in Cancer

8.2.1   Inhibition of the BCR-ABL Tyrosine Kinase

The tyrosine-kinase (TK) inhibitor imatinib was the first targeted therapy to be approved by the United States Food and Drug Administration (FDA) for clinical use in patients with chronic myeloid leukemia (CML) [9]. CML is driven by the *BCR-ABL* mutant oncogene, produced via a chromosome translocation involving chromosomes 9 and 22. This Philadelphia translocation or chromosome (designated t(9;22)/(q34;q11)) results in the fusion of the *BCR* gene on chromosome band 22q11.2 to the *ABL* gene on chromosome band 9q34.1, to create the constitutively active hybrid BCR-ABL tyrosine kinase [10]. Imatinib selectively inhibits BCR-ABL, and first-line therapy with imatinib induced durable responses in CML patients, with an overall survival (OS) of 89% and a median follow-up of 60 months [11].

Imatinib also targets the TK activity of platelet-derived growth factor receptor (PDGFR) and c-KIT, a stem cell growth factor receptor. Approximately, 70–80% of gastrointestinal stromal tumors (GIST) harbor c-KIT activating mutations and an additional 5–8% have activating mutations in the kinase PDGFRα subunit [12]. Phase III clinical studies have shown that imatinib can achieve disease control in 70–85% of GIST patients with a median progression-free survival (PFS) of 20–24 months [12–15].

8.2.2   Inhibition of the EGFR Family of Receptor Tyrosine Kinases

EGFR belongs to the ERBB/HER family of receptor tyrosine kinases (RTKs) and is frequently mutated and overexpressed in different types of human cancers [16]. Activating mutations in EGFR are present in 10–20% of NSCLC patients, conferring sensitivity to the EGFR inhibitors gefitinib and erlotinib [6, 17]. Compared to chemotherapy alone, both gefitinib and erlotinib have shown significant benefits in response and PFS as first-line treatment for EGFR-mutant NSCLC (i.e. median

PFS 9.7 months for erlotinib vs. 5.2 months for standard chemotherapy) [5, 6]. The EGFR-inhibitory antibodies cetuximab and panitumumab are also FDA-approved for the treatment of KRAS wild-type colorectal cancer patients [18, 19].

The EGFR homolog ERBB2/HER2 is overexpressed in 20–25% of all breast cancers, and patients with HER2+ breast cancer are treated with HER2 inhibitors, including the monoclonal antibodies trastuzumab and pertuzumab, the TK inhibitor lapatinib and the antibody-drug conjugate trastuzumab-DM1 [20–23]. A Phase III study of HER2+ early breast cancer patients, with a median follow-up of 11 years, showed that 1 year of trastuzumab therapy after adjuvant chemotherapy improved long-term disease-free survival, compared to the observation group (Hazard Ratio (HR) 0.76, 95% confidence interval (CI) 0.68–0.86)) [24]. Trastuzumab is also used to treat HER2+ metastatic gastric and gastroesophageal junction cancer, and HER2 inhibition in combination with chemotherapy increased the median OS to 13.8 months, compared to 11.1 months for chemotherapy alone [25].

8.2.3 Inhibiting ALK and ROS Rearrangements in NSCLC

A subset of NSCLCs is driven by rearrangements involving the anaplastic lymphoma kinase (*ALK*) gene or the receptor tyrosine kinase gene *ROS1*. Treatment of patients with locally advanced or metastatic ALK-positive NSCLC with the TK inhibitor crizotinib increased the response rate to 65%, compared to 20% with chemotherapy [26]. Crizotinib also showed marked antitumor activity in patients with advanced ROS1-rearranged NSCLC with an objective response rate of 72% [27].

8.2.4 Inhibition of BRAF^{V600} in Metastatic Melanoma

Mutations that constitutively activate the BRAF kinase occur in around 50% of cutaneous melanomas (Fig. 8.1). The most prevalent mutation affects valine 600 and leads to V600E, and less frequently to the V600K/R/D missense mutations [28, 29]. The selective BRAF^{V600} inhibitors vemurafenib, dabrafenib and second-generation inhibitor encorafenib improve the PFS and OS of patients with advanced BRAF^{V600}-mutant melanoma [7, 30, 31]. In particular, vemurafenib resulted in a median PFS of 6.9 months and a median OS of 13.6 months compared to a PFS of 1.6 months and an OS of 9.7 months for dacarbazine [30]. Similarly, treatment of BRAF^{V600}-mutant metastatic melanoma patients with the BRAF inhibitor dabrafenib led to a PFS of 5.1 months compared to 2.7 months for dacarbazine [8]. Encorafenib has shown superior activity compared to vemurafenib in BRAF^{V600}-mutant metastatic melanoma with a PFS of 9.6 months for encorafenib monotherapy, compared to 7.3 months in vemurafenib monotherapy [32].

The combination of selective BRAF inhibitors with inhibitors of the downstream BRAF effector kinases MEK1/2 are currently the standard of care for patients with

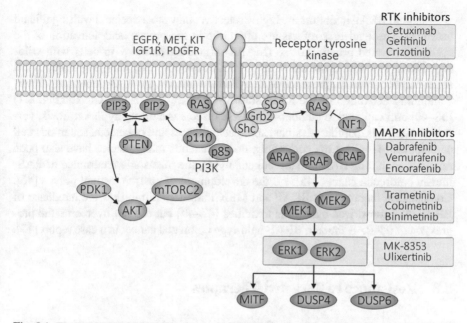

Fig. 8.1 The MAPK and PI3K signaling networks. Receptor tyrosine kinase signaling induces activation and membrane localization of the RAS GTPase which induces the activation of mitogen-activated protein kinase (MAPK) and phosphoinositide 3-kinase (PI3K) pathways. MAPK activation involves dimerization of the ARAF, BRAF and CRAF kinase homologues. These RAF proteins bind to and phosphorylate downstream kinases MEK1 and MEK2, which subsequently phosphorylate and activate the downstream effector kinases, ERK1 and ERK2. ERK regulates multiple proteins including the transcription of the microphthalmia-associated transcription factor (MITF) and the MAPK negative regulator phosphatases, DUSP4 and DUSP6. Activated PI3K (complex of p110 and p85 subunits) phosphorylates phospholipid phosphatidylinositol-4,5-bisphosphate (PIP2) forming phosphatidyl-3,4,5-trisphosphate (PIP3) at the plasma membrane. AKT is one of the major downstream effectors of PI3K, and it undergoes complete activation upon phosphorylation by PDK1 and by the mammalian target of rapamycin (mTOR) complex 2 (mTORC2). Active AKT phosphorylates over 100 different substrates, many shared with the ERK signaling cascade (MNK, MYC, TCF, RSK, BAD, rS6, eIF4E). The phosphatase and tensin homologue (PTEN) inhibits PI3K signaling and AKT activity by dephosphorylating PIP3 into PIP2. Example RTKs, MAPK and RTK inhibitors are also shown. *EGFR* epidermal growth factor receptor, *PDGFR* platelet-derived growth factor receptor, *IGF1R* insulin-like growth factor 1 receptor

advanced BRAF^{V600}-mutant melanoma. Several allosteric MEK inhibitors have been developed, including trametinib, binimetinib and cobimetinib (reviewed in [33]). Melanoma patient outcomes are consistently improved with combination therapy compared to BRAF inhibitor monotherapy. For instance, the risk of death was reduced with combination dabrafenib plus trametinib vs. dabrafenib alone (HR 0.63; 95% CI, 0.42–0.94) [34], and encorafenib plus binimetinib vs. vemurafenib alone (HR 0.61; 95% CI, 0.47–0.79) [35]. Despite consistent improvements in the response of patients to combination BRAF and MEK inhibitors, the effects are short-lived and, within a year, the majority of patients develop resistance to these targeted therapies [36].

Although BRAF inhibitors are highly selective, they are associated with significant toxicities. These adverse effects are often due to the paradoxical activation of the mitogen-activated protein kinase (MAPK) signaling pathway in cells with wild-type BRAF and with upstream RAS or RTK activation (Fig. 8.1) [37]. Paradoxical activation occurs in the presence of BRAF inhibitors via the RAS-dependent dimerization and activation of the RAF isoforms, ARAF, BRAF and CRAF (Fig. 8.1) [38–40] and can lead to cutaneous adverse effects including hyperkeratosis, verrucous keratosis, papillary lesions, keratoacanthomas and cutaneous squamous cell carcinomas [41–43]. Less commonly, non-cutaneous malignancies have also been reported, including RAS-mutant leukemia [44], the metastatic recurrence of RAS-mutant colorectal cancer [45] and the development of gastrointestinal polyps [46]. Combination therapy with BRAF and MEK inhibitors diminishes the incidence of BRAF inhibitor-driven cutaneous toxicities [47–49] but did not overcome the progression of a KRAS-mutant, BRAF-wild-type colorectal cancer in a case report [45].

8.3 Resistance to Targeted Therapies

Response to targeted therapies is often associated with intra-patient and inter-patient heterogeneity, and there is substantial variability in the kinetics of response for individual metastases within each patient [37]. Similarly, resistance to therapy is also heterogeneous, and the proportion of metastases progressing in an individual can range from 6 to 100% [50]. Recent modelling predicts that radiographically detectable lesions harbor at least ten resistant sub-clones [51], and thus resistance is thought to arise via the selection and expansion of small populations (sub-clones) of tumor cells with pre-existing alterations that confer treatment resistance [37]. Thus, the concepts of intrinsic resistance, where a patient fails to respond to therapy from the onset of treatment, and acquired resistance where a patient initially responds but ultimately progresses on treatment [33], may reflect the size and number of the pre-existing resistant tumor sub-clones. It is also worth noting that the efficacy of combination therapies will depend on whether single mutations confer resistance to the combination of drugs [52].

In metastatic melanoma patients, approximately 50% of patients with BRAF^{V600}-mutant melanoma show intrinsic resistance and do not meet RECIST[1] criteria [53] for response to BRAF inhibitor monotherapy. For the 50% of melanoma patients who initially respond to BRAF inhibition, almost all will eventually acquire resistance, with 50% of patients progressing within 6–8 months of treatment with vemurafenib

---

[1] Response evaluation criteria in solid tumors (RECIST) is a set of guidelines used in the assessment of the change in tumor burden. It recommends evaluation of a maximum of five lesions (maximum two per organ) as target lesions. In addition, a pathological lymph node requires a short axis diameter of ≥ 15 mm to be assessable as target lesion. A complete response (CR) is disappearance of all target lesions or reduction of lymph node short axis to <10 mm, partial response (PR) is at least 30% decrease in the sum of diameters of target lesions and progressive disease (PD) is at least a 20% increase in the sum of diameters of target lesions or the appearance of new lesions and an absolute increase of at least 5 mm. Stable disease is defined as neither PR or PD.

or dabrafenib [7, 8, 49]. The use of combination BRAF and MEK inhibitors has improved response rates to 69% of patients with BRAF^{V600}-mutant melanoma and delayed progression by almost 3 months [49], but this combination therapy will eventually fail in most patients [54].

Resistance to targeted therapies is common in most cancer types, and although diverse resistance mechanisms have been defined, these can be classified into three categories:

1. Secondary alterations within the drug target;
2. Re-activation of oncogene-regulated signaling; and
3. Activation of alternative, compensatory signaling pathways [55].

In the case of BRAF^{V600}-mutant melanoma, progression on BRAF inhibitor monotherapy or combination BRAF and MEK inhibitor treatment predominantly reactivates the MAPK signaling cascade [56–58]. Resistance mechanisms that are independent of MAPK signaling account for only 11% of all identified genetic resistance mechanisms [56]. Resistant pathways can be activated by genomic alterations or via non-genomic mechanisms that reprogram the transcriptome and methylome [59]. A summary of the multiple mechanisms of resistance to BRAF and MEK inhibitors in BRAF^{V600}-mutant melanoma is detailed in Table 8.1.

8.3.1 Secondary Alterations Within the Drug Target

Resistance to small molecule kinase inhibitors, such as imatinib in CML and EGFR inhibitors in NSCLC are commonly associated with the acquisition of mutations in the target RTK which prevent drug binding. Mutations affecting a small gatekeeper residue within the ATP-binding domain of RTKs are the most frequent clinical resistance mutations in BCR-ABL, c-KIT, PDGFRß and EGFR [60]. Resistance to BRAF inhibitors is more complicated than the other inhibitors. Although missense mutations that diminish drug binding have not been detected, alterations affecting mutant BRAF are common in resistance. For instance, amplification of the mutant *BRAF* allele occurs in 8–36% of melanomas resistant to BRAF or BRAF/MEK inhibitors [57, 58, 61]. Further, alternate splicing of mutant BRAF leads to BRAF^{V600} variants that lack the C-terminal RAS-binding domain and are prone to forming homodimers which have diminished affinity for BRAF inhibitors [39, 57, 61, 62].

8.3.2 Re-activation of Oncogene-Regulated Signaling

One of the most common downstream effector pathways of oncogenic RTK signaling is the MAPK cascade, which promotes cell proliferation, survival, migration and angiogenesis [37]. Resistance to BRAF and MEK inhibitors in melanoma frequently involves re-activation of MAPK signaling via distinct mechanisms including:

Table 8.1 Mechanisms of acquired resistance to BRAF and MEK inhibitor therapies in BRAF[V600]-mutant melanoma

Mechanism	Type of alteration	References
Secondary alterations within the drug target		
MAPK re-activation	*BRAF* gene amplification	[57, 58, 61]
	BRAF alternative splicing	[39, 57, 61, 62]
Re-activation of oncogene-regulated signaling		
MAPK re-activation	CRAF, ARAF overexpression	[63, 64]
	NRAS activating mutations	[56, 57, 65]
	MEK1/2 activating mutations	[56, 58, 66]
	RTK overexpression (IGF1R, MET, PDGFRβ, EGFR)	[59, 60, 63, 67, 68]
	Overexpression of alternative kinases COT and PAKs	[69, 70]
	Inhibition of negative feedback regulators DUSP4 and DUSP6 (through *STAG2/3* mutation)	[59, 71]
	Loss of function mutations in RAS negative regulator *NF1*	[72]
Activation of alternative, compensatory signaling pathways		
PI3K/AKT signaling	*NRAS, KRAS* activating mutations	[56, 65]
	RTK overexpression (IGF1R, MET, PDGFRβ, EGFR)	[59, 60, 63, 67, 68]
	AKT1/3 activating mutations	[56, 65]
	PIK3CA and PIK3CG activating mutations	[65]
	Loss of function mutations in negative regulatory genes *PTEN, PIK3R2, PHLPP1*	[65]
Alterations in cell differentiation state	Dysregulation of the regulator of differentiation MITF	[81, 82, 88, 89]
Epigenetic mechanisms	Aberrant methylation of MET and LEF1	[59]
Immune escape	Overexpression of immune checkpoint regulator PD-L1	[91, 92]

  i. The overexpression of BRAF homologues CRAF and ARAF, which enables a switch in RAF isoform usage within the MAPK cascade [63, 64].

 ii. Activating mutations in NRAS, the upstream MAPK regulator. NRAS mutations occur in approximately 30% of BRAF[V600]-mutant melanomas with acquired resistance to BRAF and MEK inhibitors [56, 57, 65].

iii. Mutational activation of the BRAF effector kinases, MEK1 and MEK2, occur in approximately 7% of BRAF inhibitor-resistant and 27% of BRAF/MEK inhibitor-resistant melanomas [56, 58]. Many of these mutations lead to increased RAF-independent MEK kinase activity and reactivation of MAPK signaling [33]. Preexisting MEK1[P124]-mutations also diminish the response to BRAF inhibitor therapy [66].

 iv. Overexpression of upstream RTKs, including IGF1R, MET, PDGFRß, EGFR [59, 60, 63, 67, 68].

  v. Overexpression of alternate kinases, including MAP3K8/Cancer Osaka Thyroid (COT) kinase and p21-activated serine/threonine kinases (PAKs), occurs in a small subset of melanoma tissues from patients who have progressed on BRAF inhibitor therapy [69, 70].

  vi. Direct and indirect inhibition of negative feedback regulators of MAPK signaling. For instance, loss of function mutations in the ERK phosphatase DUSP4 and downregulation of the homologue DUSP6 via loss of cohesin complex components STAG2 and STAG3 promote MAPK reactivation [59, 71].

  vii. Loss of function mutations in the RAS inhibitor neurofibromin 1 (NF1) can also activate the upstream regulator RAS, driving resistance to BRAF inhibitor through activation of CRAF [72].

Similarly, activating mutations and gene amplifications in MAPK pathway genes, including BRAF and RAS, have also been found in colorectal cancer and NSCLC patients who developed resistance to EGFR-targeted therapies (reviewed in [73, 74]).

8.3.3   Activation of Alternative Compensatory Signaling Pathways

Compensatory activation of alternate signaling pathways has also been shown to contribute to targeted therapy resistance. In particular, the activation of the phosphoinositide 3-kinase (PI3K) pathway (Fig. 8.1) may contribute to BRAF inhibitor resistance in approximately 20% of $BRAF^{V600}$-mutant melanomas. PI3K activation is associated with gain of function NRAS and KRAS mutations [56, 65] and upregulation of RTKs, including PDGFRβ, EGFR, IGF1R and MET [59, 60, 63, 67, 68]. An additional 4% of BRAF inhibitor-resistant melanomas display genetic alterations, including oncogenic AKT1/3 mutations, loss of function PTEN mutations and putative functional mutations in other PI3K regulatory genes (i.e. *PIK3CA*, *PIK3CG*, *PHLPP1* and *PIK3R2*) that activate only the PI3K/AKT network [65]. Recent data suggest that acquired activation of PI3K signaling does not enable melanoma proliferative capacity in response to combination BRAF and MEK inhibition, but instead permits the survival of tumor subclones and the selection of MAPK activating mutations [75].

Induction of additional signaling pathways via the amplification or upregulation of alternative RTKs is also common in tumors that develop resistance to EGFR, HER2 and ALK-targeted therapies (reviewed in [55]). For instance, activation of HER2 and HER3 is frequent in NSCLC that develop resistance to both EGFR and ALK-targeted therapies [74, 76]. Another example is the amplification of MET in NSCLC tumors that have developed resistance to EGFR-targeted therapies [77]. Mutations in members of the PI3K pathway, including PIK3CA and PTEN, have also been found in EGFR-amplified colorectal cancer, EGFR-mutant NSCLC and HER2-amplified breast cancer (reviewed in [73, 74, 78]).

Alterations in genes that regulate the cell differentiation state of tumor cells are also associated with the development of resistance to targeted therapies. Slow-cycling tumor cells have been described as an important determinant of resistance to chemotherapies, targeted therapies and immunotherapies [79]. In melanoma, downregulation of the microphthalmia-associated transcription factor (MITF), a regulator of differentiation [80], is predictive of a slow-cycling, dedifferentiated and invasive phenotype which is highly resistant to BRAF/MEK inhibitors [81, 82]. This phenotype displays activation of multiple cascades, including the concurrent upregulation of several RTKs, including AXL, EGFR and PDGRFß, activation of MAPK, PI3K and WNT signaling and may involve overexpression of the chromatin-remodelling factor JARID1B [79, 81–84]. Interestingly, ectopically expressed MITF is also associated with BRAF inhibitor resistance in a subset of melanomas. The MAPK pathway tightly regulates MITF expression, and oncogenic BRAF signaling promotes MITF transcription in melanoma (Fig. 8.1) [85]. The accumulation of MITF promotes the expression of anti-apoptotic genes including *BCL2A1* and *BCL2* and cooperates with oncogenic BRAF to transform melanocytes [86, 87]. Thus, *MITF* gene amplification can confer BRAF inhibitor resistance, and this can occur in the presence of sustained MAPK inhibition [88, 89]. A recent study has shown that constitutively activation of the Aryl hydrocarbon Receptor (AhR) transcription factor also promotes a dedifferentiated phenotype in melanoma cells leading to resistance to BRAF inhibitor therapy [90].

Resistance to targeted therapies can also be driven by non-genomic mechanisms of tumor escape, including epigenetic and immune mechanisms. An integrated transcriptome-methylome analysis of melanoma tumors that progressed on targeted therapy with BRAF/MEK inhibitors has found aberrant methylation of CpG sites within tumor cells leading to the altered expression of drivers of acquired resistance that include MET up-regulation, LEF1 down-regulation and YAP1 pathway signature enrichment [59]. The authors also found recurrent transcriptional changes in multiple immune pathways suggesting that, in a subset of patients, immune evasion due to loss of antigen presentation and T-cell deficiency/exhaustion co-evolve with the acquisition of MAPK inhibitor resistance [59].

Studies regarding immune mechanisms of resistance to targeted therapies have shown that tumors with resistance to BRAF inhibitors upregulate the expression of programmed cell death protein-ligand 1 (PD-L1) [91, 92], an immunosuppressive ligand that binds to the immune checkpoint receptor programmed cell death protein 1 (PD-1). PD-1 is expressed by both B- and T-cells and is induced by interferon-γ stimulation, leading to suppression of immune activity. Additional studies have found that expression of PD-L1 by tumor cells and tumor-infiltrating lymphocytes are altered in patients that develop resistance to MAPK inhibitor therapies, and this is dependent on the expression of PD-L1 in tumors before treatment [93]. It has also been demonstrated that immune cell infiltration is not sufficient for tumor response to MAPK inhibitors although immune escape is common in resistance to these targeted therapies [94].

Likewise, activation of the PD-1/PD-L1 immune checkpoint has been shown to contribute to immune escape in other tumor types, including EGFR-mutant [95] and ALK-rearranged [96] NSCLC. Increased expression of PD-L1 has been associated to resistance to EGFR-targeted therapies in NSCLC patients [97] and PD-L1 was shown to confer resistance to EGFR-targeted therapy in NSCLC cells via upregulation of YAP1 expression [98]. In contrast, EGFR inhibitor-resistant cells that have undergone epithelial-to-mesenchymal transition, an established mechanism of resistance [99], showed reduced expression of PD-L1 [100], suggesting that the contribution of PD-L1 to targeted therapy resistance is cell context-dependent.

8.4   Emerging Therapies to Overcome Resistance to Targeted Therapy

Short-lived patient responses to targeted therapies have led to intensive research into novel combination therapies that could circumvent or overcome the development of treatment resistance. The combination of BRAF and MEK inhibitors in patients with advanced $BRAF^{V600}$-mutant melanoma delays drug resistance by a few months, reduces paradoxical MAPK pathway activation and associated skin toxicities and prolongs patient survival compared to BRAF inhibitor monotherapy [34]. Although combination BRAF and MEK inhibition is the current standard of care for patients with $BRAF^{V600}$-mutant metastatic melanoma, 50% of patients treated with this combination therapy relapse within the first 10 months of treatment [58, 101].

Our increasing knowledge of the mechanisms of acquired resistance offers a number of second-line therapeutic opportunities for patients who relapse on combination BRAF/MEK inhibition.

8.4.1   Intermittent Drug Dosing

Preclinical modelling of BRAF inhibitor resistance in melanoma revealed that abnormally elevated MAPK signaling can become a fitness deficit for a tumor and may become lethal in the absence of the drug. As a result, the intermittent dosing of BRAF inhibitors promoted the rapid regression of vemurafenib-resistant melanoma (with $BRAF^{V600E}$ amplification) in mice and significantly delayed the onset of resistance in primary human xenografts. The underlying mechanism of drug dependency is thought to reflect the level of MAPK activity, that becomes toxic in the absence of the dampening effect of BRAF inhibitors [102].

The potential efficacy of intermittent dosing was shown in a BRAF-mutant melanoma patient who developed NRAS-mutant leukemia while on a BRAF inhibitor. When the drug was discontinued, the melanoma regressed while the leukemia continued to expand [44]. Furthermore, a multi-institutional retrospective study confirmed that almost 40% of melanoma patients who discontinued BRAF inhibitor-based therapy after progression, responded to rechallenge therapy with combination BRAF/MEK inhibitors [103]. In another report, however, discontinuation of BRAF inhibitor-based treatment in two $BRAF^{V600}$ melanoma patients led to accelerated disease progression [104]. The potential benefits of intermittent BRAF/MEK inhibitor dosing in melanoma are currently being investigated in a randomized phase II clinical trial, comparing continuous drug treatment after an 8-week lead-in period to an intermittent drug schedule (5 weeks on, 3 weeks off; NCT02196181). In another phase II clinical trial, 21.4% of RAS/BRAF wild-type metastatic colorectal cancer patients progressing on EGFR-targeting antibody cetuximab plus irinotecan, responded to drug rechallenge after second-line oxaliplatin and bevacizumab treatment (NCT02296203) [105].

8.4.2   Next Generation Inhibitors

Next generation BRAF inhibitors, dubbed "paradox breakers", that selectively inhibit mutant BRAF, while preventing BRAF-CRAF dimerization and the concomitant paradoxical activation of MAPK activity have been developed. The inhibitors CCT196969 and CCT241161 are paradox breaker pan-RAF inhibitors that inhibit both BRAF and CRAF, as well as SRC kinases, and are active against both BRAF-mutant and NRAS-mutant melanomas. These inhibitors have been able to inhibit the growth of melanomas that had developed resistance to vemurafenib and dabrafenib/trametinib combination treatment [106]. The paradox breakers PLX8394 and PLX7904 also inhibited the growth of vemurafenib-resistant melanoma cells in pre-clinical studies, overcoming mechanisms of resistance to first-generation RAF inhibitors, such as dimerization-mediated resistance and secondary NRAS mutations [107, 108]. An ongoing early phase clinical trial is testing the use of PLX8394 in refractory solid tumors, in combination with cobicistat, an inhibitor of cytochrome P450 3A (CYP3A) used to enhance PLX8394 exposure (NCT02428712). In a phase I clinical trial, three BRAF^{V600}-mutant patients (23%) (colorectal cancer, glioma and ovarian) have shown partial responses, and in a phase II trial, three patients (30%) had stable disease [109].

Traditional allosteric MEK inhibitors such as trametinib, cobimetinib and binimetinib bind at a site outside the MEK1/2 ATP-binding pocket and modulate kinase activity in an allosteric manner [110]. The next generation MEK inhibitors E6201 and MAP855 function by competing for ATP binding to MEK1/2, and have shown activity in melanoma cells with MEK1/2 mutations that confer resistance to the traditional allosteric MEK inhibitors like trametinib [111, 112]. The ATP-competitive MEK inhibitor E6201 has been tested in early-stage clinical trials on patients with advanced solid tumors [113] and is presently being evaluated in melanoma patients with central nervous system metastases (NCT03332589).

It is important to note that there are currently no FDA-approved targeted therapies that can overcome resistance to the first-line combination of BRAF and MEK inhibitors in BRAF^{V600} mutant melanoma. However, this is not the case for other cancer types, and a summary of FDA-approved targeted therapies used to overcome resistance is summarized in Table 8.2.

Inhibitors that target "gatekeeper" mutations in RTKs have also been developed. The BCR-ABL inhibitor ponatinib has shown anti-leukemic activity in CML patients carrying the "gatekeeper" T315I mutation, with 70% of patients with the

Table 8.2 Overcoming secondary resistance to targeted therapy by targeting acquired mutations or bypass pathway activation

Cancer type	Oncogenic mutation or overexpression	Pathway involved	Therapeutic options	Response rate/PFS	Resistance mechanism	FDA-approved targeted therapy to overcome resistance	Response rate/PFS	References
Breast cancer	HER2 amplification or overexpression	MAPK, PI3K/AKT	Trastuzumab Lapatinib	50%/7.4 months 24%/28.4 weeks	Altered receptor-antibody interaction or further activation of downstream pathways[a]	Trastuzumab-emtansine (TDM-1)	43.6%/9.6 months	[20, 23, 197, 198]
CML	BCR-ABL1 fusion gene	MAPK, JAK/STAT, PI3K/AKT	Imatinib Dasatinib	CCR rate 66%[b] 77%[b]	Resistant BCR-ABL gene mutation or amplification BCR-ABL T315I	Nilotinib Ponatinib	CCR rate 31%[b]	[199–202]
GIST	c-KIT mutation	SCF/c-KIT	Imatinib	53.7%[b]	Mutations in the ATP-binding site (exons 13/14) or activation loop (exons 17/18)	Sunitinib	34-58%/5.1–19.4 months	[15, 203]
NSCLC	EGFR exon 19 deletions or exon 21 (L858R) substitution	MAPK, PI3K/AKT, and PLC-γ1-PKC	Gefitinib Erlotinib	74%/10.8 months 78%/9.4 months	EGFR T790M[c] Other mechanisms: MET or HER2 amplification, EMT, PIK3CA mutation	Osimertinib	71%/10.1 months	[4, 6, 116, 204]
	ALK rearrangement	JAK/STAT, PI3K/AKT	Crizotinib	74%/10.9 months	Secondary mutations within ALK-TK domain, EMLA4-ALK amplification, alternative signaling pathways[d]	Alectinib Ceritinib	48%[b] 56%[b]	[205–209]

(continued)

Table 8.2 (continued)

Cancer type	Oncogenic mutation or overexpression	Pathway involved	Therapeutic options	Response rate/PFS	Resistance mechanism	FDA-approved targeted therapy to overcome resistance	Response rate/PFS	References
Renal cell carcinoma	*VHL* gene mutation or silencing	VHL/HIF/VEGF	Sunitinib Pazopanib	24%/9.5 months 31%/8.4 months	Restoration of angiogenesis through the activation of VEGF independent pathways	Cabozantinib Everolimus	17%/7.4 months 3%/3.9 months	[210–212]

ALK anaplastic lymphoma kinase, *ATP* adenosine triphosphate, *BCR-ABL1* Breakpoint cluster region-Abelson 1, *CCR* complete cytological response, *EGFR* Epidermal growth factor receptor, *EMT* Epithelial-mesenchymal transition, *HIF* Hypoxia-inducible factor, *HER2* Human epidermal growth factor receptor 2, *JAK* Janus kinase, *MAPK* Mitogen-activated protein kinase, *PI3K* Phosphoinositide 3-kinase, *PKC* Protein kinase C, *PLC-γ1* Phospholipase C-γ1, *SCF* Stem cell factor, *STAT* Signal Transducer and Activator of Transcription, *TK* tyrosine kinase, *VHL* Von-Hippel-Lindau, *VEGF* Vascular endothelial growth factor

[a]Activation of downstream pathways occurs by increasing signaling from other members of the HER family or other receptors or constitutive activation of downstream elements

[b]Progression-free survival not reported

[c]Mutation confirmation is required in the clinical setting to access second-generation targeted therapy following failure of initial therapy

[d]Alternative signaling pathways include EGFR, c-KIT, KRAS, IGF1R

T315I mutation showing cytogenetic response [114], and this has led to its accelerated approval by the FDA [115]. The EGFR inhibitors osimertinib, WZ4002 and rociletinib are next-generation drugs that can irreversibly inhibit the gatekeeper mutation EGRF^{T790M} [74]. Furthermore, osimertinib has demonstrated superior efficacy compared to platinum-based chemotherapy in a phase III trial in NSCLC patients with the acquired resistance mutation EGFR^{T790M} [116] (Table 8.2).

Sym004, a mixture of the antibodies futuximab and modotuximab that bind to nonoverlapping epitopes of the EGFR extracellular domain, has also recently been tested in a phase II randomized clinical trial in colorectal cancer patients with acquired resistance to anti-EGFR therapy. Sym004 treatment did not improve OS in an unselected patient population, when compared with investigators' treatment of choice, but showed an improvement in OS of patients that were triple-negative for RAS, BRAF and EGFR-extracellular domain mutations [117].

8.4.3 Novel Combination Inhibitors Targeting MAPK Signaling

Combination drugs targeting oncogenic pathways have led to improved patient responses and survival compared to single-agent therapies. However, acquired resistance remains a significant limitation to combination therapies, presumably because single mutations confer resistance to the combination of drugs. For instance, mutations activating NRAS or MEK1/2, and BRAF copy number gains can promote resistance to single-agent BRAF inhibitors, MEK inhibitor monotherapy and combination BRAF/MEK inhibitors in melanoma [58]. There is interest in the inhibition of the downstream MAP kinase, ERK (extracellular signal-regulated kinase), and several inhibitors of ERK are currently being developed. Preclinical studies have confirmed that ERK inhibitors exhibit activity in *in vitro* and *in vivo* models of BRAF and MEK inhibitor resistance [118–120]. In preclinical models of colorectal cancer resistant to BRAF, EGFR and MEK inhibitors, ERK inhibition, in combination with BRAF and EGFR inhibition, led to decreased cell growth *in vitro* and to tumor regression *in vivo* [121]. In early phase clinical trials, the ERK inhibitor MK-8353 was well tolerated and exhibited antitumor activity in patients with BRAF^{V600}-mutant melanoma [122]. Similarly, the ERK inhibitor ulixertinib had an acceptable safety profile and exhibited clinical activity in NRAS and BRAF^{V600} and non-V600-mutant BRAF solid-tumour malignancies in a phase I clinical trial [123]. Further clinical trials will be required to determine the efficacy of ERK inhibitors in combination with BRAF or MEK inhibitors.

An alternative strategy to inhibit MAPK signaling involves targeting chaperone proteins. The Heat Shock Protein 90 (HSP90) is an adenosine triphosphate (ATP)–dependent molecular chaperone that has a critical role in the folding, aggregation and stability of many client proteins, including the oncoproteins AKT, MEK, MET, BRAF, CRAF and EGFR [124, 125]. Cancer cells are often more dependent on

HSP90 activity as mutant oncoproteins can be misfolded and require HSP90-mediated correction. Thus, several HSP90 inhibitors have been developed and these show activity in preclinical models of cancer with alterations affecting EGFR, ALK, KRAS, MET and BRAF (reviewed in [124]). This class of drugs was first tested in phase I trials in 1999, and the results in unselected patients have been generally disappointing. The focus of new clinical trials involves the rational combination of HSP90 inhibitors in distinct cancer molecular subtypes, including combination with BRAF and MEK inhibitors in BRAF^{V600}-mutant melanoma [126] (NCT02097225, NCT02721459).

Another important MAPK scaffolding protein that binds to RAF, MEK and ERK and mediates signal transduction is the IQ motif-containing GTPase activating protein 1 (IQGAP1). In a pre-clinical study, pharmacological targeting of IQGAP1 using a cell-permeable peptide that blocks the IQGAP1-ERK1/2 interaction suppressed tumor cell proliferation in mouse models and bypassed acquired resistance to the BRAF inhibitor vemurafenib in BRAF^{V600} melanoma cell lines [127]. Additional studies will be needed to evaluate the clinical significance of these findings.

Acquired resistance to EGFR-targeted therapies has been linked with the occurrence of mutations in KRAS, NRAS and BRAF and consequent reactivation of MAPK signaling [73, 128]. MAPK inhibition using MEK inhibitors, therefore, represents a promising strategy to overcome resistance to EGFR-targeted therapies and several clinical trials are currently ongoing in both NSCLC and CRC to evaluate the use of MEK inhibitors in combination with both chemotherapy and targeted therapies (reviewed in [129]). Triple therapy using the MEK inhibitor trametinib, the BRAF inhibitor dabrafenib and the anti-EGFR panitumumab has recently shown promising results in CRC patients with BRAF^{V600E} [130].

8.4.4 Inhibition of the PI3K Pathway

The PI3K signaling pathway is frequently activated, either via specific mutation in effector kinases or overexpression of RTKs, during the development of resistance to various targeted therapies. Selective inhibitors targeting the PI3K pathway have been developed, including pan-PI3K and isoform-specific PI3K-inhibitors, as well as AKT and mTOR inhibitors [131]. Even though inhibitors of this signaling pathway have shown limited efficacy as single-agents in advanced solid tumors, such as breast and NSCLC [131], combination therapies using PI3K inhibitors together with inhibitors of other signaling pathways are being explored to overcome resistance to targeted therapies.

The PI3K pathway is activated in over 20% of melanomas displaying acquired resistance to BRAF inhibition [65] and thus is an attractive target for salvaging patients who have progressed on BRAF inhibitors [36]. Pre-clinical studies in

BRAF^{V600}-mutant cells have shown that pan-PI3K inhibitors synergize with combination inhibition of MEK and BRAF to suppress tumor cell proliferation. Further, pan-PI3K inhibition was more effective at suppressing the proliferation of BRAF^{V600}-mutant melanoma cells, compared with inhibitors of individual PI3K isoforms or inhibitors of mTORC1/2 [132]. The dual inhibition of MAPK and PI3K signaling may be synergistic in inhibiting the growth and survival of BRAF^{V600}-mutant melanoma cells because abrogation of oncogenic BRAF activity stimulates the phosphorylation and activation of AKT and mTOR [133].

Multiple *in vitro* studies have shown that treatment of resistant cells with PI3K pathway inhibitors differentially and partially overcome resistance to BRAF/MEK inhibitors. For instance, in one study the concurrent blockade of the MAPK and PI3K pathways differentially suppressed melanoma cell growth but did not promote melanoma cell death [134–136]. In contrast, in PTEN-null and IGF1R-upregulated melanoma cells with resistance to BRAF inhibition, the dual blockade of MAPK and PI3K induced potent cell death [137]. The differential activity of PI3K/MAPK inhibitors in BRAF inhibitor resistance is poorly understood, and appears cell-dependent, rather than merely reflecting the mechanism of BRAF inhibitor resistance. For instance, patient-derived melanoma cell lines with BRAF inhibitor resistance driven by activating NRAS mutations varied in their response to combination inhibition of MAPK and PI3K pathways [134]. Nevertheless, the enhanced anti-tumor activity of combined targeting of MAPK and PI3K pathways was also demonstrated *in vivo*. Mice bearing trametinib-resistant tumors that received a combination of dabrafenib, trametinib and the PI3K/mTOR inhibitor GSK2126458 showed sustained tumor growth inhibition [138].

Despite some promising pre-clinical data, clinical trials testing the combination of PI3K pathway inhibitors with BRAF and MEK inhibitors have so far been disappointing. In phase I clinical trials, inhibitors of the PI3K-AKT-mTOR pathway were found to be associated with a higher risk of infection [139]. Another study evaluating the MEK inhibitor trametinib in combination with the AKT inhibitor afuresertib in patients with solid tumors, showed that continuous dosing of trametinib/afuresertib combination was poorly tolerated and consequently the study was closed for enrollment [140]. In this study only one BRAF wild-type melanoma patient had a partial response [140]. Multiple studies testing the combination of drugs targeting the MAPK and PI3K pathways are currently ongoing and will help determine the potential of this combined therapy in melanoma.

Activation of the PI3K pathway has also been shown to lead to resistance to HER2-targeted therapy in breast cancer patients [78]. In the BOLERO-3 clinical trial, women with HER2-positive, trastuzumab-resistant, advanced breast carcinoma who had previously received taxane therapy, showed trastuzumab sensitivity when it was combined with the mTOR inhibitor everolimus. The combination of everolimus with trastuzumab plus vinorelbine significantly prolonged PFS but led to significant adverse effects [141].

8.4.5 Combination Inhibition of Receptor Tyrosine Kinases

Combination inhibition of RTKs is a promising, alternative strategy to circumvent resistance by inhibiting multiple downstream signaling pathways and abrogating the rebound-signaling activation that results from BRAF inhibition. In BRAF mutant cells, the dual inhibition of BRAF and either HGF or MET resulted in the reversal of stromal cell-mediated drug resistance [68]. Sorafenib is a multi-kinase inhibitor that inhibits tumor proliferation by targeting multiple kinases including the vascular endothelial growth factor receptors VEGFR1, VEGFR2, VEGFR3 and PDGFR and c-KIT, as well as RAF kinases [142]. Despite the disappointing results of a 2006 phase II clinical trial that found little or no anti-tumor activity for sorafenib in advanced melanoma patients as a single-agent [143], this drug is now being tested as a combination treatment. An ongoing clinical trial is investigating the combination of vemurafenib with crizotinib or sorafenib in patients with BRAF-mutated advanced cancers. Preliminary data from this trial indicate that these combinations are well tolerated and show encouraging activity in patients previously treated with BRAF/MEK inhibitors [144].

HGF/MET inhibitors have also shown efficacy in EGFR-resistant NSCLC cells that developed resistance due to MET amplification and the combination of the MET inhibitor crizotinib and the EGFR inhibitor gefitinib potently decreased cell viability [145]. Additionally, several clinical studies using other HGF/MET inhibitors showed some improvement in therapeutic efficacy when combined with EGFR-inhibitors (reviewed in [146]), but further studies are warranted.

8.4.6 Alternative Combination Treatments

As previously mentioned, MITF amplification confers resistance to both BRAF and MEK inhibitors in melanoma [88]. A drug-repurposing screen identified the HIV protease inhibitor nelfinavir as an inhibitor of MITF and nelfinavir suppressed MITF expression and sensitized melanoma cells with NRAS mutations or BRAF and NRAS mutations to MEK inhibitors [147]. A clinical trial is currently testing the combination of nelfinavir, hypofractionated radiation therapy and immunotherapies in advanced cancer patients, including patients with recurrent melanoma (NCT03050060).

Inhibitors of the cyclin-dependent kinases CDK4/6 are effective at blocking cell cycle progression and are being explored in combination with BRAF/MEK inhibitors in melanoma. Combination of palbociclib, a CDK4/6 inhibitor, with BRAF and MEK inhibitors has have shown superior activity, compared to BRAF/MEK inhibition in preclinical models of naive melanoma [148, 149]. In BRAF/MEK inhibitor-resistant melanoma, the combination of CDK4/6, BRAF and MEK inhibitors have produced conflicting results. For instance, the combination of palbociclib with dabrafenib and trametinib, resensitized BRAF/MEK-resistant melanoma, leading to decreased tumor growth in xenograft models [149], whereas in another report BRAF inhibitor-resistant cells did not respond to combination BRAF/MEK inhibitor therapy with palbociclib [148]. A phase Ib/II clinical trial is currently evaluating the triple combination therapy with encorafenib, binimetinib and the CDK4/6 inhibitor ribociclib in patients with BRAF^{V600}-mutant solid tumors (NCT01543698). Preliminary data showed that this triple combination therapy led to overall response rates of 52.4% with increased toxicity [150].

Inhibition of regulatory mechanisms that affect cellular homeostasis can also be an alternative strategy to overcoming resistance to targeted therapies. In melanoma cells, inhibition of the deubiquitinating enzyme USP14 with the drug b-AP15 overcomes resistance to BRAF inhibitors. USP14 inhibition in melanoma cells promoted the accumulation of poly-ubiquitinated proteins and chaperones, mitochondrial dysfunction, endoplasmic reticulum stress, production of reactive oxygen species and consequent cell death [151]. In NSCLC cells, treatment with the small-molecule compound M-COPA (2-methylcoprophilinamide), which disrupts the Golgi apparatus, inhibited cell growth *in vitro* and had an anti-tumor effect in xenograft models of NSCLC cells resistant to EGFR inhibitors [152].

Epigenetic mechanisms can also contribute to MAPK inhibitor resistance by affecting the expression of genes that drive resistance to these therapies [59, 153, 154]. Therefore, the pharmacological inhibition of DNA methyltransferases (DNMTs) or histone deacetylases (HDACs) might re-establish the expression of aberrantly silenced genes, leading to the inhibition of some mechanisms of resistance [155]. Indeed, it has been shown that combined treatment of BRAF inhibitor-resistant cell lines with the BRAF inhibitor encorafenib and the pan-HDAC inhibitor panobinostat restored BRAF inhibitor sensitivity in cells with acquired resistance characterized by lack of MAPK pathway reactivation [156]. Nevertheless, results from phase I clinical trials found that panobinostat is not active as a single agent in the treatment of metastatic melanoma [157], but this agent is currently being studied for use in combination with decitabine (a DNMT inhibitor) and chemotherapy [158]. Another phase I clinical study also analyzed the combination of vemurafenib with subcutaneous administration of the chemotherapy decitabine. This combination treatment was demonstrated to be safe and exhibited activity in BRAF^{V600}-mutant metastatic melanoma [158]. Future studies exploring the combination of MAPK inhibition and epigenetic therapies in melanoma are needed to evaluate the potential of this approach.

In NSCLC, epigenetic alterations have also been linked with the acquisition of resistance to targeted therapies and with the acquisition of a mesenchymal phenotype after EGFR-targeted therapies [159, 160]. In pre-clinical studies, combination treatment using the HDAC inhibitor MPT0E028 and erlotinib was able to enhance erlotinib-induced cell death in EGFR-TKI-resistant cells [161]. Clinical trials have also explored the combination of HDAC inhibitor vorinostat and EGFR-targeted therapies but showed no clinical benefit [162, 163]. Nevertheless, biomarker analysis in the vorinostat/gefitinib combination treatment suggests that this combination may be more effective in patients with EGFR-mutant NSCLC by enhancing EGFR phosphorylation and in patients with a deletion polymorphism in the pro-apoptotic gene *BIM* [162]. This polymorphism has previously been shown to confer resistance to TK inhibitors in EGFR-mutant NSCLC [164]. A clinical trial is currently testing the potential of the vorinostat/gefitinib combination therapy in EGFR-mutant patients resistant to EGFR inhibitors, that possess the *BIM* deletion polymorphism (NCT02151721).

8.4.7   Combination Treatments with Immunotherapy

The tumor microenvironment and particularly tumor-infiltrating lymphocytes play an important role in the response of melanomas to targeted therapy [165]. Patients treated with BRAF inhibitor-based therapy showed significant tumor infiltration of CD4+ and CD8+ lymphocytes early during treatment [93, 166, 167] and increased numbers of intra-tumoral CD8+ lymphocytes correlated with a reduction in tumor size and an increase in necrosis in post-treatment biopsies [166]. Moreover, treatment with BRAF and MEK inhibitors leads to increased expression of melanoma antigens and is associated with a reduction in the immunosuppressive cytokines IL-6 and IL-8 [168]. As discussed above, there is compelling evidence that BRAF inhibition leads to an increase in the expression of PD-L1 by tumor cells [91–94], a target of immune checkpoint therapies. Despite some pre-clinical studies pointing to a T-cell inhibitory effect of MEK inhibition [91, 169], trametinib treatment has been shown to have minimal inhibitory effects on circulating immune cells. This treatment can enhance the efficacy and tumor infiltration of CD8+ effective cells [170].

Modern cancer immunotherapies focus on the augmentation of cell-mediated immunity using monoclonal antibodies targeting key regulators, or checkpoints [171]. Antibody inhibitors of the immune checkpoints, CTLA4 (cytotoxic T-lymphocyte-associated Protein 4) and PD-1 (programmed cell death protein 1) have dramatically improved the survival of patients with high-risk melanoma [172–175]. The anti-CTLA4 antibody ipilimumab was the first immunotherapy to lead to an improvement in median OS from 6.4 months among patients receiving a gp100 vaccine to 10.1 months among patients receiving ipilimumab [172]. The anti-PD-1 antibodies nivolumab and pembrolizumab led to further improvements in survival rates, with nivolumab treatment leading to an improved PFS of 5.1 months compared to 2.2 months with chemotherapy [173] and pembrolizumab showing a PFS of 5.5 months in bi-weekly treatment compared with 2.8 months with ipilimumab [174]. In another study, the combination of PD-1 and CTLA4 inhibitors, substantially improved PFS (11.5 months) compared with either anti-PD-1 (6.9 months) or anti-CTLA4 (2.9 months) monotherapy [175].

Pre-clinical studies using a $BRAF^{V600E}/PTEN^{-/-}$ syngeneic tumor graft immunocompetent mouse model have shown that administration of anti-PD-1 or antibodies against the PD-1 ligand, PD-L1, together with a BRAF inhibitor led to an enhanced response, significantly prolonging survival and slowing tumor growth, as well as significantly increasing the number and activity of tumor-infiltrating lymphocytes

[176]. Another study using a syngeneic BRAF^{V600E}-driven melanoma mouse model has also shown that combination therapy using dabrafenib, trametinib and anti-PD-1 provided superior anti-tumor activity than either single anti-PD-1 or BRAF inhibitor/MEK inhibitor combination [177]. Altogether, the clinical and mouse model data, combined with evidence obtained in other types of cancer models, suggest that pharmacological inhibition of the MAPK pathway can potentiate the effect of immune checkpoint inhibition [178], providing the rationale for the use of a combination of targeted and immunotherapies for melanoma treatment.

Despite the compelling data from clinical and pre-clinical studies, there is a concern that these combination therapies may result in significant toxicities. Indeed, a phase I trial of the concurrent administration of the BRAF inhibitor vemurafenib and the CTLA4-blocking antibody ipilimumab in patients with advanced melanoma resulted in a high-frequency of dose-limiting hepatotoxicity that resulted in the closure of the study [179].

The optimal timing and sequence of targeted and immune-stimulating treatment also need to be determined. Prolonged treatment with MAPK inhibitors can lead to the selection of resistant tumor cells with evidence of transcriptional reprogramming associated with signatures of mesenchymal transition [180]. Moreover, transcriptomic analysis of paired biopsies of melanoma patients has shown that half of the melanomas with acquired resistance to MAPK inhibition displayed CD8+ T-cell deficiency and exhaustion, which can lead to cross-resistance to salvage immunotherapy [59]. Indeed, recent clinical data confirm that anti-PD-1 is less effective as salvage therapy in patients who have progressed on MAPK inhibitor therapy; rapid death (defined as occurring within 3 months) was significantly higher in BRAF^{V600}-mutant melanoma patients post targeted therapy, compared to melanoma patients failing chemotherapy or anti-CTLA4 [181]. Nevertheless, the sequential use of targeted and immune therapy, in patients with BRAF-mutant advanced melanoma is being addressed in a randomized phase III clinical trial (NCT02224781).

The early use of targeted therapies and the impact on the host immune system is also being explored. For instance, neoadjuvant followed by adjuvant combination dabrafenib and trametinib in patients with high-risk, surgically resectable melanoma led to an improved PFS, and transcriptional profiling of baseline tumors revealed upregulation of cytotoxic T-cell genes in patients who showed a complete pathological response. Tumors of patients that did not achieve complete pathological response presented higher levels of CD8+ T-cells expressing the negative immunomodulators PD-1, TIM-3, and LAG-3 [182]. These patients could benefit from subsequent treatment with immunotherapies that target these regulators.

A series of clinical trials are currently underway to explore the safety of concomitant administration of BRAF plus MEK and PD-1 or PDL-1 inhibition (NCT02130466, NCT02967692, NCT02908672). Data from these clinical trials will lead to the future reshaping of the standard of care for advanced melanoma patients.

In NSCLC, immune-checkpoint inhibitors have had promising results, with a recent study showing that single-agent treatment with the anti-PD-1 pembrolizumab was associated with significantly longer PFS and OS in patients with advanced

NSCLC and PD-L1 expression on at least 50% of tumor cells, compared to chemotherapy [183]. Nevertheless, combination treatments using EGFR-targeted therapy and anti-PD-1 have resulted in disappointing results, with two early phase clinical trials evaluating the use of combined EGFR-targeted therapy and the anti-PD-L1 antibody durvalumab showing no advantage compared to EGFR-monotherapy (reviewed in [184]). Nevertheless, a phase I clinical trial testing the combination of erlotinib and nivolumab has shown an acceptable safety profile and durable responses in patients with EGFR-mutant, TKI-treated NSCLC [185]. Additional trials are currently underway to examine the potential of combination immune-checkpoint and RTK inhibitors to overcome targeted therapy resistance in NSCLC [186].

Adoptive cell therapy (ACT) is a personalized cancer immunotherapy that involves administration of autologous tumor-specific immune cells and has shown promising results in multiple tumor types [187]. Several studies involving ACT using naturally occurring tumor-reactive lymphocytes have mediated durable responses, with complete regression in 24% of patients and a median survival rate of more than 3 years [188]. A recent pilot study evaluating the co-administration of vemurafenib and ACT in metastatic melanoma patients has shown that this treatment is well tolerated and can generate favorable clinical responses. Seven of 11 patients experienced an objective clinical response, and two patients had a complete response of more than 3 years [189]. Further clinical studies are needed to evaluate the potential of the combination of ACT and targeted therapies.

8.5　Limitations and Future Directions

The introduction of molecularly targeted therapies for the treatment of cancer patients with specific oncogenic driver mutations has had a substantial clinical impact and improved the outcomes of patients with various tumor types. Examples of cancers where breakthrough improvements in response rates have been achieved include BCR-ABL-translocated CML, HER2-amplified breast cancer, EGFR-mutant, EMLA4-ALK fusion or ROS-rearranged NSCLC and BRAF^{V600}-mutant melanoma [4, 6–8, 20, 22, 26, 27, 190, 191]. Nevertheless, the majority of patients treated with targeted therapies will eventually relapse due to the development of resistance mechanisms that lead to reactivation of primary oncogene-regulated signaling or via alternative signaling pathways. Preclinical and clinical data have shown that overcoming resistance will involve multiple strategies, including drug holidays, alternating drug treatments, optimized sequencing, administering next-generation molecular targeted inhibitors that may overcome resistance mutations and incorporating new classes of drugs that target alternate signaling pathways.

Despite evidence suggesting that immunotherapies may prove less useful as salvage, rather than first-line therapies in melanoma patients [192], additional work is required on the timing and selection of optimal drug sequencing with other targeted therapies, chemotherapy and immunotherapy in melanoma and other cancer types. Alternating drug treatments will require a precise and rapid analytical pipeline to monitor patient response and resistance in real time. With the development of highly sensitive digital droplet PCR and next-generation sequencing of circulating tumor DNA, regular monitoring of patients is now feasible [193, 194]. The potential to accurately select the best treatment based on drug screening of patient-derived tumor organoids is attractive and is currently being incorporated into clinical trial designs for colorectal cancer and other tumor types (NCT02732860). However, this type of intervention is expensive and unlikely to be effective in most cancers, with further challenges in obtaining sufficient tumor material in patients with tumors that are difficult to biopsy.

The rationale that lower cancer burden may produce durable responses is based on significant clinical data, with smaller melanoma metastases more likely to undergo complete response to targeted therapies [50]. Therefore, another potential strategy to overcome resistance may be to treat patients earlier in the treatment paradigm, that is, in the adjuvant or neoadjuvant setting. Recent adjuvant and neoadjuvant clinical trials using the combination of BRAF/MEK inhibitors have demonstrated improvement in recurrence-free survival [182, 195] and in cancers such as GIST and HER2-positive breast cancer, targeted therapy in the adjuvant setting is the standard of care [145, 196].

In summary, the integration of novel therapeutic salvage approaches will be required to achieve more durable responses and ultimately, to improve survival for patients treated with targeted therapies. These approaches would include next-generation targeted agents, new combination therapies and readjustment of drug timing and sequencing, combined with improved clinical trial design, treatment of earlier stage cancer patients and sensitive real-time monitoring of patient responses.

Conflict of Interest   No potential conflicts of interest to disclose.

Funding: This work was supported by funding from NHMRC project grants 1130423 and 1093017. HR is supported by an NHMRC Research Fellowship.

References

1. Sawyers C. Targeted cancer therapy. Nature. 2004;432(7015):294–7. https://doi.org/10.1038/nature03095.
2. Weinstein IB. Cancer. Addiction to oncogenes-the Achilles heal of cancer. Science. 2002;297(5578):63–4. https://doi.org/10.1126/science.1073096.
3. Vogelstein B, Papadopoulos N, Velculescu VE, Zhou S, Diaz LA Jr, Kinzler KW. Cancer genome landscapes. Science. 2013;339(6127):1546–58. https://doi.org/10.1126/science.1235122.
4. Maemondo M, Inoue A, Kobayashi K, Sugawara S, Oizumi S, Isobe H, et al. Gefitinib or chemotherapy for non-small-cell lung cancer with mutated EGFR. N Engl J Med. 2010;362(25):2380–8. https://doi.org/10.1056/NEJMoa0909530.
5. Mok TS, Wu YL, Thongprasert S, Yang CH, Chu DT, Saijo N, et al. Gefitinib or carboplatin-paclitaxel in pulmonary adenocarcinoma. N Engl J Med. 2009;361(10):947–57. https://doi.org/10.1056/NEJMoa0810699.
6. Rosell R, Carcereny E, Gervais R, Vergnenegre A, Massuti B, Felip E, et al. Erlotinib versus standard chemotherapy as first-line treatment for European patients with advanced

EGFR mutation-positive non-small-cell lung cancer (EURTAC): a multicentre, open-label, randomised phase 3 trial. Lancet Oncol. 2012;13(3):239–46. https://doi.org/10.1016/S1470-2045(11)70393-X.

7. Chapman PB, Hauschild A, Robert C, Haanen JB, Ascierto P, Larkin J, et al. Improved survival with vemurafenib in melanoma with BRAF V600E mutation. N Engl J Med. 2011;364(26):2507–16. https://doi.org/10.1056/NEJMoa1103782.

8. Hauschild A, Grob JJ, Demidov LV, Jouary T, Gutzmer R, Millward M, et al. Dabrafenib in BRAF-mutated metastatic melanoma: a multicentre, open-label, phase 3 randomised controlled trial. Lancet. 2012;380(9839):358–65. https://doi.org/10.1016/S0140-6736(12)60868-X.

9. Druker BJ, Sawyers CL, Kantarjian H, Resta DJ, Reese SF, Ford JM, et al. Activity of a specific inhibitor of the BCR-ABL tyrosine kinase in the blast crisis of chronic myeloid leukemia and acute lymphoblastic leukemia with the Philadelphia chromosome. N Engl J Med. 2001;344(14):1038–42. https://doi.org/10.1056/NEJM200104053441402.

10. Ren R. Mechanisms of BCR-ABL in the pathogenesis of chronic myelogenous leukaemia. Nat Rev Cancer. 2005;5(3):172–83. https://doi.org/10.1038/nrc1567.

11. Druker BJ, Guilhot F, O'Brien SG, Gathmann I, Kantarjian H, Gattermann N, et al. Five-year follow-up of patients receiving imatinib for chronic myeloid leukemia. N Engl J Med. 2006;355(23):2408–17. https://doi.org/10.1056/NEJMoa062867.

12. Corless CL, Barnett CM, Heinrich MC. Gastrointestinal stromal tumours: origin and molecular oncology. Nat Rev Cancer. 2011;11(12):865–78. https://doi.org/10.1038/nrc3143.

13. Verweij J, Casali PG, Zalcberg J, LeCesne A, Reichardt P, Blay JY, et al. Progression-free survival in gastrointestinal stromal tumours with high-dose imatinib: randomised trial. Lancet. 2004;364(9440):1127–34. https://doi.org/10.1016/s0140-6736(04)17098-0.

14. Blanke CD, Rankin C, Demetri GD, Ryan CW, von Mehren M, Benjamin RS, et al. Phase III randomized, intergroup trial assessing imatinib mesylate at two dose levels in patients with unresectable or metastatic gastrointestinal stromal tumors expressing the kit receptor tyrosine kinase: S0033. J Clin Oncol. 2008;26(4):626–32. https://doi.org/10.1200/jco.2007.13.4452.

15. Demetri GD, von Mehren M, Blanke CD, Van den Abbeele AD, Eisenberg B, Roberts PJ, et al. Efficacy and safety of imatinib mesylate in advanced gastrointestinal stromal tumors. N Engl J Med. 2002;347(7):472–80. https://doi.org/10.1056/NEJMoa020461.

16. Yarden Y, Pines G. The ERBB network: at last, cancer therapy meets systems biology. Nat Rev Cancer. 2012;12(8):553–63. https://doi.org/10.1038/nrc3309.

17. Lynch TJ, Bell DW, Sordella R, Gurubhagavatula S, Okimoto RA, Brannigan BW, et al. Activating mutations in the epidermal growth factor receptor underlying responsiveness of non-small-cell lung cancer to gefitinib. N Engl J Med. 2004;350(21):2129–39. https://doi.org/10.1056/NEJMoa040938.

18. Bokemeyer C, Van Cutsem E, Rougier P, Ciardiello F, Heeger S, Schlichting M, et al. Addition of cetuximab to chemotherapy as first-line treatment for KRAS wild-type metastatic colorectal cancer: pooled analysis of the CRYSTAL and OPUS randomised clinical trials. Eur J Cancer. 2012;48(10):1466–75. https://doi.org/10.1016/j.ejca.2012.02.057.

19. Price TJ, Peeters M, Kim TW, Li J, Cascinu S, Ruff P, et al. Panitumumab versus cetuximab in patients with chemotherapy-refractory wild-type KRAS exon 2 metastatic colorectal cancer (ASPECCT): a randomised, multicentre, open-label, non-inferiority phase 3 study. Lancet Oncol. 2014;15(6):569–79. https://doi.org/10.1016/S1470-2045(14)70118-4.

20. Slamon DJ, Leyland-Jones B, Shak S, Fuchs H, Paton V, Bajamonde A, et al. Use of chemotherapy plus a monoclonal antibody against HER2 for metastatic breast cancer that overexpresses HER2. N Engl J Med. 2001;344(11):783–92. https://doi.org/10.1056/nejm200103153441101.

21. Baselga J, Cortes J, Kim SB, Im SA, Hegg R, Im YH, et al. Pertuzumab plus trastuzumab plus docetaxel for metastatic breast cancer. N Engl J Med. 2012;366(2):109–19. https://doi.org/10.1056/NEJMoa1113216.

22. Blackwell KL, Burstein HJ, Storniolo AM, Rugo H, Sledge G, Koehler M, et al. Randomized study of Lapatinib alone or in combination with trastuzumab in women with ErbB2-positive, trastuzumab-refractory metastatic breast cancer. J Clin Oncol. 2010;28(7):1124–30. https://doi.org/10.1200/jco.2008.21.4437.

23. Verma S, Miles D, Gianni L, Krop IE, Welslau M, Baselga J, et al. Trastuzumab emtansine for HER2-positive advanced breast cancer. N Engl J Med. 2012;367(19):1783–91. https://doi.org/10.1056/NEJMoa1209124.

24. Cameron D, Piccart-Gebhart MJ, Gelber RD, Procter M, Goldhirsch A, de Azambuja E, et al. 11 years' follow-up of trastuzumab after adjuvant chemotherapy in HER2-positive early breast cancer: final analysis of the HERceptin adjuvant (HERA) trial. Lancet. 2017;389(10075):1195–205. https://doi.org/10.1016/s0140-6736(16)32616-2.

25. Bang YJ, Van Cutsem E, Feyereislova A, Chung HC, Shen L, Sawaki A, et al. Trastuzumab in combination with chemotherapy versus chemotherapy alone for treatment of HER2-positive advanced gastric or gastro-oesophageal junction cancer (ToGA): a phase 3, open-label, randomised controlled trial. Lancet. 2010;376(9742):687–97. https://doi.org/10.1016/S0140-6736(10)61121-X.

26. Shaw AT, Kim DW, Nakagawa K, Seto T, Crino L, Ahn MJ, et al. Crizotinib versus chemotherapy in advanced ALK-positive lung cancer. N Engl J Med. 2013;368(25):2385–94. https://doi.org/10.1056/NEJMoa1214886.

27. Shaw AT, Ou SH, Bang YJ, Camidge DR, Solomon BJ, Salgia R, et al. Crizotinib in ROS1-rearranged non-small-cell lung cancer. N Engl J Med. 2014;371(21):1963–71. https://doi.org/10.1056/NEJMoa1406766.

28. Akbani R, Akdemir Kadir C, Aksoy BA, Albert M, Ally A, Amin Samirkumar B, et al. Genomic classification of cutaneous melanoma. Cell. 2015;161(7):1681–96. https://doi.org/10.1016/j.cell.2015.05.044.

29. Menzies AM, Haydu LE, Visintin L, Carlino MS, Howle JR, Thompson JF, et al. Distinguishing clinicopathologic features of patients with V600E and V600K BRAF-mutant metastatic melanoma. Clin Cancer Res. 2012;18(12):3242–9. https://doi.org/10.1158/1078-0432.ccr-12-0052.

30. McArthur GA, Chapman PB, Robert C, Larkin J, Haanen JB, Dummer R, et al. Safety and efficacy of vemurafenib in BRAF(V600E) and BRAF(V600K) mutation-positive melanoma (BRIM-3): extended follow-up of a phase 3, randomised, open-label study. Lancet Oncol. 2014;15(3):323–32. https://doi.org/10.1016/S1470-2045(14)70012-9.

31. Koelblinger P, Thuerigen O, Dummer R. Development of encorafenib for BRAF-mutated advanced melanoma. Curr Opin Oncol. 2018;30(2):125–33. https://doi.org/10.1097/CCO.0000000000000426.

32. Dummer R, Ascierto PA, Gogas HJ, Arance A, Mandala M, Liszkay G, et al. Encorafenib plus binimetinib versus vemurafenib or encorafenib in patients with BRAF-mutant melanoma (COLUMBUS): a multicentre, open-label, randomised phase 3 trial. Lancet Oncol. 2018;19(5):603–15. https://doi.org/10.1016/S1470-2045(18)30142-6.

33. Lim SY, Menzies AM, Rizos H. Mechanisms and strategies to overcome resistance to molecularly targeted therapy for melanoma. Cancer. 2017;123(S11):2118–29. https://doi.org/10.1002/cncr.30435.

34. Long GV, Flaherty KT, Stroyakovskiy D, Gogas H, Levchenko E, de Braud F, et al. Dabrafenib plus trametinib versus dabrafenib monotherapy in patients with metastatic BRAF V600E/K-mutant melanoma: long-term survival and safety analysis of a phase 3 study. Ann Oncol. 2017;28(7):1631–9. https://doi.org/10.1093/annonc/mdx176.

35. Dummer R, Ascierto PA, Gogas HJ, Arance A, Mandala M, Liszkay G, et al. Overall survival in patients with BRAF-mutant melanoma receiving encorafenib plus binimetinib versus vemurafenib or encorafenib (COLUMBUS): a multicentre, open-label, randomised, phase 3 trial. Lancet Oncol. 2018;19(10):1315–27. https://doi.org/10.1016/s1470-2045(18)30497-2.

36. Arozarena I, Wellbrock C. Overcoming resistance to BRAF inhibitors. Ann Transl Med. 2017;5(19):387. https://doi.org/10.21037/atm.2017.06.09.

37. Ahronian LG, Corcoran RB. Strategies for monitoring and combating resistance to combination kinase inhibitors for cancer therapy. Genome Med. 2017;9(1):37. https://doi.org/10.1186/s13073-017-0431-3.

38. Heidorn SJ, Milagre C, Whittaker S, Nourry A, Niculescu-Duvas I, Dhomen N, et al. Kinase-dead BRAF and oncogenic RAS cooperate to drive tumor progression through CRAF. Cell. 2010;140(2):209–21. https://doi.org/10.1016/j.cell.2009.12.040.

39. Poulikakos PI, Zhang C, Bollag G, Shokat KM, Rosen N. RAF inhibitors transactivate RAF dimers and ERK signalling in cells with wild-type BRAF. Nature. 2010;464(7287):427–30. https://doi.org/10.1038/nature08902.

40. Hatzivassiliou G, Song K, Yen I, Brandhuber BJ, Anderson DJ, Alvarado R, et al. RAF inhibitors prime wild-type RAF to activate the MAPK pathway and enhance growth. Nature. 2010;464(7287):431–5. https://doi.org/10.1038/nature08833.

41. Oberholzer PA, Kee D, Dziunycz P, Sucker A, Kamsukom N, Jones R, et al. RAS mutations are associated with the development of cutaneous squamous cell tumors in patients treated with RAF inhibitors. J Clin Oncol. 2012;30(3):316–21. https://doi.org/10.1200/JCO.2011.36.7680.

42. Su F, Viros A, Milagre C, Trunzer K, Bollag G, Spleiss O, et al. RAS mutations in cutaneous squamous-cell carcinomas in patients treated with BRAF inhibitors. N Engl J Med. 2012;366(3):207–15. https://doi.org/10.1056/NEJMoa1105358.

43. Gibney GT, Messina JL, Fedorenko IV, Sondak VK, Smalley KS. Paradoxical oncogenesis—the long-term effects of BRAF inhibition in melanoma. Nat Rev Clin Oncol. 2013;10(7):390–9. https://doi.org/10.1038/nrclinonc.2013.83.

44. Callahan MK, Rampal R, Harding JJ, Klimek VM, Chung YR, Merghoub T, et al. Progression of RAS-mutant leukemia during RAF inhibitor treatment. N Engl J Med. 2012;367(24):2316–21. https://doi.org/10.1056/NEJMoa1208958.

45. Andrews MC, Behren A, Chionh F, Mariadason J, Vella LJ, Do H, et al. BRAF inhibitor-driven tumor proliferation in a KRAS-mutated colon carcinoma is not overcome by MEK1/2 inhibition. J Clin Oncol. 2013;31(35):e448–51. https://doi.org/10.1200/jco.2013.50.4118.

46. Amaravadi RK, Hamilton KE, Ma X, Piao S, Portillo AD, Nathanson KL, et al. Multiple gastrointestinal polyps in patients treated with BRAF inhibitors. Clin Cancer Res. 2015;21(23):5215–21. https://doi.org/10.1158/1078-0432.ccr-15-0469.

47. Carlos G, Anforth R, Clements A, Menzies AM, Carlino MS, Chou S, et al. Cutaneous toxic effects of BRAF inhibitors alone and in combination with MEK inhibitors for metastatic melanoma. JAMA Dermatol. 2015;151(10):1103–9. https://doi.org/10.1001/jamadermatol.2015.1745.

48. Robert C, Karaszewska B, Schachter J, Rutkowski P, Mackiewicz A, Stroiakovski D, et al. Improved overall survival in melanoma with combined dabrafenib and trametinib. N Engl J Med. 2015;372(1):30–9. https://doi.org/10.1056/NEJMoa1412690.

49. Long GV, Stroyakovskiy D, Gogas H, Levchenko E, de Braud F, Larkin J, et al. Dabrafenib and trametinib versus dabrafenib and placebo for Val600 BRAF-mutant melanoma: a multicentre, double-blind, phase 3 randomised controlled trial. Lancet. 2015;386(9992):444–51. https://doi.org/10.1016/s0140-6736(15)60898-4.

50. Menzies AM, Haydu LE, Carlino MS, Azer MW, Carr PJ, Kefford RF, et al. Inter- and intra-patient heterogeneity of response and progression to targeted therapy in metastatic melanoma. PLoS One. 2014;9(1):e85004. https://doi.org/10.1371/journal.pone.0085004.

51. Bozic I, Nowak MA. Timing and heterogeneity of mutations associated with drug resistance in metastatic cancers. Proc Natl Acad Sci U S A. 2014;111(45):15964–8. https://doi.org/10.1073/pnas.1412075111.

52. Bozic I, Reiter JG, Allen B, Antal T, Chatterjee K, Shah P, et al. Evolutionary dynamics of cancer in response to targeted combination therapy. elife. 2013;2:e00747. https://doi.org/10.7554/eLife.00747.

53. Eisenhauer EA, Therasse P, Bogaerts J, Schwartz LH, Sargent D, Ford R, et al. New response evaluation criteria in solid tumours: revised RECIST guideline (version 1.1). Eur J Cancer. 2009;45(2):228–47. https://doi.org/10.1016/j.ejca.2008.10.026.

54. Long GV, Weber JS, Infante JR, Kim KB, Daud A, Gonzalez R, et al. Overall survival and durable responses in patients with BRAF V600-mutant metastatic melanoma receiving Dabrafenib combined with Trametinib. J Clin Oncol. 2016;34(8):871–8. https://doi.org/10.1200/jco.2015.62.9345.

55. Pagliarini R, Shao W, Sellers WR. Oncogene addiction: pathways of therapeutic response, resistance, and road maps toward a cure. EMBO Rep. 2015;16(3):280–96. https://doi.org/10.15252/embr.201439949.
56. Johnson DB, Menzies AM, Zimmer L, Eroglu Z, Ye F, Zhao S, et al. Acquired BRAF inhibitor resistance: a multicenter meta-analysis of the spectrum and frequencies, clinical behaviour, and phenotypic associations of resistance mechanisms. Eur J Cancer. 2015;51(18):2792–9. https://doi.org/10.1016/j.ejca.2015.08.022.
57. Rizos H, Menzies AM, Pupo GM, Carlino MS, Fung C, Hyman J, et al. BRAF inhibitor resistance mechanisms in metastatic melanoma: spectrum and clinical impact. Clin Cancer Res. 2014;20(7):1965–77. https://doi.org/10.1158/1078-0432.CCR-13-3122.
58. Long GV, Fung C, Menzies AM, Pupo GM, Carlino MS, Hyman J, et al. Increased MAPK reactivation in early resistance to dabrafenib/trametinib combination therapy of BRAF-mutant metastatic melanoma. Nat Commun. 2014;5:5694. https://doi.org/10.1038/ncomms6694.
59. Hugo W, Shi H, Sun L, Piva M, Song C, Kong X, et al. Non-genomic and immune evolution of melanoma acquiring MAPKi resistance. Cell. 2015;162(6):1271–85. https://doi.org/10.1016/j.cell.2015.07.061.
60. Zhang J, Yang PL, Gray NS. Targeting cancer with small molecule kinase inhibitors. Nat Rev Cancer. 2009;9(1):28–39. https://doi.org/10.1038/nrc2559.
61. Shi H, Moriceau G, Kong X, Lee MK, Lee H, Koya RC, et al. Melanoma whole-exome sequencing identifies (V600E)B-RAF amplification-mediated acquired B-RAF inhibitor resistance. Nat Commun. 2012;3:724. https://doi.org/10.1038/ncomms1727.
62. Poulikakos PI, Persaud Y, Janakiraman M, Kong X, Ng C, Moriceau G, et al. RAF inhibitor resistance is mediated by dimerization of aberrantly spliced BRAF(V600E). Nature. 2011;480(7377):387–90. https://doi.org/10.1038/nature10662.
63. Villanueva J, Vultur A, Lee JT, Somasundaram R, Fukunaga-Kalabis M, Cipolla AK, et al. Acquired resistance to BRAF inhibitors mediated by a RAF kinase switch in melanoma can be overcome by cotargeting MEK and IGF-1R/PI3K. Cancer Cell. 2010;18(6):683–95. https://doi.org/10.1016/j.ccr.2010.11.023.
64. Montagut C, Sharma SV, Shioda T, McDermott U, Ulman M, Ulkus LE, et al. Elevated CRAF as a potential mechanism of acquired resistance to BRAF inhibition in melanoma. Cancer Res. 2008;68(12):4853–61. https://doi.org/10.1158/0008-5472.CAN-07-6787.
65. Shi H, Hugo W, Kong X, Hong A, Koya RC, Moriceau G, et al. Acquired resistance and clonal evolution in melanoma during BRAF inhibitor therapy. Cancer Discov. 2014;4(1):80–93. https://doi.org/10.1158/2159-8290.CD-13-0642.
66. Carlino MS, Fung C, Shahheydari H, Todd JR, Boyd SC, Irvine M, et al. Preexisting MEK1P124 mutations diminish response to BRAF inhibitors in metastatic melanoma patients. Clin Cancer Res. 2015;21(1):98–105. https://doi.org/10.1158/1078-0432.ccr-14-0759.
67. Nazarian R, Shi H, Wang Q, Kong X, Koya RC, Lee H, et al. Melanomas acquire resistance to B-RAF(V600E) inhibition by RTK or N-RAS upregulation. Nature. 2010;468(7326):973–7. https://doi.org/10.1038/nature09626.
68. Straussman R, Morikawa T, Shee K, Barzily-Rokni M, Qian ZR, Du J, et al. Tumour microenvironment elicits innate resistance to RAF inhibitors through HGF secretion. Nature. 2012;487(7408):500–4. https://doi.org/10.1038/nature11183.
69. Johannessen CM, Boehm JS, Kim SY, Thomas SR, Wardwell L, Johnson LA, et al. COT drives resistance to RAF inhibition through MAP kinase pathway reactivation. Nature. 2010;468(7326):968–72. https://doi.org/10.1038/nature09627.
70. Lu H, Liu S, Zhang G, Bin W, Zhu Y, Frederick DT, et al. PAK signalling drives acquired drug resistance to MAPK inhibitors in BRAF-mutant melanomas. Nature. 2017;550(7674):133–6. https://doi.org/10.1038/nature24040.
71. Shen CH, Kim SH, Trousil S, Frederick DT, Piris A, Yuan P, et al. Loss of cohesin complex components STAG2 or STAG3 confers resistance to BRAF inhibition in melanoma. Nat Med. 2016;22(9):1056–61. https://doi.org/10.1038/nm.4155.
72. Whittaker SR, Theurillat JP, Van Allen E, Wagle N, Hsiao J, Cowley GS, et al. A genome-scale RNA interference screen implicates NF1 loss in resistance to RAF inhibition. Cancer Discov. 2013;3(3):350–62. https://doi.org/10.1158/2159-8290.cd-12-0470.

73. Bardelli A, Siena S. Molecular mechanisms of resistance to cetuximab and panitumumab in colorectal cancer. J Clin Oncol. 2010;28(7):1254–61. https://doi.org/10.1200/jco.2009.24.6116.

74. Kuwano M, Sonoda K, Murakami Y, Watari K, Ono M. Overcoming drug resistance to receptor tyrosine kinase inhibitors: learning from lung cancer. Pharmacol Ther. 2016;161:97–110. https://doi.org/10.1016/j.pharmthera.2016.03.002.

75. Irvine M, Stewart A, Pedersen B, Boyd S, Kefford R, Rizos H. Oncogenic PI3K/AKT promotes the step-wise evolution of combination BRAF/MEK inhibitor resistance in melanoma. Oncogene. 2018;7(9):72. https://doi.org/10.1038/s41389-018-0081-3.

76. Tanizaki J, Okamoto I, Okabe T, Sakai K, Tanaka K, Hayashi H, et al. Activation of HER family signaling as a mechanism of acquired resistance to ALK inhibitors in EML4-ALK-positive non-small cell lung cancer. Clin Cancer Res. 2012;18(22):6219–26. https://doi.org/10.1158/1078-0432.ccr-12-0392.

77. Bean J, Brennan C, Shih JY, Riely G, Viale A, Wang L, et al. MET amplification occurs with or without T790M mutations in EGFR mutant lung tumors with acquired resistance to gefitinib or erlotinib. Proc Natl Acad Sci U S A. 2007;104(52):20932–7. https://doi.org/10.1073/pnas.0710370104.

78. Wilks ST. Potential of overcoming resistance to HER2-targeted therapies through the PI3K/Akt/mTOR pathway. Breast (Edinburgh, Scotland). 2015;24(5):548–55. https://doi.org/10.1016/j.breast.2015.06.002.

79. Ahn A, Chatterjee A, Eccles MR. The slow cycling phenotype: a growing problem for treatment resistance in melanoma. Mol Cancer Ther. 2017;16(6):1002–9. https://doi.org/10.1158/1535-7163.mct-16-0535.

80. Kawakami A, Fisher DE. The master role of microphthalmia-associated transcription factor in melanocyte and melanoma biology. Lab Invest. 2017;97(6):649–56. https://doi.org/10.1038/labinvest.2017.9.

81. Konieczkowski DJ, Johannessen CM, Abudayyeh O, Kim JW, Cooper ZA, Piris A, et al. A melanoma cell state distinction influences sensitivity to MAPK pathway inhibitors. Cancer Discov. 2014;4(7):816–27. https://doi.org/10.1158/2159-8290.cd-13-0424.

82. Muller J, Krijgsman O, Tsoi J, Robert L, Hugo W, Song C, et al. Low MITF/AXL ratio predicts early resistance to multiple targeted drugs in melanoma. Nat Commun. 2014;5:5712. https://doi.org/10.1038/ncomms6712.

83. Roesch A, Vultur A, Bogeski I, Wang H, Zimmermann KM, Speicher D, et al. Overcoming intrinsic multidrug resistance in melanoma by blocking the mitochondrial respiratory chain of slow-cycling JARID1B(high) cells. Cancer Cell. 2013;23(6):811–25. https://doi.org/10.1016/j.ccr.2013.05.003.

84. Ji Z, Erin Chen Y, Kumar R, Taylor M, Jenny Njauw CN, Miao B, et al. MITF modulates therapeutic resistance through EGFR signaling. J Invest Dermatol. 2015;135(7):1863–72. https://doi.org/10.1038/jid.2015.105.

85. Wellbrock C, Rana S, Paterson H, Pickersgill H, Brummelkamp T, Marais R. Oncogenic BRAF regulates melanoma proliferation through the lineage specific factor MITF. PLoS One. 2008;3(7):e2734. https://doi.org/10.1371/journal.pone.0002734.

86. Haq R, Yokoyama S, Hawryluk EB, Jonsson GB, Frederick DT, McHenry K, et al. BCL2A1 is a lineage-specific antiapoptotic melanoma oncogene that confers resistance to BRAF inhibition. Proc Natl Acad Sci U S A. 2013;110(11):4321–6. https://doi.org/10.1073/pnas.1205575110.

87. McGill GG, Horstmann M, Widlund HR, Du J, Motyckova G, Nishimura EK, et al. Bcl2 regulation by the melanocyte master regulator Mitf modulates lineage survival and melanoma cell viability. Cell. 2002;109(6):707–18.

88. Van Allen EM, Wagle N, Sucker A, Treacy DJ, Johannessen CM, Goetz EM, et al. The genetic landscape of clinical resistance to RAF inhibition in metastatic melanoma. Cancer Discov. 2014;4(1):94–109. https://doi.org/10.1158/2159-8290.Cd-13-0617.

89. Garraway LA, Widlund HR, Rubin MA, Getz G, Berger AJ, Ramaswamy S, et al. Integrative genomic analyses identify MITF as a lineage survival oncogene amplified in malignant melanoma. Nature. 2005;436(7047):117–22. https://doi.org/10.1038/nature03664.

90. Corre S, Tardif N, Mouchet N, Leclair HM, Boussemart L, Gautron A, et al. Sustained activation of the aryl hydrocarbon receptor transcription factor promotes resistance to BRAF-inhibitors in melanoma. Nat Commun. 2018;9(1):4775. https://doi.org/10.1038/s41467-018-06951-2.

91. Jiang X, Zhou J, Giobbie-Hurder A, Wargo J, Hodi FS. The activation of MAPK in melanoma cells resistant to BRAF inhibition promotes PD-L1 expression that is reversible by MEK and PI3K inhibition. Clin Cancer Res. 2013;19(3):598–609. https://doi.org/10.1158/1078-0432.ccr-12-2731.

92. Atefi M, Avramis E, Lassen A, Wong DJ, Robert L, Foulad D, et al. Effects of MAPK and PI3K pathways on PD-L1 expression in melanoma. Clin Cancer Res. 2014;20(13):3446–57. https://doi.org/10.1158/1078-0432.ccr-13-2797.

93. Kakavand H, Wilmott JS, Menzies AM, Vilain R, Haydu LE, Yearley JH, et al. PD-L1 expression and tumor-infiltrating lymphocytes define different subsets of MAPK inhibitor-treated melanoma patients. Clin Cancer Res. 2015;21(14):3140–8. https://doi.org/10.1158/1078-0432.ccr-14-2023.

94. Kakavand H, Rawson RV, Pupo GM, Yang JYH, Menzies AM, Carlino MS, et al. PD-L1 expression and immune escape in melanoma resistance to MAPK inhibitors. Clin Cancer Res. 2017;23(20):6054–61. https://doi.org/10.1158/1078-0432.ccr-16-1688.

95. Akbay EA, Koyama S, Carretero J, Altabef A, Tchaicha JH, Christensen CL, et al. Activation of the PD-1 pathway contributes to immune escape in EGFR-driven lung tumors. Cancer Discov. 2013;3(12):1355–63. https://doi.org/10.1158/2159-8290.cd-13-0310.

96. Ota K, Azuma K, Kawahara A, Hattori S, Iwama E, Tanizaki J, et al. Induction of PD-L1 expression by the EML4-ALK oncoprotein and downstream signaling pathways in non-small cell lung cancer. Clin Cancer Res. 2015;21(17):4014–21. https://doi.org/10.1158/1078-0432.ccr-15-0016.

97. Su S, Dong ZY, Xie Z, Yan LX, Li YF, Su J, et al. Strong programmed death ligand 1 expression predicts poor response and de novo resistance to EGFR tyrosine kinase inhibitors among NSCLC patients with EGFR mutation. J Thorac Oncol. 2018;13:1668–75. https://doi.org/10.1016/j.jtho.2018.07.016.

98. Tung JN, Lin PL, Wang YC, Wu DW, Chen CY, Lee H. PD-L1 confers resistance to EGFR mutation-independent tyrosine kinase inhibitors in non-small cell lung cancer via upregulation of YAP1 expression. Oncotarget. 2018;9(4):4637–46. https://doi.org/10.18632/oncotarget.23161.

99. Sequist LV, Waltman BA, Dias-Santagata D, Digumarthy S, Turke AB, Fidias P, et al. Genotypic and histological evolution of lung cancers acquiring resistance to EGFR inhibitors. Sci Transl Med. 2011;3(75):75ra26. https://doi.org/10.1126/scitranslmed.3002003.

100. Suda K, Rozeboom L, Rivard CJ, Yu H, Ellison K, Melnick MAC, et al. Therapy-induced E-cadherin downregulation alters expression of programmed death ligand-1 in lung cancer cells. Lung Cancer (Amsterdam, Netherlands). 2017;109:1–8. https://doi.org/10.1016/j.lungcan.2017.04.010.

101. Long GV, Eroglu Z, Infante J, Patel S, Daud A, Johnson DB, et al. Long-term outcomes in patients with BRAF V600-mutant metastatic melanoma who received dabrafenib combined with trametinib. J Clin Oncol. 2018;36(7):667–73. https://doi.org/10.1200/jco.2017.74.1025.

102. Das Thakur M, Salangsang F, Landman AS, Sellers WR, Pryer NK, Levesque MP, et al. Modelling vemurafenib resistance in melanoma reveals a strategy to forestall drug resistance. Nature. 2013;494(7436):251–5. https://doi.org/10.1038/nature11814.

103. Valpione S, Carlino MS, Mangana J, Mooradian MJ, McArthur G, Schadendorf D, et al. Rechallenge with BRAF-directed treatment in metastatic melanoma: a multi-institutional retrospective study. Eur J Cancer. 2018;91:116–24. https://doi.org/10.1016/j.ejca.2017.12.007.

104. Carlino MS, Vanella V, Girgis C, Giannarelli D, Guminski A, Festino L, et al. Cessation of targeted therapy after a complete response in BRAF-mutant advanced melanoma: a case series. Br J Cancer. 2016;115(11):1280–4. https://doi.org/10.1038/bjc.2016.321.

105. Rossini D, Cremolini C, Re MD, Lonardi S, Busico A, Rofi E, et al. Abstract CT088: efficacy of anti-EGFR rechallenge in *RAS* and *BRAF* wt metastatic colorectal cancer: clinical and translational results of the phase II CRICKET study by GONO. Cancer Res. 2018;78(13 Suppl):CT088-CT. https://doi.org/10.1158/1538-7445.am2018-ct088.

106. Girotti MR, Lopes F, Preece N, Niculescu-Duvaz D, Zambon A, Davies L, et al. Paradox-breaking RAF inhibitors that also target SRC are effective in drug-resistant BRAF mutant melanoma. Cancer Cell. 2015;27(1):85–96. https://doi.org/10.1016/j.ccell.2014.11.006.

107. Zhang C, Spevak W, Zhang Y, Burton EA, Ma Y, Habets G, et al. RAF inhibitors that evade paradoxical MAPK pathway activation. Nature. 2015;526(7574):583–6. https://doi.org/10.1038/nature14982.

108. Le K, Blomain ES, Rodeck U, Aplin AE. Selective RAF inhibitor impairs ERK1/2 phosphorylation and growth in mutant NRAS, vemurafenib-resistant melanoma cells. Pigment Cell Melanoma Res. 2013;26(4):509–17. https://doi.org/10.1111/pcmr.12092.

109. Janku F, Vaishampayan UN, Khemka V, Bhatty M, Sherman EJ, Tao J, et al. Phase 1/2 precision medicine study of the next-generation BRAF inhibitor PLX8394. J Clin Oncol. 2018;36(15_Suppl):2583. https://doi.org/10.1200/JCO.2018.36.15_suppl.2583.

110. Caunt CJ, Sale MJ, Smith PD, Cook SJ. MEK1 and MEK2 inhibitors and cancer therapy: the long and winding road. Nat Rev Cancer. 2015;15(10):577–92. https://doi.org/10.1038/nrc4000.

111. Gao Y, Chang MT, McKay D, Na N, Zhou B, Yaeger R, et al. Allele-specific mechanisms of activation of MEK1 mutants determine their properties. Cancer Discov. 2018;8(5):648–61. https://doi.org/10.1158/2159-8290.cd-17-1452.

112. Narita Y, Okamoto K, Kawada MI, Takase K, Minoshima Y, Kodama K, et al. Novel ATP-competitive MEK inhibitor E6201 is effective against vemurafenib-resistant melanoma harboring the MEK1-C121S mutation in a preclinical model. Mol Cancer Ther. 2014;13(4):823–32. https://doi.org/10.1158/1535-7163.mct-13-0667.

113. Tibes R, Borad MJ, Dutcus CE, Reyderman L, Feit K, Eisen A, et al. Safety, pharmacokinetics, and preliminary efficacy of E6201 in patients with advanced solid tumours, including melanoma: results of a phase 1 study. Br J Cancer. 2018;118(12):1580–5. https://doi.org/10.1038/s41416-018-0099-5.

114. Cortes JE, Kim DW, Pinilla-Ibarz J, le Coutre P, Paquette R, Chuah C, et al. A phase 2 trial of ponatinib in Philadelphia chromosome-positive leukemias. N Engl J Med. 2013;369(19):1783–96. https://doi.org/10.1056/NEJMoa1306494.

115. Yang K, Fu LW. Mechanisms of resistance to BCR-ABL TKIs and the therapeutic strategies: a review. Crit Rev Oncol Hematol. 2015;93(3):277–92. https://doi.org/10.1016/j.critrevonc.2014.11.001.

116. Mok TS, Wu YL, Ahn MJ, Garassino MC, Kim HR, Ramalingam SS, et al. Osimertinib or platinum-pemetrexed in EGFR T790M-positive lung cancer. N Engl J Med. 2017;376(7):629–40. https://doi.org/10.1056/NEJMoa1612674.

117. Montagut C, Argiles G, Ciardiello F, Poulsen TT, Dienstmann R, Kragh M, et al. Efficacy of Sym004 in patients with metastatic colorectal cancer with acquired resistance to anti-EGFR therapy and molecularly selected by circulating tumor DNA analyses: a phase 2 randomized clinical trial. JAMA Oncol. 2018;4(4):e175245. https://doi.org/10.1001/jamaoncol.2017.5245.

118. Carlino MS, Todd JR, Gowrishankar K, Mijatov B, Pupo GM, Fung C, et al. Differential activity of MEK and ERK inhibitors in BRAF inhibitor resistant melanoma. Mol Oncol. 2014;8(3):544–54. https://doi.org/10.1016/j.molonc.2014.01.003.

119. Germann UA, Furey BF, Markland W, Hoover RR, Aronov AM, Roix JJ, et al. Targeting the MAPK signaling pathway in cancer: promising preclinical activity with the novel selective ERK1/2 inhibitor BVD-523 (Ulixertinib). Mol Cancer Ther. 2017;16(11):2351–63. https://doi.org/10.1158/1535-7163.mct-17-0456.

120. Morris EJ, Jha S, Restaino CR, Dayananth P, Zhu H, Cooper A, et al. Discovery of a novel ERK inhibitor with activity in models of acquired resistance to BRAF and MEK inhibitors. Cancer Discov. 2013;3(7):742–50. https://doi.org/10.1158/2159-8290.cd-13-0070.
121. Hazar-Rethinam M, Kleyman M, Han GC, Liu D, Ahronian LG, Shahzade HA, et al. Convergent therapeutic strategies to overcome the heterogeneity of acquired resistance in BRAF(V600E) colorectal cancer. Cancer Discov. 2018;8(4):417–27. https://doi.org/10.1158/2159-8290.Cd-17-1227.
122. Moschos SJ, Sullivan RJ, Hwu WJ, Ramanathan RK, Adjei AA, Fong PC, et al. Development of MK-8353, an orally administered ERK1/2 inhibitor, in patients with advanced solid tumors. JCI insight. 2018;3(4) https://doi.org/10.1172/jci.insight.92352.
123. Sullivan RJ, Infante JR, Janku F, Wong DJL, Sosman JA, Keedy V, et al. First-in-class ERK1/2 inhibitor ulixertinib (BVD-523) in patients with MAPK mutant advanced solid tumors: results of a phase I dose-escalation and expansion study. Cancer Discov. 2018;8(2):184–95. https://doi.org/10.1158/2159-8290.cd-17-1119.
124. Chatterjee S, Bhattacharya S, Socinski MA, Burns TF. HSP90 inhibitors in lung cancer: promise still unfulfilled. Clin Adv Hematol Oncol. 2016;14(5):346–56.
125. Neckers L, Workman P. Hsp90 molecular chaperone inhibitors: are we there yet? Clin Cancer Res. 2012;18(1):64–76. https://doi.org/10.1158/1078-0432.ccr-11-1000.
126. Eroglu Z, Chen YA, Gibney GT, Weber JS, Kudchadkar RR, Khushalani NI, et al. Combined BRAF and HSP90 inhibition in patients with unresectable BRAF(V600E)-mutant melanoma. Clin Cancer Res. 2018;24:5516–24. https://doi.org/10.1158/1078-0432.ccr-18-0565.
127. Jameson KL, Mazur PK, Zehnder AM, Zhang J, Zarnegar B, Sage J, et al. IQGAP1 scaffold-kinase interaction blockade selectively targets RAS-MAP kinase-driven tumors. Nat Med. 2013;19(5):626–30. https://doi.org/10.1038/nm.3165.
128. Ercan D, Xu C, Yanagita M, Monast CS, Pratilas CA, Montero J, et al. Reactivation of ERK signaling causes resistance to EGFR kinase inhibitors. Cancer Discov. 2012;2(10):934–47. https://doi.org/10.1158/2159-8290.cd-12-0103.
129. Martinelli E, Morgillo F, Troiani T, Ciardiello F. Cancer resistance to therapies against the EGFR-RAS-RAF pathway: the role of MEK. Cancer Treat Rev. 2017;53:61–9. https://doi.org/10.1016/j.ctrv.2016.12.001.
130. Corcoran RB, Andre T, Atreya CE, Schellens JHM, Yoshino T, Bendell JC, et al. Combined BRAF, EGFR, and MEK inhibition in patients with BRAF(V600E)-mutant colorectal cancer. Cancer Discov. 2018;8(4):428–43. https://doi.org/10.1158/2159-8290.cd-17-1226.
131. Fruman DA, Rommel C. PI3K and cancer: lessons, challenges and opportunities. Nat Rev Drug Discov. 2014;13(2):140–56. https://doi.org/10.1038/nrd4204.
132. Sweetlove M, Wrightson E, Kolekar S, Rewcastle GW, Baguley BC, Shepherd PR, et al. Inhibitors of pan-PI3K signaling synergize with BRAF or MEK inhibitors to prevent BRAF-mutant melanoma cell growth. Front Oncol. 2015;5:135. https://doi.org/10.3389/fonc.2015.00135.
133. Sanchez-Hernandez I, Baquero P, Calleros L, Chiloeches A. Dual inhibition of (V600E) BRAF and the PI3K/AKT/mTOR pathway cooperates to induce apoptosis in melanoma cells through a MEK-independent mechanism. Cancer Lett. 2012;314(2):244–55. https://doi.org/10.1016/j.canlet.2011.09.037.
134. Atefi M, von Euw E, Attar N, Ng C, Chu C, Guo D, et al. Reversing melanoma cross-resistance to BRAF and MEK inhibitors by co-targeting the AKT/mTOR pathway. PLoS One. 2011;6(12):e28973. https://doi.org/10.1371/journal.pone.0028973.
135. Greger JG, Eastman SD, Zhang V, Bleam MR, Hughes AM, Smitheman KN, et al. Combinations of BRAF, MEK, and PI3K/mTOR inhibitors overcome acquired resistance to the BRAF inhibitor GSK2118436 dabrafenib, mediated by NRAS or MEK mutations. Mol Cancer Ther. 2012;11(4):909–20. https://doi.org/10.1158/1535-7163.MCT-11-0989.
136. Shi H, Kong X, Ribas A, Lo RS. Combinatorial treatments that overcome PDGFRbeta-driven resistance of melanoma cells to V600EB-RAF inhibition. Cancer Res. 2011;71(15):5067–74. https://doi.org/10.1158/0008-5472.can-11-0140.

137. Paraiso KH, Xiang Y, Rebecca VW, Abel EV, Chen YA, Munko AC, et al. PTEN loss confers BRAF inhibitor resistance to melanoma cells through the suppression of BIM expression. Cancer Res. 2011;71(7):2750–60. https://doi.org/10.1158/0008-5472.can-10-2954.

138. Villanueva J, Infante JR, Krepler C, Reyes-Uribe P, Samanta M, Chen HY, et al. Concurrent MEK2 mutation and BRAF amplification confer resistance to BRAF and MEK inhibitors in melanoma. Cell Rep. 2013;4(6):1090–9. https://doi.org/10.1016/j.celrep.2013.08.023.

139. Rafii S, Roda D, Geuna E, Jimenez B, Rihawi K, Capelan M, et al. Higher risk of infections with PI3K-AKT-mTOR pathway inhibitors in patients with advanced solid tumors on phase I clinical trials. Clin Cancer Res. 2015;21(8):1869–76. https://doi.org/10.1158/1078-0432.ccr-14-2424.

140. Tolcher AW, Patnaik A, Papadopoulos KP, Rasco DW, Becerra CR, Allred AJ, et al. Phase I study of the MEK inhibitor trametinib in combination with the AKT inhibitor afuresertib in patients with solid tumors and multiple myeloma. Cancer Chemother Pharmacol. 2015;75(1):183–9. https://doi.org/10.1007/s00280-014-2615-5.

141. Andre F, O'Regan R, Ozguroglu M, Toi M, Xu B, Jerusalem G, et al. Everolimus for women with trastuzumab-resistant, HER2-positive, advanced breast cancer (BOLERO-3): a randomised, double-blind, placebo-controlled phase 3 trial. Lancet Oncol. 2014;15(6):580–91. https://doi.org/10.1016/s1470-2045(14)70138-x.

142. Mangana J, Levesque MP, Karpova MB, Dummer R. Sorafenib in melanoma. Expert Opin Investig Drugs. 2012;21(4):557–68. https://doi.org/10.1517/13543784.2012.665872.

143. Eisen T, Ahmad T, Flaherty KT, Gore M, Kaye S, Marais R, et al. Sorafenib in advanced melanoma: a phase II randomised discontinuation trial analysis. Br J Cancer. 2006;95(5):581–6. https://doi.org/10.1038/sj.bjc.6603291.

144. Sakamuri D, Kato S, Huang HJ, Naing A, Holley VR, Patel S, et al. 404PDose escalation study of vemurafenib with crizotinib or sorafenib in patient with BRAF-mutated advance cancers. Ann Oncol. 2017;28(Suppl_5):mdx367.037. https://doi.org/10.1093/annonc/mdx367.037.

145. Crystal AS, Shaw AT, Sequist LV, Friboulet L, Niederst MJ, Lockerman EL, et al. Patient-derived models of acquired resistance can identify effective drug combinations for cancer. Science. 2014;346(6216):1480–6. https://doi.org/10.1126/science.1254721.

146. Pasquini G, Giaccone G. C-MET inhibitors for advanced non-small cell lung cancer. Expert Opin Investig Drugs. 2018;27(4):363–75. https://doi.org/10.1080/13543784.2018.1462336.

147. Smith MP, Brunton H, Rowling EJ, Ferguson J, Arozarena I, Miskolczi Z, et al. Inhibiting drivers of non-mutational drug tolerance is a salvage strategy for targeted melanoma therapy. Cancer Cell. 2016;29(3):270–84. https://doi.org/10.1016/j.ccell.2016.02.003.

148. Martin CA, Cullinane C, Kirby L, Abuhammad S, Lelliott EJ, Waldeck K, et al. Palbociclib synergizes with BRAF and MEK inhibitors in treatment naive melanoma but not after the development of BRAF inhibitor resistance. Int J Cancer. 2018;142(10):2139–52. https://doi.org/10.1002/ijc.31220.

149. Harris AL, Lee SE, Dawson LK, Marlow LA, Edenfield BH, Durham WF, et al. Targeting the cyclin dependent kinase and retinoblastoma axis overcomes standard of care resistance in BRAF (V600E) -mutant melanoma. Oncotarget. 2018;9(13):10905–19. https://doi.org/10.18632/oncotarget.23649.

150. Ascierto PA, Bechter O, Wolter P, Lebbe C, Elez E, Miller WH, et al. A phase Ib/II dose-escalation study evaluating triple combination therapy with a BRAF (encorafenib), MEK (binimetinib), and CDK 4/6 (ribociclib) inhibitor in patients (pts) with BRAF V600-mutant solid tumors and melanoma. J Clin Oncol. 2017;35(15_Suppl):9518. https://doi.org/10.1200/JCO.2017.35.15_suppl.9518.

151. Didier R, Mallavialle A, Ben Jouira R, Domdom MA, Tichet M, Auberger P, et al. Targeting the proteasome-associated deubiquitinating enzyme USP14 impairs melanoma cell survival and overcomes resistance to MAPK-targeting therapies. Mol Cancer Ther. 2018;17(7):1416–29. https://doi.org/10.1158/1535-7163.Mct-17-0919.

152. Ohashi Y, Okamura M, Katayama R, Fang S, Tsutsui S, Akatsuka A, et al. Targeting the Golgi apparatus to overcome acquired resistance of non-small cell lung cancer cells to

EGFR tyrosine kinase inhibitors. Oncotarget. 2018;9(2):1641–55. https://doi.org/10.18632/oncotarget.22895.

153. Strub T, Ghiraldini FG, Carcamo S, Li M, Wroblewska A, Singh R, et al. SIRT6 haploin-sufficiency induces BRAF(V600E) melanoma cell resistance to MAPK inhibitors via IGF signalling. Nat Commun. 2018;9(1):3440. https://doi.org/10.1038/s41467-018-05966-z.

154. Song C, Piva M, Sun L, Hong A, Moriceau G, Kong X, et al. Recurrent tumor cell-intrinsic and -extrinsic alterations during MAPKi-induced melanoma regression and early adaptation. Cancer Discov. 2017;7(11):1248–65. https://doi.org/10.1158/2159-8290.cd-17-0401.

155. Mattia G, Puglisi R, Ascione B, Malorni W, Care A, Matarrese P. Cell death-based treat-ments of melanoma: conventional treatments and new therapeutic strategies. Cell Death Dis. 2018;9(2):112. https://doi.org/10.1038/s41419-017-0059-7.

156. Gallagher SJ, Gunatilake D, Beaumont KA, Sharp DM, Tiffen JC, Heinemann A, et al. HDAC inhibitors restore BRAF-inhibitor sensitivity by altering PI3K and survival signal-ling in a subset of melanoma. Int J Cancer. 2018;142(9):1926–37. https://doi.org/10.1002/ijc.31199.

157. Ibrahim N, Buchbinder EI, Granter SR, Rodig SJ, Giobbie-Harder A, Becerra C, et al. A phase I trial of panobinostat (LBH589) in patients with metastatic melanoma. Cancer Med. 2016;5(11):3041–50. https://doi.org/10.1002/cam4.862.

158. Xia C, Leon-Ferre R, Laux D, Deutsch J, Smith BJ, Frees M, et al. Treatment of resistant metastatic melanoma using sequential epigenetic therapy (decitabine and panobinostat) com-bined with chemotherapy (temozolomide). Cancer Chemother Pharmacol. 2014;74(4):691–7. https://doi.org/10.1007/s00280-014-2501-1.

159. Bronte G, Bravaccini S, Bronte E, Burgio MA, Rolfo C, Delmonte A, et al. Epithelial-to-mesenchymal transition in the context of epidermal growth factor receptor inhibition in non-small-cell lung cancer. Biol Rev Camb Philos Soc. 2018;93(4):1735–46. https://doi.org/10.1111/brv.12416.

160. Duruisseaux M, Esteller M. Lung cancer epigenetics: from knowledge to applications. Semin Cancer Biol. 2018;51:116–28. https://doi.org/10.1016/j.semcancer.2017.09.005.

161. Chen MC, Chen CH, Wang JC, Tsai AC, Liou JP, Pan SL, et al. The HDAC inhibitor, MPT0E028, enhances erlotinib-induced cell death in EGFR-TKI-resistant NSCLC cells. Cell Death Dis. 2013;4:e810. https://doi.org/10.1038/cddis.2013.330.

162. Han JY, Lee SH, Lee GK, Yun T, Lee YJ, Hwang KH, et al. Phase I/II study of gefitinib (Iressa((R))) and vorinostat (IVORI) in previously treated patients with advanced non-small cell lung cancer. Cancer Chemother Pharmacol. 2015;75(3):475–83. https://doi.org/10.1007/s00280-014-2664-9.

163. Reguart N, Rosell R, Cardenal F, Cardona AF, Isla D, Palmero R, et al. Phase I/II trial of vorinostat (SAHA) and erlotinib for non-small cell lung cancer (NSCLC) patients with epidermal growth factor receptor (EGFR) mutations after erlotinib progression. Lung Cancer (Amsterdam, Netherlands). 2014;84(2):161–7. https://doi.org/10.1016/j.lungcan.2014.02.011.

164. Ng KP, Hillmer AM, Chuah CT, Juan WC, Ko TK, Teo AS, et al. A common BIM deletion polymorphism mediates intrinsic resistance and inferior responses to tyrosine kinase inhibi-tors in cancer. Nat Med. 2012;18(4):521–8. https://doi.org/10.1038/nm.2713.

165. Welsh SJ, Rizos H, Scolyer RA, Long GV. Resistance to combination BRAF and MEK inhibition in metastatic melanoma: where to next? Eur J Cancer. 2016;62:76–85. https://doi.org/10.1016/j.ejca.2016.04.005.

166. Wilmott JS, Long GV, Howle JR, Haydu LE, Sharma RN, Thompson JF, et al. Selective BRAF inhibitors induce marked T-cell infiltration into human metastatic melanoma. Clin Cancer Res. 2012;18(5):1386–94. https://doi.org/10.1158/1078-0432.Ccr-11-2479.

167. Cooper ZA, Frederick DT, Juneja VR, Sullivan RJ, Lawrence DP, Piris A, et al. BRAF inhibition is associated with increased clonality in tumor-infiltrating lymphocytes. Oncoimmunology. 2013;2(10):e26615. https://doi.org/10.4161/onci.26615.

168. Frederick DT, Piris A, Cogdill AP, Cooper ZA, Lezcano C, Ferrone CR, et al. BRAF inhibition is associated with enhanced melanoma antigen expression and a more favorable tumor microenvironment in patients with metastatic melanoma. Clin Cancer Res. 2013;19(5):1225–31. https://doi.org/10.1158/1078-0432.Ccr-12-1630.

169. Vella LJ, Pasam A, Dimopoulos N, Andrews M, Knights A, Puaux AL, et al. MEK inhibition, alone or in combination with BRAF inhibition, affects multiple functions of isolated normal human lymphocytes and dendritic cells. Cancer Immunol Res. 2014;2(4):351–60. https://doi.org/10.1158/2326-6066.Cir-13-0181.

170. Liu L, Mayes PA, Eastman S, Shi H, Yadavilli S, Zhang T, et al. The BRAF and MEK inhibitors dabrafenib and trametinib: effects on immune function and in combination with immunomodulatory antibodies targeting PD-1, PD-L1, and CTLA-4. Clin Cancer Res. 2015;21(7):1639–51. https://doi.org/10.1158/1078-0432.ccr-14-2339.

171. Pardoll DM. The blockade of immune checkpoints in cancer immunotherapy. Nat Rev Cancer. 2012;12(4):252–64. https://doi.org/10.1038/nrc3239.

172. Hodi FS, O'Day SJ, McDermott DF, Weber RW, Sosman JA, Haanen JB, et al. Improved survival with ipilimumab in patients with metastatic melanoma. N Engl J Med. 2010;363(8):711–23. https://doi.org/10.1056/NEJMoa1003466.

173. Robert C, Long GV, Brady B, Dutriaux C, Maio M, Mortier L, et al. Nivolumab in previously untreated melanoma without BRAF mutation. N Engl J Med. 2015;372(4):320–30. https://doi.org/10.1056/NEJMoa1412082.

174. Robert C, Schachter J, Long GV, Arance A, Grob JJ, Mortier L, et al. Pembrolizumab versus Ipilimumab in advanced melanoma. N Engl J Med. 2015;372(26):2521–32. https://doi.org/10.1056/NEJMoa1503093.

175. Larkin J, Chiarion-Sileni V, Gonzalez R, Grob JJ, Cowey CL, Lao CD, et al. Combined nivolumab and Ipilimumab or monotherapy in untreated melanoma. N Engl J Med. 2015;373(1):23–34. https://doi.org/10.1056/NEJMoa1504030.

176. Cooper ZA, Juneja VR, Sage PT, Frederick DT, Piris A, Mitra D, et al. Response to BRAF inhibition in melanoma is enhanced when combined with immune checkpoint blockade. Cancer Immunol Res. 2014;2(7):643–54. https://doi.org/10.1158/2326-6066.Cir-13-0215.

177. Hu-Lieskovan S, Mok S, Homet Moreno B, Tsoi J, Robert L, Goedert L, et al. Improved antitumor activity of immunotherapy with BRAF and MEK inhibitors in BRAF(V600E) melanoma. Sci Transl Med. 2015;7(279):279ra41. https://doi.org/10.1126/scitranslmed.aaa4691.

178. Gotwals P, Cameron S, Cipolletta D, Cremasco V, Crystal A, Hewes B, et al. Prospects for combining targeted and conventional cancer therapy with immunotherapy. Nat Rev Cancer. 2017;17(5):286–301. https://doi.org/10.1038/nrc.2017.17.

179. Ribas A, Hodi FS, Callahan M, Konto C, Wolchok J. Hepatotoxicity with combination of vemurafenib and ipilimumab. N Engl J Med. 2013;368(14):1365–6. https://doi.org/10.1056/NEJMc1302338.

180. Hugo W, Zaretsky JM, Sun L, Song C, Moreno BH, Hu-Lieskovan S, et al. Genomic and transcriptomic features of response to anti-PD-1 therapy in metastatic melanoma. Cell. 2016;165(1):35–44. https://doi.org/10.1016/j.cell.2016.02.065.

181. Amini-Adle M, Khanafer N, Le-Bouar M, Duru G, Dalle S, Thomas L. Ineffective anti PD-1 therapy after BRAF inhibitor failure in advanced melanoma. BMC Cancer. 2018;18(1):705. https://doi.org/10.1186/s12885-018-4618-9.

182. Amaria RN, Prieto PA, Tetzlaff MT, Reuben A, Andrews MC, Ross MI, et al. Neoadjuvant plus adjuvant dabrafenib and trametinib versus standard of care in patients with high-risk, surgically resectable melanoma: a single-centre, open-label, randomised, phase 2 trial. Lancet Oncol. 2018;19(2):181–93. https://doi.org/10.1016/s1470-2045(18)30015-9.

183. Reck M, Rodriguez-Abreu D, Robinson AG, Hui R, Csoszi T, Fulop A, et al. Pembrolizumab versus chemotherapy for PD-L1-positive non-small-cell lung cancer. N Engl J Med. 2016;375(19):1823–33. https://doi.org/10.1056/NEJMoa1606774.

184. Karachaliou N, Gonzalez-Cao M, Sosa A, Berenguer J, Bracht JWP, Ito M, et al. The combination of checkpoint immunotherapy and targeted therapy in cancer. Ann Transl Med. 2017;5(19):388. https://doi.org/10.21037/atm.2017.06.47.

185. Gettinger S, Hellmann MD, Chow LQM, Borghaei H, Antonia S, Brahmer JR, et al. Nivolumab plus erlotinib in patients with EGFR-mutant advanced NSCLC. J Thorac Oncol. 2018;13(9):1363–72. https://doi.org/10.1016/j.jtho.2018.05.015.

186. Moya-Horno I, Viteri S, Karachaliou N, Rosell R. Combination of immunotherapy with tar-geted therapies in advanced non-small cell lung cancer (NSCLC). Ther Adv Med Oncol. 2018;10:1758834017745012. https://doi.org/10.1177/1758834017745012.

187. Rosenberg SA, Restifo NP. Adoptive cell transfer as personalized immunotherapy for human cancer. Science. 2015;348(6230):62–8. https://doi.org/10.1126/science.aaa4967.

188. Goff SL, Dudley ME, Citrin DE, Somerville RP, Wunderlich JR, Danforth DN, et al. Randomized, prospective evaluation comparing intensity of lymphodepletion before adop-tive transfer of tumor-infiltrating lymphocytes for patients with metastatic melanoma. J Clin Oncol. 2016;34(20):2389–97. https://doi.org/10.1200/jco.2016.66.7220.

189. Deniger DC, Kwong ML, Pasetto A, Dudley ME, Wunderlich JR, Langhan MM, et al. A pilot trial of the combination of vemurafenib with adoptive cell therapy in patients with meta-static melanoma. Clin Cancer Res. 2017;23(2):351–62. https://doi.org/10.1158/1078-0432. Ccr-16-0906.

190. Druker BJ. Circumventing resistance to kinase-inhibitor therapy. N Engl J Med. 2006;354(24):2594–6. https://doi.org/10.1056/NEJMe068073.

191. Das Thakur M, Stuart DD. The evolution of melanoma resistance reveals therapeutic oppor-tunities. Cancer Res. 2013;73(20):6106–10. https://doi.org/10.1158/0008-5472.can-13-1633.

192. Ascierto PA, Margolin K. Ipilimumab before BRAF inhibitor treatment may be more beneficial than vice versa for the majority of patients with advanced melanoma. Cancer. 2014;120(11):1617–9. https://doi.org/10.1002/cncr.28622.

193. Lee JH, Long GV, Boyd S, Lo S, Menzies AM, Tembe V, et al. Circulating tumour DNA pre-dicts response to anti-PD1 antibodies in metastatic melanoma. Ann Oncol. 2017;28(5):1130–6. https://doi.org/10.1093/annonc/mdx026.

194. Gray ES, Rizos H, Reid AL, Boyd SC, Pereira MR, Lo J, et al. Circulating tumor DNA to monitor treatment response and detect acquired resistance in patients with metastatic mela-noma. Oncotarget. 2015;6(39):42008–18. https://doi.org/10.18632/oncotarget.5788.

195. Long GV, Hauschild A, Santinami M, Atkinson V, Mandala M, Chiarion-Sileni V, et al. Adjuvant dabrafenib plus trametinib in stage III BRAF-mutated melanoma. N Engl J Med. 2017;377(19):1813–23. https://doi.org/10.1056/NEJMoa1708539.

196. Piccart-Gebhart MJ, Procter M, Leyland-Jones B, Goldhirsch A, Untch M, Smith I, et al. Trastuzumab after adjuvant chemotherapy in HER2-positive breast cancer. N Engl J Med. 2005;353(16):1659 72. https://doi.org/10.1056/NEJMoa052306.

197. Gajria D, Chandarlapaty S. HER2-amplified breast cancer: mechanisms of trastuzumab resis-tance and novel targeted therapies. Expert Rev Anticancer Ther. 2011;11(2):263–75. https://doi.org/10.1586/era.10.226.

198. Gomez HL, Doval DC, Chavez MA, Ang PC, Aziz Z, Nag S, et al. Efficacy and safety of lapatinib as first-line therapy for ErbB2-amplified locally advanced or metastatic breast can-cer. J Clin Oncol. 2008;26(18):2999–3005. https://doi.org/10.1200/jco.2007.14.0590.

199. Cortes JE, Kantarjian H, Shah NP, Bixby D, Mauro MJ, Flinn I, et al. Ponatinib in refractory Philadelphia chromosome-positive leukemias. N Engl J Med. 2012;367(22):2075–88. https://doi.org/10.1056/NEJMoa1205127.

200. Gorre ME, Mohammed M, Ellwood K, Hsu N, Paquette R, Rao PN, et al. Clinical resistance to STI-571 cancer therapy caused by BCR-ABL gene mutation or amplification. Science. 2001;293(5531):876–80. https://doi.org/10.1126/science.1062538.

201. Kantarjian H, Shah NP, Hochhaus A, Cortes J, Shah S, Ayala M, et al. Dasatinib versus imatinib in newly diagnosed chronic-phase chronic myeloid leukemia. N Engl J Med. 2010;362(24):2260–70. https://doi.org/10.1056/NEJMoa1002315.

202. Kantarjian HM, Giles F, Gattermann N, Bhalla K, Alimena G, Palandri F, et al. Nilotinib (formerly AMN107), a highly selective BCR-ABL tyrosine kinase inhibitor, is effective in patients with Philadelphia chromosome-positive chronic myelogenous leukemia in chronic

phase following imatinib resistance and intolerance. Blood. 2007;110(10):3540–6. https://doi.org/10.1182/blood-2007-03-080689.

203. Heinrich MC, Maki RG, Corless CL, Antonescu CR, Harlow A, Griffith D, et al. Primary and secondary kinase genotypes correlate with the biological and clinical activity of sunitinib in imatinib-resistant gastrointestinal stromal tumor. J Clin Oncol. 2008;26(33):5352–9. https://doi.org/10.1200/jco.2007.15.7461.

204. Yu HA, Arcila ME, Rekhtman N, Sima CS, Zakowski MF, Pao W, et al. Analysis of tumor specimens at the time of acquired resistance to EGFR-TKI therapy in 155 patients with EGFR-mutant lung cancers. Clin Cancer Res. 2013;19(8):2240–7. https://doi.org/10.1158/1078-0432.ccr-12-2246.

205. Shaw AT, Kim DW, Mehra R, Tan DS, Felip E, Chow LQ, et al. Ceritinib in ALK-rearranged non-small-cell lung cancer. N Engl J Med. 2014;370(13):1189–97. https://doi.org/10.1056/NEJMoa1311107.

206. Shaw AT, Gandhi L, Gadgeel S, Riely GJ, Cetnar J, West H, et al. Alectinib in ALK-positive, crizotinib-resistant, non-small-cell lung cancer: a single-group, multicentre, phase 2 trial. Lancet Oncol. 2016;17(2):234–42. https://doi.org/10.1016/s1470-2045(15)00488-x.

207. Friboulet L, Li N, Katayama R, Lee CC, Gainor JF, Crystal AS, et al. The ALK inhibitor ceritinib overcomes crizotinib resistance in non-small cell lung cancer. Cancer Discov. 2014;4(6):662–73. https://doi.org/10.1158/2159-8290.cd-13-0846.

208. Katayama R, Shaw AT, Khan TM, Mino-Kenudson M, Solomon BJ, Halmos B, et al. Mechanisms of acquired crizotinib resistance in ALK-rearranged lung cancers. Sci Transl Med. 2012;4(120):120ra17. https://doi.org/10.1126/scitranslmed.3003316.

209. Solomon BJ, Mok T, Kim DW, Wu YL, Nakagawa K, Mekhail T, et al. First-line crizotinib versus chemotherapy in ALK-positive lung cancer. N Engl J Med. 2014;371(23):2167–77. https://doi.org/10.1056/NEJMoa1408440.

210. Morais C. Sunitinib resistance in renal cell carcinoma. J Kidney Cancer VHL. 2014;1(1):1–11. https://doi.org/10.15586/jkcvhl.2014.7.

211. Choueiri TK, Escudier B, Powles T, Tannir NM, Mainwaring PN, Rini BI, et al. Cabozantinib versus everolimus in advanced renal cell carcinoma (METEOR): final results from a randomised, open-label, phase 3 trial. Lancet Oncol. 2016;17(7):917–27. https://doi.org/10.1016/s1470-2045(16)30107-3.

212. Motzer RJ, Hutson TE, Cella D, Reeves J, Hawkins R, Guo J, et al. Pazopanib versus sunitinib in metastatic renal-cell carcinoma. N Engl J Med. 2013;369(8):722–31. https://doi.org/10.1056/NEJMoa1303989.

Chapter 9
Targeting Epigenetic Regulators in Cancer to Overcome Resistance to Targeted Therapy

Mukesh Verma and Vineet Kumar

Abstract Resistance to cancer therapy is an ongoing challenge, and there is a need to seek out non-traditional approaches such as targeting epigenetic components for cancer therapy. Epigenomics provides essential tools not only for therapeutic intervention but also as predictors of drug response. Unlike alteration of genetic components, where the structure of a gene is changed, such as mutations, deletions, additions, and single nucleotide polymorphisms, epigenetics changes gene expression without altering the genetic sequence. Furthermore, several epigenetic changes are reversible, and as a result, drugs have been developed that can reverse the epigenetic changes associated with different cancers. These epigenetic drugs target DNA methyltransferases, histone deacetylases and proteins associated with post-transcriptionally modified histones. Epigenetic regulators represent potential therapeutic targets as they often have binding domains that lend themselves well to small molecule inhibition. Here, we discuss factors that contribute to the development of resistance to targeted therapy and how epigenetic regulators can be utilized to overcome this resistance. We provide examples of several cancer types for which conventional targeted therapy has limited effects, but improved treatment outcomes are observed following epigenetic reprogramming of gene expression patterns, including modification of histones and DNA. Results from clinical trials have indicated the efficacy of epigenetic drugs as cancer therapy, mainly when administered in combination with traditional anticancer drugs. These promising data suggest that epigenetic drugs have great potential in controlling and treating cancer.

M. Verma (✉)
Methods and Technologies Branch, Epidemiology and Genomics Research Program, Division of Cancer Control and Population Sciences, National Cancer Institute, National Institutes of Health, Bethesda, MD, USA
e-mail: vermam@mail.nih.gov

V. Kumar (✉)
Department of Physiology, National University of Singapore, Singapore, Singapore
e-mail: phcvk@nus.edu.sg

© Springer Nature Switzerland AG 2019
M. R. Szewczuk et al. (eds.), *Current Applications for Overcoming Resistance to Targeted Therapies*, Resistance to Targeted Anti-Cancer Therapeutics 20,
https://doi.org/10.1007/978-3-030-21477-7_9

Keywords Biomarker · Epigenetics · Epidemiology · Histones · Methylation · Treatment

Abbreviations

AUC	Area under curve
CDKN1	Cyclin-dependent kinase inhibitor 1
CRC	Colorectal cancer
CRPC	Castration resistant prostate cancer
CSCs	Cancer stem cells
DNMTs	DNA methyltransferases
EMT	Epithelial-to-mesenchymal transition
EZH2	Enhancer of zeste homolog 2
HATs	Histone acetyltransferases
HCC	Hepatocellular carcinoma
HDAC	Histone deacetylase
HER2	Human epidermal growth factor receptor
HY-PDT	Hypericin-mediated photodynamic therapy
KMTs	Histone lysine methyltransferases
LINE	Long interspersed nuclear elements
miRs	Micro RNAs
NaPB	3-[4,5-Dimethylthiazol-2-yl]-2,5-diphenyltetrazolium bromide
NSCLC	Non-small cell lung cancer
oncomiR	Oncogenic miRNAs
ORR	Overall response rate
PSA	Prostate-specific antigen
RCC	Renal cell carcinoma
SAHA	Suberoylanilide hydroximic acid
SINE	Short interspersed nuclear elements
TET	Ten-eleven translocation protein family
TSA	Trichostatin A
VEGF	Vascular endothelial growth factor
VPA	Valproic acid

9.1 Introduction: The Landscape of Epigenetics

Cancer epigenetics is very complicated, primarily because gene silencing by epigenetics varies in different tumour types [1–5]. Both genetics and epigenetics contribute to cancer development, and multicellular organisms cannot develop and function without the interaction between the epigenome and the genome [6]. While genetics provides a repertoire of the genetic potential of an organism, epigenetics regulate gene expression and dictate how much of this genetic potential is actualized. As such, epigenetic alterations are far more dynamic than genetic changes, which cannot be reversed. That being said, the main regulatory components of the epigenome include DNA methylation (mostly in the promoter region), histone post-translation modifications, non-histone proteins such as the polycomb repressor complex, noncoding RNAs (mainly microRNAs), and alterations in chromatin conformation, providing accessibility to transcription factors and other factors needed for gene transcription [7–9].

Chromatin comprises both a DNA and a protein scaffold. The basic structure of chromatin, also called a nucleosome, consists of two copies of each of the four histone proteins, namely H2A, H2B, H3, and H4, in the form of an octamer [2, 10–12]. DNA wraps around the octamer to neutralize the basic charge of the DNA, providing stability to the genome. Histone H1 is a linker and functions as a scaffolding protein [13]. Histone proteins respond to the microenvironment and post-translational modifications such as acetylation, butylation, phosphorylation, ubiquitination, and methylation, which can modulate non-covalent interactions between DNA and histones [14, 15].

In regards to cancer development, aberrant epigenetic profiling and impaired gene expression are first modifications that occur and specifically affect oncogenes and tumour suppressor genes. These epigenetic changes are outlined below.

9.1.1 Histone Acetylation

Acetylation of histones is the most common form of epigenetic modification and increases chromatin accessibility through alteration of the overall histone charge and reductions in the DNA-histone interaction. Histone lysine methyltransferases (KMTs), histone acetyltransferases (HATs), and DNA methyltransferases (DNMTs) generate covalent marks called 'writers" which are then interpreted by the methyl-CpG-binding domain (MBD) proteins called "readers." Almost all epigenetic marks can be erased by "erasers" including histone deacetylases (HDACs), histone demethylases (KDMs) and other enzymes (ten-eleven translocation (TET) family of 5-methylcytosine oxidases). KMTs and lysine demethylases (KDMs) are particularly crucial epigenetic histone modifiers of cancer gene expression and have been shown to have broader implications as both potential therapeutic targets and in the understanding of cancer progression. For example, in prostate cancer, lysine methyltransferases SUV39H1 (KMT1A) and SETDB1 (KMT1E) were shown to enhance prostate cancer cell migration and invasion, and as such have been considered potential epigenetic therapeutic targets [16]. Additionally, lysine-specific demethylase 1 (LSD1/KDM1A) worked as an oncogene in prostate and other cancers [17, 18]. Conversely, lysine demethylase 5 (KDM5) loss was associated with resistance to docetaxel in prostate cancer [19]. Overall, histone modifications are an integral part of epigenetic regulation and work in combination with other epigenetic components.

9.1.2 DNA Methylation and Aberrations in Epigenetic Regulation in Cancer

An additional component of the epigenome is the modulation of gene expression through DNA methylation. Methylation of cytosine in the promoter region of a DNA strand results in silencing downstream genes which may contribute to tumour development and drug resistance [20–24]. DNA methylation occurs through the addition of a methyl group to the fifth carbon of cytosine (5-methyl cytosine) by a DNA methyltransferase enzyme and exclusively occurs within the CpG dinucleotide. The process of DNA methylation is dynamic and reversible and can be easily altered by external stimuli. Gene transcription can be stopped or repressed by DNA methylation by inhibiting the binding of the transcription machinery.

Aberrant DNA methylation is a hallmark of cancer. Most studies in cancer and methylation have been conducted in the promoter region, however, even within a single promoter region, not all CpG Sites, called CpG islands, are functionally equivalent. Transcriptional silencing is often controlled by methylation of one or more parts of the promoter. Identifying the precise location of clinically relevant CpG islands is useful for developing treatment strategies for cancer.

DNA methylation is an actively regulated process that involves a balance between methylation (by DNA methyltransferases) and demethylation (by demethylases). DNMT1, DNMT3A, and DNMT3B are the main DNA methyltransferases, with DNMT1 maintaining methylation levels and DNMT3A and DNMT3B initiating *de novo* methylation. Demethylation of DNA involves oxidation of 5-methyl-cytosine to 5-methyl-hydroxy-cytosine which in turn is removed by DNA machinery and replication. The oxidation step occurs due to the activity of Ten-eleven Translocation (TET) protein families, with TET1 working in the promoter region and TET2 working in the main body of the gene. Individual gene methylation was initially studied in cancer, but current research focuses on genome-wide methylation due to the development of microarray and methylation sequencing technologies.

Part of the genome is already methylated, particularly repeat sequences, Short Interspersed Nuclear Elements (SINEs) and Long Interspersed Nuclear Elements (LINEs), which provide stability to the genome. However, during cancer development, SINEs and LINEs are hypomethylated due to the activity of demethylating enzymes. Common genes which get inactivated due to methylation are summarized in Table 9.1 [13, 15, 22]. Promoters of some types of cancers, such as colorectal cancer (CRC), exhibit a CpG island methylator phenotype (CIMP) which is characterized by the increased prevalence of CpG islands in methylation profiling [25]. CRC tumours with CIMP show distinct molecular features and are tightly associated with BRAF mutations and increased DNMT3b expression. BRAF is an important oncogene in the regulation of cell proliferation and apoptosis. As outlined above, methylation patterns significantly contribute to the development of cancer and are viable therapeutic targets.

Table 9.1 Genes inactivated by methylation in various cancer types

Cancer type	Genes inactivated due to methylation
Bladder cancer	APC, RARB2, RASSF1A, JUP, DAL1, and DAPK1
Brain cancer	TIMP3 and PCDHA8
Breast cancer	NDRG2 and HOXD1
Cervical cancer	DKK3, PCTH, and SFRP1
Colorectal cancer	PTGIS, PTGFR, EBN2, p14, ARF, and AKR1B1
Endometrial cancer	APC, RASF1A, MGM2, and hMLH1
Esophageal cancer	PTK2, RDN1, and UBL3
Gastric cancer	NGRT2, RASGRF1, and CDH1
Lung cancer	F2RL3
Renal cancer	PITx1, FOXE3, TWF2, EHBPL1 and RIN1

9.1.3 MicroRNAs and Their Role in Modifying Gene Expression

MicroRNAs (miRNAs) and non-coding RNAs (small interfering RNAs, small nucleolar RNAs, and piwi-interacting RNAs) are essential components of epigenetics that mediate gene expression. About 1400 human miRNAs have been identified to date (miRBase—http://www.mirbase.org/cgi-bin/browse.pl), and approximately 30–40% of genes are regulated by miRNAs [13, 26–29]. About 40% of the total miRNAs in humans are clustered, and each cluster typically regulates a common pathway. miRNAs are a class of non-coding RNAs that act post-transcriptionally and affect gene expression and are reported to contribute to the development of resistance to anticancer drugs. For example, resistance to 5-fluorouracil is mediated by miR-21, miR-27a/b, and miR-155, and resistance to docetaxel is mediated by miR-98, miR-192, miR-194, miR-200b, miR-212, and miR-424 [30]. High-throughput technologies have been developed which can identify differential miRNA profiles in tumours.

Due to the abnormal miRNA expression observed during cancer development, it is possible that these miRNAs can be therapeutically targeted [31]. Mechanistically, the expression of miRNAs can be regulated by methylation and histone modifications. More specifically, expression of miRNAs which inactivate tumour suppressor genes can be reversed through treatment with epigenetic drugs such as demethylating or acetylating agents. Thus, oncogenic miRNAs (oncomiR) can be targeted by epigenetics to reduce or inhibit cancer cell proliferation [31–35].

The biosynthesis of miRNAs requires specific processing before active miRNAs are synthesized. The processed miRNA comes from its precursor primary miRNA (primiRNA) which can have different secondary structures with loops of 60–80 nucleotides [36, 37]. These loops are recognized by a nuclear RNase III endonucle-ase called DORSHA in association with a protein called DGCR-8 and a pre-miRNA with two 3′ nucleotides overhang is generated. The pre-miRNA is transported from the nucleus to the cytoplasm with the help of two proteins, exoportion 5 and Ran-GTP. Finally, RNase III DICER cleaves the pre-miRNA into its mature and func-tional miRNA of 22–25 nucleotides, which is very stable in the cytoplasm. Each tumour type has a specific miRNA profile, making them excellent targets for diag-nosis and prognosis [31, 38–41].

9.1.4   Current Therapeutic Options for Targeting the Epigenome in Cancer

In cancer, plasticity refers to the ability of a given genotype to confer a variety of phenotypes due to interaction with external and internal environmental fac-tors. These factors interact with epigenetic components and may lead to several disorders. Thus, individuals with epigenetic alterations and their associated disorders may not respond to therapy. Understanding personalized genomics and epigenomics might help in designing a precise treatment plan for each patient. Longitudinal follow-ups at different time points will be needed for such approaches. A few projects, such as the National Institutes of Health Roadmap Epigenomics Mapping Consortium, the International Human Epigenomic Consortium, the European Community Initiative BLUEPRINT, the Encyclopedia of DNA Elements, and the Cancer Genomic Atlas, have pro-vided large amounts of data which have helped in our understanding of how epigenetic and genetic mechanisms regulate physiological and pathological gene expression [6].

Currently, DNA methylation inhibitors are the standard of care for certain hema-tologic malignancies, and several new drugs that target histone modifications are being tested in clinical trials [3, 6, 42]. Two main categories of epigenetic inhibitors are hypomethylating agents (such as decitabine, a DNA methyltransferase inhibitor) and histone deacetylase inhibitors (such as panobinostat) [22, 42]. Several other epigenetic drugs and their activities are summarized in Table 9.2. Epigenetic regula-tors have been utilized in the treatment of hematologic malignancies such as myelo-dysplastic syndrome and acute myelogenic leukemia. However, this approach has several challenges in the treatment of solid tumours [43–47]. Some of the chal-lenges include identifying a specific miRNA targeted therapy in tumours and avoid-ing adverse side effects. For example, in CLL patients with 13q deletion, higher levels of BCL2, which controls apoptosis, were observed due to the loss of miR-15a/miR-16-1. In the same patients, higher levels of tumour suppressor protein TP53 were also observed, resulting in a different phenotype [39]. The goal is to find out what amount of miRNA expression is needed to have an optimal clinical outcome.

Table 9.2 Targets and FDA approval status of epigenetic drugs

Name of drug	Therapeutic target	Cancer type	FDA approval	Refs
Belinostat	HDAC inhibitor	Works on different cancers, not specific for one tumour type	Yes	[163]
FK228	A cyclic peptide HDAC inhibitor which is specific for HDAC1	Works on different cancers, not specific for one tumour type	No	[164]
Suberoylanilide hydroxamic acid [165] (SAHA)	HDAC inhibitor	Acts on all types of cancers, phase III for lung cancer	Yes	[166, 167]
Panobinostat	HDAC inhibitor	Acts on all types of cancers	Yes	[164, 168, 169]
Zebularine	DNA methyltransferase inhibitor	Suitable for childhood medulloblastoma treatment	Yes	[6]
BET inhibitors (JQ1 and trametinib in combination)	DNA methyltransferase inhibitor	Works for colorectal cancer by reducing cell proliferation mediated by MYC downregulation	No	[167]
5-Azacytidine (Azacytidine), trade name Vidaza	Demethylating agent	Phase II for leukemia, lung, and colorectal cancer	Yes	[164, 168, 169]
5-Aza-2'deoxycytidine (decitabine), trade name Dacogen	Demethylating agent	Being used for Phase II for leukemia	Yes	[6, 168, 169]
4-Phenyl butyric acid (PBA)	HDAC inhibitor	Phase II for leukemia, lung cancer, lymphoma, multiple myeloma, and plasma cell neoplasm, prostate cancer	No	[167]
Valproic acid (VPA)	HDAC inhibitor	For leukemia and head and neck cancer	Yes	[166–169]
Trichostatin (TSA)	HDAC inhibitor	For different cancers	Yes	[6, 164]

Insufficient miRNA expression will not be enough for antitumor activity, and excess expression may result in unintended consequences, given that a single miRNA can influence many genes. An additional challenge is related to the use of miRNA therapy in personalized medicine. This would require that a specific preferred route of drug administration and duration of action are identified for specific miRNAs and specific patients. Once those above are addressed, miRNA therapy presents as a promising therapy either as a single agent or in combination with other conventional anticancer agents.

9.1.5 Overview of the Role of Epigenetics in the Development of Drug Resistance

Although there have been several drugs and therapies developed with some success for the treatment of cancer, the development of resistance remains to be a critical challenge, primarily due to the unknown underlying mechanisms of acquiring resistance to therapy. For example, trastuzumab is the standard treatment for HER-2 positive metastatic breast cancer, but 25–30% of patients undergoing first-line of treatment do not respond to this therapy due to the acquisition of resistance [32]. In attempts to overcome this resistance, targeting epigenetic components has been proposed due to the pivotal role played by epigenetics in regulating the malignant phenotype [48–50]. Panja et al. have developed an integrative epigenome analysis to predict response to androgen-deprivation therapy in prostate cancer and identified a panel that can be utilized to pre-screen patients and identify individuals that are classified as high-risk non-responders to therapy [51].

Additionally, a new epigenomic approach has recently been developed to identify cisplatin-resistant cells during cancer therapy [50]. Cisplatin is the most widely used therapeutic agent for solid tumours, including lung, ovarian, testis, and head and neck cancer. A recent report by Sharma et al. identified dynamic modifications as a novel non-mutational mechanism of drug resistance reversible by HDAC inhibitors [52]. Among HDAC isoforms, benzamide works on class 1 HDAC isoform whereas hydroxamic acid works on both class 1 and 2 HDAC isoforms. Although the underlying role of epigenetics in the development of drug resistance is currently being elucidated, this area of research has seen an exponential increase in the number of publications reporting on epigenetic regulators in targeted therapy resistance and are summarized in Table 9.3.

9.2 Therapeutic Resistance and Epigenetic Approaches in Treating Different Cancers

Response rates to treatment regimens have been shown to vary in patients and not surprisingly, 100% therapeutic efficacy has not been achieved for any tumour type. As discussed above, this is due to drug resistance limiting the potency of both conventional chemotherapeutic agents and biological agents [30, 38, 53]. Although some success has been achieved in hematologic malignancies, attempts are being made to develop alternative treatment options for solid cancers using single inhibitors or a combination of inhibitors of cancer development and progression. This section focuses on resistance to targeted therapy in several cancer types as dictated by epigenetic modifications to the cancer genome. As an extension of this, the current advancements in therapeutically targeting the epigenome are discussed with a focus on how to overcome resistance to therapy. Additionally, the obstacles of

Table 9.3 Literature in the field of epigenetic therapy and drug resistance

Terms used	Number of publications
Epigenetics	25,653
Cancer	3,697,125
Cancer epigenetics	10,235
Cancer therapy	670,057
Cancer drug resistance	116,792
Cancer therapy resistance	56,995
Epigenetics and cancer therapy	2262
Resistance to epigenetic therapy	1580
Epigenetic regulators in cancer	1466
Epigenetic regulators in cancer therapy	380
Histone inhibitors in cancer therapy	4763
Methylation inhibitors in cancer therapy	1560
Combination of epigenetic inhibitors in cancer therapy	517

The PubMed search was conducted in July 2018 using the indicated terms. The analysis indicates that the number of publications in epigenetic regulators in resistance to targeted drug therapy is much less than in drug resistance

targeting epigenetic regulators and potential solutions to overcome these challenges are discussed in order to improve patient outcomes.

9.2.1 Breast Cancer

Breast cancer is among the most heterogeneous type of cancer and is classified broadly into several subtypes, many of which acquire a resistant phenotype following treatment with radiation and chemotherapy [32]. As such, determining whether patients will be responsive to conventional or targeted therapies is an important avenue to explore, particularly as it relates to the epigenome and the resulting modifications that contribute to the development of resistance. With respect to the predictive potential of epigenetics, Gampenrieder et al. recently identified methylation loci which could distinguish between responders and non-responders to bevacizumab, an anti-VEGF therapy administered to patients with metastatic breast cancer, with a high predictive response (overall response rate (ORR) of 40, $p < 0.001$ and an area under curve (AUC) of 0.91) in metastatic breast cancer therapy [54]. Earlier studies where other biomarkers (e.g. plasma levels of VEGF-A or VEGFR-2, tissue markers such as the VEGFR co-receptor neuropilin-1, single nucleotide polymorphisms in VEGF-A, or clinical markers including treatment-induced hypertension) were tested to predict response to treatment were not as useful as the methylation markers identified in the study above.

Furthermore, with respect to miRNA, Li et al. demonstrated the importance of miRNA where serum miRNA signatures (e.g. miR-940 from the tumour cells, and miR-451a, miR-16-5p, and miR-17-3p from immune cells) were predictive of the efficacy of trastuzumab, an anti-HER-2 receptor antibody, in HER-2-positive breast cancer patients and could serve as a predictive marker for survival [32]. miRNAs identified by Li et al. were shown to target signalling molecules that contribute to trastuzumab resistance directly. Additionally, the miR-200 group of miRNAs (miR-200a, miR-200b, miR-200c, miR-141, and miR-141) have also been shown to regulate epithelial-to-mesenchymal transition (EMT) and could be viable therapeutic targets [55].

Epigenetic targets have also been explored in the treatment of breast cancer. Recently, the process of histone acetylation was targeted, where HDACs were used in combination with hypericin-mediated photodynamic therapy (HY-PDT) [56]. HY-PDT is considered to be a minimally invasive treatment [57], but HY-PDT alone contributed to the development of resistance. In the first combination, HY-PDT was combined with suberoylanilide hydroximic acid (SAHA) and trichostatin (inhibitors of all classes of HDACs), and in the second combination, HY-PDT was combined with short-chain fatty acids valproic acid and sodium phenylbutyrate (inhibitors of nuclear HDACs) [58]. Both combinations attenuated HY-PDT treatment with similar potency. Interestingly, tumour suppressor gene cyclin-dependent kinase inhibitor 1A (CDKN1A), which is involved in chromatin modulation was strongly expressed in the second combination. This was a surprising revelation because 3-[4,5-Dimethylthiazol-2-yl]-2,5-diphenyltetrazolium bromide (NaPB) is known to regulate CDKN1a by acetylating enhancer and promoter elements but not the histones or DNA methylation. Taken collectively, these studies provide promising insight into the role of epigenetic modification in the development of resistance to treatment and ultimately in applying epigenetic approaches in targeted breast cancer therapy [59].

9.2.2 Cervical Cancer

Approximately 0.6% of women will be diagnosed with cervical cancer in the United States. The number of new cases of cervical cancer was 7.4 per 100,000 women per year, and the number of deaths was 2.3 per 100,000 per year (https://seer.cancer.gov/registries/). The primary risk factor for cervical cancer is the human papillomavirus infection. Although epigenetic therapy has not yet been applied in the clinical treatment of cervical cancer, methylation profiling of *MYOD1*, *ESR1*, and *hTERT*, have provided insight in predicting the response of invasive cervical cancer patients treated with standard chemotherapy and radiation [60]. As a result, it was determined that chemoradiation, compared to radiation alone, demonstrated significant improvements in the treatment of cervical cancer. Chen et al. further confirmed the importance of methylation, with oxaliplatin resistance in cervical cancer cells found to be the result of global hypermethylation [61]. Demethylating agents where then used in order to overcome resistance. miRNA maturation has also been proposed to contribute to the development of drug resistance in cervical cancer, oral squamous cell carcinoma and breast cancer [30]. For example, Sannigarhi et al. observed an increased sensitization of Has-miR-139-3p in HPV-16 positive cervical cancer [33]. Additionally, the influence of MDR1 methylation on the curative effect of intervention embolism chemotherapy was also demonstrated in cervical cancer [62].

Although the application of epigenetics is currently in a state of infancy concerning cervical cancer, aspects of the epigenome have shown to play a significant role in the development of resistance. Methylation profiling at different stages of cervical cancer development should be determined to help predict response to therapy. Moreover, epidemiological studies with a temporal collection of data should be conducted to evaluate the association of profiling as a predictor of response to therapy.

9.2.3 Colon Cancer

There are an estimated 97,000 new cases of colon cancer and 50,600 deaths from colon cancer expected in the United States. Recently, epigenetic therapy was tested in colon cancer using different HDACs due to their minimal toxicity and a few reports of sensitizing cells to other treatments [58]. He et al. demonstrated that methylation of SFNL11 is a marker of poor prognosis and cisplatin resistance in colorectal cancer [63]. Reactivation of the expression of CDKN1A through the application of HDAC inhibitors reduced resistance to hypericin-mediated photodynamic therapy in colorectal cancer [58]. Photodynamic therapy involves a combination of light, oxygen, and non-toxic photosensitizer and is considered an alternative minimally invasive method of cancer treatment. In another study, upregulation of Nrf2 (a basic leucine zipper that regulates expression of antioxidant proteins) in 5-fluorouracil-resistant cells was achieved by treatment with DNA demethylase and histone methyltransferase [64]. Colon cancer stem cells develop resistance to chemotherapeutics, but Fesler et al. proposed that selected miRNAs can overcome this resistance and reduce the plasticity of colon cancer stem cells [65]. MiR-206 was found to regulate 5-fluorouracil resistance by targeting Bcl-2 activity [40].

Furthermore, demethylating inhibitors were found to be effective in eliminating resistance to camptothecin in colon cancer [66]. Recently, microarray profiling of the whole methylome of colon cancer indicated differential epigenetic regulation in serrated adenocarcinoma, which might be useful in explaining the weak immune response that is characteristic of serrated adenocarcinoma [67]. This method of profiling will also help in identifying potential targets for treating this cancer type which otherwise lacks molecular targeted therapy. Thus, demethylating agents and miRNA therapy, have potential in the treatment of colon cancer, which when followed by periodic evaluation, may lead to earlier identification and better management of the disease.

9.2.4 Glioblastoma

Glioblastoma is a malignant grade IV tumour where a large portion of tumour cells are in the dividing phase. A tumour is mainly made up of abnormal astrocytic cells but also contains a mix of different cell types. Generally, glioblastoma initially grows slowly, but can progressively become more aggressive. Although chemotherapy is the standard of care for the treatment of glioblastoma, it has had a marginal rate of success, primarily due to the limited permeability of the blood-brain barrier to drugs [68]. This has led to temozolomide treatment becoming a more viable option as it has demonstrated some success [69]. However, it is known that several histone demethylase genes are overexpressed in glioblastoma in comparison to normal brain cells, and their expression is further increased during the development of temozolomide resistance [70]. This is particularly significant because temozolomide treatment was especially effective in patients in which hypermethylation resulted in MGMT (a DNA repair gene) inactivation. Further research showed that antagomic miR-21 and miR-10b pretreatment of glioblastoma-sensitized cells and lower doses of temozolomide were found to be more effective than temozolomide alone [71].

Concerning the importance of miRNA, Cheng et al. found that miR-132 was capable of inducing resistance to temozolomide and promoting a cancer stem cell phenotype by acting on tumour suppressor gene TUSC3 [72]. Additionally, miR-181b affected temozolomide efficacy by targeting the epidermal growth factor receptor (EGFR) on glioblastoma cells [73]. Banelli et al. further demonstrated that small molecules targeting histone demethylase genes inhibited the growth of temozolomide-resistant glioblastoma cells [74]. Taken collectively, there is evidence on the importance of targeting epigenetic modifications on resistant phenotypes in order to improve response to therapy, and this area of research should continue to be explored.

9.2.5 Hepatocellular Carcinoma

In liver cancer or hepatocellular carcinoma (HCC), hepatitis B infection plays a significant role in the development and progression of cancer. Current treatment options can control disease progression, but resistance can develop as a result of covalently closed circular viral DNA, which is decorated with histones and non-histone proteins [75]. Although additional research is needed to eliminate epigenetically regulated therapy resistance in HCC, several examples demonstrate the importance of epigenetics in both the development of resistance and as a therapeutic target. For example, histone acetyltransferase-1 was shown to induce cisplatin resistance in HCC [76]. In contrast, concerning miRNA, miR-9 was able to enhance the sensitivity of epithelial phenotype cells of hepatocellular carcinoma to cetuximab through regulation of a transcription factor eIF-5A-2 [77]. MiR-122 downregulated expression of the multidrug resistance (MDR) gene in HCC [78], whereas miR-221 is associated with sorafenib resistance [79]. Tang et al. demonstrated RNAi-mediated EZH2 depletion resulted in a decrease in MDR expression and sensitization of HCC cells [80].

9.2.6   Leukemia

Epigenetic regulators have been utilized for the treatment of hematologic malignancies including myelodysplastic syndrome (MDS) and acute myeloid leukemia (AML); however, in solid tumours, this approach has several challenges. MDS shows several mutations located in epigenetic regulatory genes, specifically DNA methyltransferases and histone methyl transferases [81]. More than 70% of AML patients have shown at least one mutation in their epigenetic regulatory genes [82]. In one clinical trial, children with AML were treated with decitabine, an inhibitor of methyltransferase, followed by standard treatment, with successful survival outcomes [43]. MDS and AML exist along a continuous disease spectrum starting with early-stage MDS which may progress to other pathologically identifiable stages called advanced MDS, AML, cured AML or resistant AML. These stages have a common feature in that they produce immature blood cells. Epigenetic-based treatments are now considered to be a useful treatment option in efforts to decrease the abnormal epigenetic alterations. However, one challenge of epigenetic therapy in leukemia, which may also be the case for other cancer types, is to tackle the challenge of combining drugs to optimize synergy and decrease the risk of antagonism or inhibition. Reliable biomarkers of the efficacy of the drugs are also needed.

9.2.7   Lung Cancer

Among all types of lung cancers, non-small cell lung cancer (NSCLC) is the most common cause of cancer-related death [83, 84]. Conventional NSCLC therapy includes radiation, surgery, and cisplatin therapy. However, the malignant cells generally acquire resistance to cisplatin chemotherapy. To overcome this resistance, a combination of immunotherapy and epigenetic inhibitors have been used, demonstrating modest success [85]. In particular, the success rate from this study can be attributed to the sequential administration of both DNMTi and HDACi which resulted in a favourable response to immunotherapy as a result of cytoplasmic double-stranded RNA-mediated interferon response.

In order to explore other avenues of therapy, different approaches have been applied. One group of investigators used a combination of radiation therapy with epigenetic inhibitor SAHA and was able to successfully inhibit EMT and stemness of NSCLC cells [86]. In another approach, Taguchi et al. applied meta-analysis of reprogrammed NSCLC to identify targets for epigenetic therapy [87]. A third group of investigators, Duruisseaux and Esteller, suggested integration of tissue-derived epigenetic biomarkers and epigenetics drugs in clinical trial design to prevent drug resistance and improve lung cancer patient outcomes [88]. Lastly, Armas-Lopez et al. reported mesenchyme homeobox2-GLI1 transcription axis and involvement of H3K27AC and H3K4me3 in drug resistance [89]. The above examples indicate that different approaches are now available for epigenetic therapy of lung cancer and epigenetic disruptions could present as reliable biomarkers for lung cancer risk assessment, early detection, disease stratification, and follow up of survival.

9.2.8 Melanoma

Melanoma is considered to be the most aggressive among all skin cancers. Early stage melanoma can be treated surgically, but metastatic melanoma treatment requires alternative approaches. As outlined above, cancer is a genetic and epigenetic disease where epigenetic modifications play a significant role in the progression and development of resistance in different tumour types including melanoma [15].

A few cancer types are responsive to single-agent treatment, but in the case of melanoma, single inhibitors are not as effective as a combination of inhibitors. For example, in BRAF (V600E) positive melanoma, vemurafenib, an inhibitor of BRAF, was determined to be ineffective when administered in combination with methyltransferase inhibitor decitabine [90]. Regarding the underlying epigenetic mechanism of melanoma progression, loss of DNA hydroxymethylation and hypermethylation of the promoter region in selected genes was demonstrated to be the underlying cause of melanoma progression. [91]. As an alternative therapeutic approach, targeting the catalytic activity of ten-eleven translocation family dioxygenase generating 5-hydroxymethylcytosine with 5-aza-2′-deoxycytidine has also shown to be efficacious [91]. Mechanistically, variants of histone H2A (H2A.Z and macroH2A) were identified to be exchanged during melanoma progression, affecting chromatin opening and cell cycle regulators, and thus, could also serve as therapeutic targets [92]. The above indicates that in addition to methylation, histone modification and chromosomal conformation changes can also contribute to the development of melanoma.

9.2.9 Multiple Myelomas

Multiple myelomas, a malignant hematologic disease characterized by the clonal proliferation of malignant plasma cells, tends to relapse in most cases. The underlying cause of relapse is attributed to cancer stem cells (CSCs) which are resistant to treatment via epigenetic regulators [93]. Every somatic cell possesses an epigenetic signature, which is obtained during lineage-specific differentiation of pluripotent stem cells and is tissue specific [94–98].

Cancer stem cells are involved in invasiveness, drug resistance, and relapse of cancer [99]. In this hematologic malignancy, it is difficult to distinguish stem cells from cancer stem cells and characterize the microenvironment in which these cells proliferate. It has been demonstrated that survival of CSCs is not a hereditary mechanism, instead involves epigenetic regulation [100]. Furthermore, epigenetic regulatory pathways such as the Hedgehog pathway, the Notch pathway, and the Wnt/beta-catenin pathway, were found to be deregulated in CSCs [101]. These pathways are involved in cell differentiation, and their deregulation contributes to metastasis and resistance to treatment [14, 102].

Furthermore, CSCs are equipped with detoxification tools such as ABC efflux transporters and aldehyde dehydrogenases which contribute to the development of resistance [102]. Markers which are expressed by these CSCs include CD24, CD34, CD44, CD133, and ADH1 [103–105]. However, the expression is unique to each cancer type. Therefore, it is challenging to stratify patients that may be at high or low risk of responding to therapy or becoming resistant to the therapy due to the heterogeneity of the disease.

As such, epigenetic changes in multiple myeloma that could potentially be targeted for better treatment outcomes include the effect of miRNAs and polycomb group of proteins (non-histone proteins), chromatin conformation, histone modifications, and methylation of DNA. Overall genome-wide hypomethylation in multiple myeloma may lead to the reactivation of transposable elements and modification of silenced genes [106]. Multiple myeloma patients treated with bortezomib showed higher global methylation and greater patient survival compared to untreated individuals [107]. In newly diagnosed patients with multiple myeloma, higher relapse was observed when hypermethylation of CDKN2A, CDKN2B, and TNF occurred [108]. An additional challenge is that during treatment, a group of stem cells remain dormant, and promote metastasis once out of their quiescent. Given the complexity of the disease, there is a need to identify factors which can activate these dormant CSCs and prevent initiation of metastasis.

9.2.10 Oropharyngeal Squamous Cell Carcinoma and Head and Neck Cancer

Infection by human papillomavirus (HPV) has been reported in head and neck squamous cell carcinoma (HNSCC) and oropharyngeal squamous cell carcinoma (OPSCC), which comprises squamous cell carcinoma of the tongue, tonsillar region, soft plate and part of pharynx (represents a significantly higher proportion of HNSCC) and has an underlying mechanism including alteration of epigenetic components [109–111]. Oropharyngeal cancer is increasing in incidence, which can be attributed to HPV infection, making men more susceptible than women for this cancer [112–114]. HNSCC develops in the mucosal epithelial lining of the oral cavity, hypopharynx, oropharynx, or larynx and this cancer is expected to affect approximately 833,000 people worldwide in 2020 [110].

The tumour microenvironment of this type of cancer is characterized by stromal fibroblasts, vasculature, immune cells, cytokine and hypoxia, all of which play a significant role in the progression and metastasis of HNSCC. Collectively, the tumour microenvironment then leads to the acquisition of cancer stem cells properties, recurrence of the disease and therapeutic resistance to treatment.

Epigenetic processes contribute to disease progression and can thus be viable therapeutic targets to treat this malignancy. For example, radiotherapy resistance was observed in HNSCC due to inactivation of *CHFR* through hypermethylation and upregulation of PARP1 [115, 116]. Furthermore, hypermethylation of genes including *DAPK*, *RASSF1*, *CCNA1*, *CDKN2A*, *APC*, *MGMT*, *TUSC3*, *CADM1*, *IGS4*, *SPDEF*, *TIMP3*, *ESR1*, *GRB7*, *RCF21*, *SFRP1* and *SFRP4* was observed, and these genes play a significant role in apoptosis, cell cycle regulation, cell fate determination, inflammation, invasion, metastasis, cell signalling and WNT signalling pathways [110]. HPV genes also get hypermethylated, especially at *L1* and *L2* genes of HPV in OPSCC patients [117, 118]. However, demethylation of HPV16 LCR (extended coding region) by 5-aza-deoxycytidine resulted in the repression of E6 and E7 followed by cell cycle arrest. An additional therapeutic target is a histone methyltransferase called enhancer of zeste homolog 2 (EZH2) which is overexpressed and is associated with poor prognosis of HNSCC and OPSCC [119, 120]. EZH2 is responsible for trimethylation at lysine 27 of histone H3. Therefore, the development of EZH2 inhibitors is a viable therapeutic option for exploring the role of epigenetics in sensitizing tumours to current therapies. The significance of these observation lies in the fact that multiple epigenetic therapy-based options are now available for the treatment of therapy-resistant tumors.

9.2.11   Ovarian Cancer

Among gynecological cancers, ovarian cancer is the leading cause of death due to late tumour diagnosis and tolerance to available drug therapy [121]. The standard treatment for ovarian cancer is platinum-based chemotherapy followed by surgery. It was observed that a set of functionally related genes which are involved in the epigenetic reprogramming of ovarian cancer are controlled by specific transcription factors [122–124]. Specifically, one transcription factor, C/EBPβ, is capable of recruiting histone methyltransferases in order to keep chromatin in an open state by methylating *H3K79*, a gene which also affects multiple drug resistance genes in ovarian cancer [125]. These investigators suggested targeting C/EBPβ to alleviate drug resistance. Additionally, epigenetic-mediated immune suppression of positive co-stimulators, 4-1BB ligand (4-1BBL/CD157) and OX-40 ligand (OX-40L/CD252) were also identified to contribute to chemoresistant ovarian cancer cells [126]. Although the application of targeting epigenetic regulators to overcome resistance to therapies is currently in its infancy, it is indisputable that epigenetics may serve as the basis of the development of diagnostic tools aiding in early detection of malignant ovarian tumours and developing new epigenetic therapeutics for treatment.

9.2.12 Pancreatic Cancer

Pancreatic cancer can form in exocrine cells, which is more common and occurs in advanced stages, as well as in neuroendocrine cells. Treatment options for this cancer depend on the stage of the disease and include surgery, radiation, chemotherapy, chemoradiation and supportive care. Aggressive pancreatic ductal adenocarcinoma (PDAC) ranks as the fourth leading cause of cancer-related deaths with a 5-year survival rate of 8% in the United States [127]. Patients undergoing treatment develop resistance likely due to the presence of a small subset of PDAC cancer stem cells which possess an aggressive phenotype.

Epigenetic therapies have been administered to treat this malignancy and have shown some promise. For example, when two HDAC inhibitors, trichostatin A (TSA) and SAHA, were used in PDAC cells, apoptosis was higher following combination therapy than TSA alone [128]. As expected, both inhibitors acted on HDAC 1, 7, and 8 and higher levels of acetylated histones (particularly H3K4me2 and H3K9me2) were observed. Furthermore, re-expression of E-cadherin mRNA and protein levels were also observed. Currently, gemcitabine is the standard chemotherapy for patients with advanced pancreatic cancer. When these HDAC inhibitors were used in combination with gemcitabine, elimination of pancreatic cancer stem cells through the modification of Oct-4, Sox-2, and Nanog was observed, indicating the potential of alternative therapy for pancreatic cancer [128]. Ma et al. used entinostat, an orally bioavailable HDAC inhibitor in combination with gemcitabine and showed inhibition of pancreatic cancer cell proliferation and increased apoptosis [129]. Another group used a demethylating agent, 5-aza-2'-deoxycytidine and 5-aza-deoxycytidine in combination with ionizing radiation to successfully eliminate pancreatic cancer stem cells [130]. Given these observations, supplementing the current standard of care therapies with inhibitors of epigenetic regulators may confer an advantage when treating this aggressive malignancy.

Another viable treatment option for pancreatic cancer that is currently being tested is dual epigenetic therapy inhibiting tumour growth due to depletion of Myc and induction of CD8+ T-cells [85]. In this study, cells were treated with azacytidine followed by different doses of histone inhibitors belonging to class 1, 2, 3, and 6. Transcriptional analysis and pathway analysis indicated that three pathways were inhibited, with the most significant effect on the myc pathway. Protein analysis indicated a reduction in myc protein and inhibition of cell proliferation. Tumours which show high myc expression display resistance to interferon gamma signalling and reduction in the activity of cytotoxic T-cells. This process highlighted the potential of epigenetic inhibitor treatment to reactivate the sensitivity of cells to interferon gamma and promote better antigen presentation. Taken collectively, therapies targeting epigenetic regulator show promise in treating pancreatic cancer.

9.2.13 Prostate Cancer

Prostate cancer is leading cancer among men. Over 90% of prostate cancer patients undergo radiation therapy, and many of these patients develop radiotoxicity [131, 132]. However, miR-121, miR-146a, and miR-155 contribute to radiation sensitivity and thus present as a viable therapeutic option [28]. Concerning chemotherapy treatment options for prostate cancer, androgen deprivation therapy is one of the most common therapies [133]. When this therapy becomes ineffective, patients develop castration-resistant prostate cancer (CRPC), which is associated with a high mortality rate [134, 135]. Long noncoding RNA HOXD-AS1 (also known as HAGLR) was found to be expressed in CRPC and correlated with tumour size, grade, metastasis, and progression-free survival [134, 136]. HOXD-AS1 is involved in the activation of genes *PLK1*, *AURKA*, *CDC25C*, *FOXM1*, and *UBE2C,* which are associated with castration resistance and the process is mediated by trimethylation of histone H3 at the lysine four positions (H3K4me3) via recruitment of another factor called WDR5 [137, 138]. Knockdown experiments of HOXD-AS1 *in vivo* and *in vitro* have been successful and provide an alternative approach for the treatment of CRPC. Epigenetics has also been applied to improving diagnostic methods. A urine-based methylation assay has been developed for the prognosis of prostate cancer which may supplement the currently used prostate-specific antigen (PSA) assay [139]. Although the application of epigenetics is relatively novel concerning prostate cancer treatment, assays based on the analysis of miRNA, methylation and histone profiling provide useful information about the possibility of redeveloping prostate cancer in patients who have developed resistance to conventional therapies.

9.2.14 Renal Cell Carcinoma

Renal cell carcinoma (RCC) is the most common kidney cancer and accounts for approximately 2% of adult malignancies [140, 141]. RCC can be divided into several subtypes, with clear cell RCC (ccRCC) having a 5-year survival rate of 10% [140, 142]. RCC tends to spread to the brain, adrenal glands, liver, bones, lymph nodes and lungs [140, 141]. Drug resistance has been observed in RCC, and epigenetic, transcriptomic, and proteomic approaches have been developed which have helped in understanding the underlying mechanisms as well as assisted in the development of new targeted therapies for this cancer [143, 144]. Oxaliplatin is often used for the treatment of RCC, but patients develop resistance to this drug mainly due to repression of organic cation transporter (OCT2) [143, 145]. Both hypermethylation of the OCT2 promoter and the absence of H3K4 methylation were observed when samples from drug-resistant patients were analyzed [145, 146]. Typically, OCT2 is activated by MYC and interacts with the E-box motif to activate histone methylation [147]. However, in RCC patients this process was stopped due to the disrupted expression of OCT2. Additional attempts have been made to sensitize RCC cells to oxaliplatin and overcome resistance to therapy through a sequential combination therapy using decitabine [145]. Concerning combination therapy, valproic acid and 5-azacytidine synergistically inhibited RCC growth and migration [148].

Typically, epigenetic regulation of RCC affects signalling pathways including, von Hippel-Lindau disease tumour suppressor hypoxia-inducible pathway, Wnt-beta-catenin pathway, and pathways implicated in EMT [149–151]. Thus, epigenetic alterations can be considered potential biomarkers for the diagnosis of RCC disease and prognosis and predictions in response to treatment.

9.2.15 Other Tumor Types

Over the past few decades, advanced-stage cancer has been associated with higher epigenetic alterations compared to genetic alterations [6, 13, 152]. Loss of 5-hydroxymethylcytosine frequently occurs in different tumour types. However, it is unknown whether the restoration of 5-hydroxymethylcytosine could have any therapeutic efficacy. The use of sodium L-ascorbate and the oxidation-resistant form L-ascorbic acid 2-phosphate sesquimagnesium has demonstrated improvement in survival of patients suffering from RCC [153].

Osteosarcoma is the most common malignant primary bone tumour in children and adults, and chemoresistance contributes to relapse and poor prognosis. Zhao et al. reported on the role of miR-20a-5p and Homo sapiens syndecan 2 (SCD2) in osteosarcoma chemoresistance [35]. The approach included RNA-seq-based miR-omic analysis of osteosarcoma cells to follow miR-20a-5p expression. Two kinds of cells were used, G-292 cells and miR-20a-5p-antagomiR transfected SJSA-1 cells. Results indicated higher miR-20a-5p levels in G-292 cells compared to SJSA-1 cells.

In bladder cancer, epigenetic perturbation of SAT1 and ASS1 genes along with altered metabolism were observed in cisplatin resistance cells [154]. Furthermore, another study indicated that decitabine augmented cytotoxicity of cisplatin and doxorubicin to bladder cancer by activating the Hippo pathway through the *RSSF1A* gene [155]. In diffuse large B-cell lymphoma, the concept of EpiScore was proposed based on the expression of a group of genes regulated epigenetically. EpiScore identified high-risk patients with diffuse large B-cell lymphoma who could benefit from epigenetic-based therapies [156]. In the case of anaplastic lymphoma kinase (ALK) positive lung cancer, resistance developed after treatment with ALK inhibitors and the underlying mechanism involved decreased levels of H3K27ac and miR-34a [34].

9.3 Challenges and Potential Solutions

Therapeutic resistance remains to be a significant problem in clinical oncology. One of the challenges in epigenetic therapy is selecting cancer patients that will most benefit from epigenetic therapy, either alone or in combination, with the highest success rates, and how to quantitatively measure response to therapy. Previously, the focus of epigenetic therapy in addressing drug resistance was on a single enzyme, such as a methyltransferase. However, enzyme cofactors have now been identified which are context-dependent and provide sequence-specific regulation of drug-resistance [157–160]. These factors could be future targets for eliminating drug resistance.

The accumulation of genetic and epigenetic alterations contributes to the self-renewal and drug-resistant capacity of CSCs mainly due to their multipotent properties [18]. Differentiation by inflammation, oncogenes, or similar approaches might present challenges to therapies exclusively targeting CSCs. However, targeting CSCs and modulating the tumour microenvironment by epigenetic approaches to augment immune attacks on cancer is a strategy worth investigating. One report on patient samples and cell lines treated with epigenetic drugs indicated an upregulation of programmed cell death protein-1 (PD-1) and other immune inhibitor ligands and receptors which might correlate with resistance to epigenetic therapies [161]. In contrast, another independent report indicated a significant role of BRD4 inhibitors in downregulating the expression of the immune inhibitory molecules, including PD-1 and demonstrates synergy with immunotherapy [162].

Overall there is a need for a more in-depth understanding of the broad effects of epigenetic inhibitor-based therapy so that we can take advantage of their antioncogenic effects and target their use for better patient outcomes. Another aspect of targeted therapy and resistance is that all cancer treatments are patient-centric and could theoretically be treated with a personalized approach to medicine. This can be achieved through longitudinal molecular profiling such as epigenomic, transcriptomic, and metabolomic, in order to identify appropriate intervention targets.

One fundamental problem with epigenetic therapy is that epigenetic processes are needed for normal development and therefore, a rigorous understanding of the effect of inhibitory functions of epigenetic drugs is necessary to design rational therapies capable of inhibiting oncogenic properties with either no or minimal effects on normal body functions.

Despite all of the hurdles discussed above, the potential for epigenetic drugs in the treatment of resistant cancers is high and clinical trials have begun to evaluate this emerging area of research (https://clinicaltrials.gov/). As discussed, miRNAs represent a promising therapeutic strategy to target drug resistance. However, their stability in body fluids and tissues, inability to reach the target tissue and their limited uptake by affected cells remains to be a challenge and requires further research and advancements in technology to overcome these limitations.

9.4 Concluding Remarks

Epigenetics is independent of the sequence of events that physically affect the condensing of chromatin and gene expression. Involvement of epigenetic regulators in cancer heterogeneity and drug resistance has opened the possibility for the development of new drugs and approaches aimed at targeting epigenetic components. Aberrations in epigenetic components, especially methylation and miRNAs, may be involved in the development of drug resistance in targeted therapy and combined therapy with epigenetic drugs has been proposed.

Chemoresistance in cancer is a significant unmet clinical obstacle which is being addressed by different alternative approaches including through targeting epigenetics. A novel approach in the treatment of cancer is dual epigenetic therapy in combination with immune checkpoint blockade in order to increase tumour response to therapy. There is a need to develop a comprehensive panel of treatment predicting factors to improve patient stratification for targeted and cytotoxic therapies so that ineffective treatments can be avoided.

Finally, we have discussed the opportunities presented by epigenetically targeted therapy to reduce resistance in different tumour types and identified key challenges that need to be tackled by researchers, clinicians, and industrial partners to translate these approaches best to improve patient outcomes.

Financial Disclosure There is no financial conflict.

References

1. Jones P. Out of Africa and into epigenetics: discovering reprogramming drugs. Nat Cell Biol. 2011;13(1):2. https://doi.org/10.1038/ncb0111-2.
2. Jones PA. Overview of cancer epigenetics. Semin Hematol. 2005;42(3 Suppl 2):S3–8.
3. Jones PA, Laird PW. Cancer epigenetics comes of age. Nat Genet. 1999;21(2):163–7. https://doi.org/10.1038/5947.
4. Jones PA, Takai D. The role of DNA methylation in mammalian epigenetics. Science. 2001;293(5532):1068–70. https://doi.org/10.1126/science.1063852.
5. Khare S, Verma M. Epigenetics of colon cancer. Methods Mol Biol. 2012;863:177–85. https://doi.org/10.1007/978-1-61779-612-8_10.
6. Jones PA, Issa JP, Baylin S. Targeting the cancer epigenome for therapy. Nat Rev Genet. 2016;17(10):630–41. https://doi.org/10.1038/nrg.2016.93.
7. Baylin SB. Tying it all together: epigenetics, genetics, cell cycle, and cancer. Science. 1997;277(5334):1948–9.
8. Baylin SB. Stem cells, cancer, and epigenetics. Cambridge: StemBook; 2008.
9. Baylin SB. Resistance, epigenetics and the cancer ecosystem. Nat Med. 2011;17(3):288–9. https://doi.org/10.1038/nm0311-288.
10. Jones B. Epigenetics: histones pass the message on. Nat Rev Genet. 2015;16(1):3. https://doi.org/10.1038/nrg3876.
11. Sharma S, Kelly TK, Jones PA. Epigenetics in cancer. Carcinogenesis. 2010;31(1):27–36. https://doi.org/10.1093/carcin/bgp220.

12. You JS, Jones PA. Cancer genetics and epigenetics: two sides of the same coin? Cancer Cell. 2012;22(1):9–20. https://doi.org/10.1016/j.ccr.2012.06.008.
13. Verma M. Epigenome-Wide Association Studies (EWAS) in cancer. Curr Genomics. 2012;13(4):308–13. https://doi.org/10.2174/138920212800793294.
14. Mishra A, Verma M. Epigenetics of solid cancer stem cells. Methods Mol Biol. 2012;863:15–31. https://doi.org/10.1007/978-1-61779-612-8_2.
15. Verma M. Genome-wide association studies and epigenome-wide association studies go together in cancer control. Future Oncol. 2016;12(13):1645–64. https://doi.org/10.2217/fon-2015-0035.
16. Yu T, Wang C, Yang J, Guo Y, Wu Y, Li X. Metformin inhibits SUV39H1-mediated migration of prostate cancer cells. Oncogene. 2017;6(5):e324. https://doi.org/10.1038/oncsis.2017.28.
17. Metzger E, Wissmann M, Yin N, Muller JM, Schneider R, Peters AH, et al. LSD1 demethylates repressive histone marks to promote androgen-receptor-dependent transcription. Nature. 2005;437(7057):436–9. https://doi.org/10.1038/nature04020.
18. Adorno-Cruz V, Kibria G, Liu X, Doherty M, Junk DJ, Guan D, et al. Cancer stem cells: targeting the roots of cancer, seeds of metastasis, and sources of therapy resistance. Cancer Res. 2015;75(6):924–9. https://doi.org/10.1158/0008-5472.CAN-14-3225.
19. Komura K, Jeong SH, Hinohara K, Qu F, Wang X, Hiraki M, et al. Resistance to docetaxel in prostate cancer is associated with androgen receptor activation and loss of KDM5D expression. Proc Natl Acad Sci U S A. 2016;113(22):6259–64. https://doi.org/10.1073/pnas.1600420113.
20. Plimack ER, Kantarjian HM, Issa JP. Decitabine and its role in the treatment of hematopoietic malignancies. Leuk Lymphoma. 2007;48(8):1472–81. https://doi.org/10.1080/10428190701471981.
21. Plimack ER, Stewart DJ, Issa JP. Combining epigenetic and cytotoxic therapy in the treatment of solid tumors. J Clin Oncol. 2007;25(29):4519–21. https://doi.org/10.1200/JCO.2007.12.6029.
22. Verma M, Maruvada P, Srivastava S. Epigenetics and cancer. Crit Rev Clin Lab Sci. 2004;41(5–6):585–607. https://doi.org/10.1080/10408360490516922.
23. Fan H, Lu X, Wang X, Liu Y, Guo B, Zhang Y, et al. Low-dose decitabine-based chemoimmunotherapy for patients with refractory advanced solid tumors: a phase I/II report. J Immunol Res. 2014;2014:371087. https://doi.org/10.1155/2014/371087.
24. Nie J, Liu L, Li X, Han W. Decitabine, a new star in epigenetic therapy: the clinical application and biological mechanism in solid tumors. Cancer Lett. 2014;354(1):12–20. https://doi.org/10.1016/j.canlet.2014.08.010.
25. Toyota M, Ahuja N, Suzuki H, Itoh F, Ohe-Toyota M, Imai K, et al. Aberrant methylation in gastric cancer associated with the CpG island methylator phenotype. Cancer Res. 1999;59(21):5438–42.
26. Chawla JP, Iyer N, Soodan KS, Sharma A, Khurana SK, Priyadarshni P. Role of miRNA in cancer diagnosis, prognosis, therapy and regulation of its expression by Epstein-Barr virus and human papillomaviruses: with special reference to oral cancer. Oral Oncol. 2015;51(8):731–7. https://doi.org/10.1016/j.oraloncology.2015.05.008.
27. Gilot D, Galibert MD. miRNA displacement as a promising approach for cancer therapy. Mol Cell Oncol. 2018;5(1):e1406432. https://doi.org/10.1080/23723556.2017.1406432.
28. Kopcalic K, Petrovic N, Stanojkovic TP, Stankovic V, Bukumiric Z, Roganovic J, et al. Association between miR-21/146a/155 level changes and acute genitourinary radiotoxicity in prostate cancer patients: a pilot study. Pathol Res Pract. 2018;215(4):626–31. https://doi.org/10.1016/j.prp.2018.12.007.
29. Yin C, Fang C, Weng H, Yuan C, Wang F. Circulating microRNAs as novel biomarkers in the diagnosis of prostate cancer: a systematic review and meta-analysis. Int Urol Nephrol. 2016;48(7):1087–95. https://doi.org/10.1007/s11255-016-1281-4.
30. Geretto M, Pulliero A, Rosano C, Zhabayeva D, Bersimbaev R, Izzotti A. Resistance to cancer chemotherapeutic drugs is determined by pivotal microRNA regulators. Am J Cancer Res. 2017;7(6):1350–71.

31. Ors-Kumoglu G, Gulce-Iz S, Biray-Avci C. Therapeutic microRNAs in human cancer. Cytotechnology. 2019;71(1):411–25. https://doi.org/10.1007/s10616-018-0291-8.

32. Li H, Liu J, Chen J, Wang H, Yang L, Chen F, et al. A serum microRNA signature predicts trastuzumab benefit in HER2-positive metastatic breast cancer patients. Nat Commun. 2018;9(1):1614. https://doi.org/10.1038/s41467-018-03537-w.

33. Sannigrahi MK, Sharma R, Singh V, Panda NK, Rattan V, Khullar M. Role of host miRNA Hsa-miR-139-3p in HPV-16-induced carcinomas. Clin Cancer Res. 2017;23(14):3884–95. https://doi.org/10.1158/1078-0432.CCR-16-2936.

34. Yun MR, Lim SM, Kim SK, Choi HM, Pyo KH, Kim SK, et al. Enhancer remodeling and microRNA alterations are associated with acquired resistance to ALK inhibitors. Cancer Res. 2018;78(12):3350–62. https://doi.org/10.1158/0008-5472.CAN-17-3146.

35. Zhao F, Pu Y, Cui M, Wang H, Cai S. MiR-20a-5p represses the multi-drug resistance of osteosarcoma by targeting the SDC2 gene. Cancer Cell Int. 2017;17:100. https://doi.org/10.1186/s12935-017-0470-2.

36. Ma J, Lin Y, Zhan M, Mann DL, Stass SA, Jiang F. Differential miRNA expressions in peripheral blood mononuclear cells for diagnosis of lung cancer. Lab Invest. 2015;95(10):1197–206. https://doi.org/10.1038/labinvest.2015.88.

37. Rachagani S, Macha MA, Menning MS, Dey P, Pai P, Smith LM, et al. Changes in microRNA (miRNA) expression during pancreatic cancer development and progression in a genetically engineered KrasG12D;Pdx1-Cre mouse (KC) model. Oncotarget. 2015;6(37):40295–309. https://doi.org/10.18632/oncotarget.5641.

38. Donzelli S, Mori F, Biagioni F, Bellissimo T, Pulito C, Muti P, et al. MicroRNAs: short non-coding players in cancer chemoresistance. Mol Cell Ther. 2014;2:16. https://doi.org/10.1186/2052-8426-2-16.

39. Fabbri M, Bottoni A, Shimizu M, Spizzo R, Nicoloso MS, Rossi S, et al. Association of a microRNA/TP53 feedback circuitry with pathogenesis and outcome of B-cell chronic lymphocytic leukemia. JAMA. 2011;305(1):59–67. https://doi.org/10.1001/jama.2010.1919

40. Meng X, Fu R. miR-206 regulates 5-FU resistance by targeting Bcl-2 in colon cancer cells. Onco Targets Ther. 2018;11:1757–65. https://doi.org/10.2147/OTT.S159093.

41. Todorova K, Metodiev MV, Metodieva G, Mincheff M, Fernandez N, Hayrabedyan S. MicroRNA-204 participates in TMPRSS2/ERG regulation and androgen receptor reprogramming in prostate cancer. Horm Cancer. 2017;8(1):28–48. https://doi.org/10.1007/s12672-016-0279-9.

42. Verma M. Cancer epigenetics: risk assessment, diagnosis, treatment, and prognosis. Preface. Methods Mol Biol. 2015;1238:v–vi.

43. Gore L, Triche TJ Jr, Farrar JE, Wai D, Legendre C, Gooden GC, et al. A multicenter, randomized study of decitabine as epigenetic priming with induction chemotherapy in children with AML. Clin Epigenetics. 2017;9:108. https://doi.org/10.1186/s13148-017-0411-x.

44. Abaza YM, Kadia TM, Jabbour EJ, Konopleva MY, Borthakur G, Ferrajoli A, et al. Phase 1 dose escalation multicenter trial of pracinostat alone and in combination with azacitidine in patients with advanced hematologic malignancies. Cancer. 2017;123(24):4851–9. https://doi.org/10.1002/cncr.30949.

45. Diyabalanage HV, Granda ML, Hooker JM. Combination therapy: histone deacetylase inhibitors and platinum-based chemotherapeutics for cancer. Cancer Lett. 2013;329(1):1–8. https://doi.org/10.1016/j.canlet.2012.09.018.

46. Suraweera A, O'Byrne KJ, Richard DJ. Combination therapy with histone deacetylase inhibitors (HDACi) for the treatment of cancer: achieving the full therapeutic potential of HDACi. Front Oncol. 2018;8:92. https://doi.org/10.3389/fonc.2018.00092.

47. Li J, Hao D, Wang L, Wang H, Wang Y, Zhao Z, et al. Epigenetic targeting drugs potentiate chemotherapeutic effects in solid tumor therapy. Sci Rep. 2017;7(1):4035. https://doi.org/10.1038/s41598-017-04406-0.

48. Baretti M, Azad NS. The role of epigenetic therapies in colorectal cancer. Curr Probl Cancer. 2018;42(6):530–47. https://doi.org/10.1016/j.currproblcancer.2018.03.001.

49. Zain J, Kaminetzky D, O'Connor OA. Emerging role of epigenetic therapies in cutaneous T-cell lymphomas. Expert Rev Hematol. 2010;3(2):187–203. https://doi.org/10.1586/ehm.10.9.
50. Vera O, Rodriguez-Antolin C, de Castro J, Karreth FA, Sellers TA, Ibanez de Caceres I. An epigenomic approach to identifying differential overlapping and cis-acting lncRNAs in cisplatin-resistant cancer cells. Epigenetics. 2018;13(3):251–63. https://doi.org/10.1080/15592294.2018.1436364.
51. Panja S, Hayati S, Epsi NJ, Parrott JS, Mitrofanova A. Integrative (epi) genomic analysis to predict response to androgen-deprivation therapy in prostate cancer. EBioMedicine. 2018;31:110–21. https://doi.org/10.1016/j.ebiom.2018.04.007.
52. Sharma SV, Lee DY, Li B, Quinlan MP, Takahashi F, Maheswaran S, et al. A chromatin-mediated reversible drug-tolerant state in cancer cell subpopulations. Cell. 2010;141(1):69–80. https://doi.org/10.1016/j.cell.2010.02.027.
53. Broxterman HJ, Gotink KJ, Verheul HM. Understanding the causes of multidrug resistance in cancer: a comparison of doxorubicin and sunitinib. Drug Resist Updat. 2009;12(4–5):114–26. https://doi.org/10.1016/j.drup.2009.07.001.
54. Gampenrieder SP, Rinnerthaler G, Hackl H, Pulverer W, Weinhaeusel A, Ilic S, et al. DNA methylation signatures predicting bevacizumab efficacy in metastatic breast cancer. Theranostics. 2018;8(8):2278–88. https://doi.org/10.7150/thno.23544.
55. Mekala JR, Naushad SM, Ponnusamy L, Arivazhagan G, Sakthiprasad V, Pal-Bhadra M. Epigenetic regulation of miR-200 as the potential strategy for the therapy against triple-negative breast cancer. Gene. 2018;641:248–58. https://doi.org/10.1016/j.gene.2017.10.018.
56. Jendzelovsky R, Jendzelovska Z, Kucharova B, Fedorocko P. Breast cancer resistance protein is the enemy of hypericin accumulation and toxicity of hypericin-mediated photodynamic therapy. Biomed Pharmacother. 2019;109:2173–81. https://doi.org/10.1016/j.biopha.2018.11.084.
57. Krammer B, Verwanger T. Molecular response to hypericin-induced photodamage. Curr Med Chem. 2012;19(6):793–8.
58. Halaburkova A, Jendzelovsky R, Koval J, Herceg Z, Fedorocko P, Ghantous A. Histone deacetylase inhibitors potentiate photodynamic therapy in colon cancer cells marked by chromatin-mediated epigenetic regulation of CDKN1A. Clin Epigenetics. 2017;9:62. https://doi.org/10.1186/s13148-017-0359-x.
59. Su Y, Hopfinger NR, Nguyen TD, Pogash TJ, Santucci-Pereira J, Russo J. Epigenetic reprogramming of epithelial mesenchymal transition in triple negative breast cancer cells with DNA methyltransferase and histone deacetylase inhibitors. J Exp Clin Cancer Res. 2018;37(1):314. https://doi.org/10.1186/s13046-018-0988-8.
60. Sood S, Patel FD, Ghosh S, Arora A, Dhaliwal LK, Srinivasan R. Epigenetic alteration by DNA methylation of ESR1, MYOD1 and hTERT gene promoters is useful for prediction of response in patients of locally advanced invasive cervical carcinoma treated by chemoradiation. Clin Oncol (R Coll Radiol). 2015;27(12):720–7. https://doi.org/10.1016/j.clon.2015.08.001.
61. Chen CC, Lee KD, Pai MY, Chu PY, Hsu CC, Chiu CC, et al. Changes in DNA methylation are associated with the development of drug resistance in cervical cancer cells. Cancer Cell Int. 2015;15:98. https://doi.org/10.1186/s12935-015-0248-3.
62. Huang Z, Zhang S, Shen Y, Liu W, Long J, Zhou S. Influence of MDR1 methylation on the curative effect of interventional embolism chemotherapy for cervical cancer. Ther Clin Risk Manag. 2016;12:217–23. https://doi.org/10.2147/TCRM.S95453.
63. He T, Zhang M, Zheng R, Zheng S, Linghu E, Herman JG, et al. Methylation of SLFN11 is a marker of poor prognosis and cisplatin resistance in colorectal cancer. Epigenomics. 2017;9(6):849–62. https://doi.org/10.2217/epi-2017-0019.
64. Kang KA, Piao MJ, Ryu YS, Kang HK, Chang WY, Keum YS, et al. Interaction of DNA demethylase and histone methyltransferase upregulates Nrf2 in 5-fluorouracil-resistant colon cancer cells. Oncotarget. 2016;7(26):40594–620. https://doi.org/10.18632/oncotarget.9745.

65. Fesler A, Guo S, Liu H, Wu N, Ju J. Overcoming chemoresistance in cancer stem cells with the help of microRNAs in colorectal cancer. Epigenomics. 2017;9(6):793–6. https://doi.org/10.2217/epi-2017-0041.

66. Miyaki Y, Suzuki K, Koizumi K, Kato T, Saito M, Kamiyama H, et al. Identification of a potent epigenetic biomarker for resistance to camptothecin and poor outcome to irinotecan-based chemotherapy in colon cancer. Int J Oncol. 2012;40(1):217–26. https://doi.org/10.3892/ijo.2011.1189.

67. Garcia-Solano J, Turpin MC, Torres-Moreno D, Huertas-Lopez F, Tuomisto A, Makinen MJ, et al. Two histologically colorectal carcinomas subsets from the serrated pathway show different methylome signatures and diagnostic biomarkers. Clin Epigenetics. 2018;10(1):141. https://doi.org/10.1186/s13148-018-0571-3.

68. Ellis HP, Greenslade M, Powell B, Spiteri I, Sottoriva A, Kurian KM. Current challenges in glioblastoma: intratumour heterogeneity, residual disease, and models to predict disease recurrence. Front Oncol. 2015;5:251. https://doi.org/10.3389/fonc.2015.00251.

69. Hegi ME, Diserens AC, Gorlia T, Hamou MF, de Tribolet N, Weller M, et al. MGMT gene silencing and benefit from temozolomide in glioblastoma. N Engl J Med. 2005;352(10):997–1003. https://doi.org/10.1056/NEJMoa043331.

70. Banelli B, Carra E, Barbieri F, Wurth R, Parodi F, Pattarozzi A, et al. The histone demethylase KDM5A is a key factor for the resistance to temozolomide in glioblastoma. Cell Cycle. 2015;14(21):3418–29. https://doi.org/10.1080/15384101.2015.1090063.

71. Malhotra M, Sekar TV, Ananta JS, Devulapally R, Afjei R, Babikir HA, et al. Targeted nanoparticle delivery of therapeutic antisense microRNAs presensitizes glioblastoma cells to lower effective doses of temozolomide in vitro and in a mouse model. Oncotarget. 2018;9(30):21478–94. https://doi.org/10.18632/oncotarget.25135.

72. Cheng ZX, Yin WB, Wang ZY. MicroRNA-132 induces temozolomide resistance and promotes the formation of cancer stem cell phenotypes by targeting tumor suppressor candidate 3 in glioblastoma. Int J Mol Med. 2017;40(5):1307–14. https://doi.org/10.3892/ijmm.2017.3124.

73. Chen Y, Li R, Pan M, Shi Z, Yan W, Liu N, et al. MiR-181b modulates chemosensitivity of glioblastoma multiforme cells to temozolomide by targeting the epidermal growth factor receptor. J Neurooncol. 2017;133(3):477–85. https://doi.org/10.1007/s11060-017-2463-3.

74. Banelli B, Daga A, Forlani A, Allemanni G, Marubbi D, Pistillo MP, et al. Small molecules targeting histone demethylase genes (KDMs) inhibit growth of temozolomide-resistant glioblastoma cells. Oncotarget. 2017;8(21):34896–910. https://doi.org/10.18632/oncotarget.16820.

75. Hong X, Kim ES, Guo H. Epigenetic regulation of hepatitis B virus covalently closed circular DNA: implications for epigenetic therapy against chronic hepatitis B. Hepatology. 2017;66(6):2066–77. https://doi.org/10.1002/hep.29479.

76. Jin X, Tian S, Li P. Histone acetyltransferase 1 promotes cell proliferation and induces cisplatin resistance in hepatocellular carcinoma. Oncol Res. 2017;25(6):939–46. https://doi.org/10.3727/096504016X14809827856524.

77. Xue F, Liang Y, Li Z, Liu Y, Zhang H, Wen Y, et al. MicroRNA-9 enhances sensitivity to cetuximab in epithelial phenotype hepatocellular carcinoma cells through regulation of the eukaryotic translation initiation factor 5A-2. Oncol Lett. 2018;15(1):813–20. https://doi.org/10.3892/ol.2017.7399.

78. Yahya SMM, Fathy SA, El-Khayat ZA, El-Toukhy SE, Hamed AR, Hegazy MGA, et al. Possible role of microRNA-122 in modulating multidrug resistance of hepatocellular carcinoma. Indian J Clin Biochem. 2018;33(1):21–30. https://doi.org/10.1007/s12291-017-0651-8.

79. Niu L, Liu L, Yang S, Ren J, Lai PBS, Chen GG. New insights into sorafenib resistance in hepatocellular carcinoma: responsible mechanisms and promising strategies. Biochim Biophys Acta. 2017;1868(2):564–70. https://doi.org/10.1016/j.bbcan.2017.10.002.

80. Tang B, Zhang Y, Liang R, Gao Z, Sun D, Wang L. RNAi-mediated EZH2 depletion decreases MDR1 expression and sensitizes multidrug-resistant hepatocellular carcinoma cells to chemotherapy. Oncol Rep. 2013;29(3):1037–42. https://doi.org/10.3892/or.2013.2222.

81. Heuser M, Yun H, Thol F. Epigenetics in myelodysplastic syndromes. Semin Cancer Biol. 2018;51:170–9. https://doi.org/10.1016/j.semcancer.2017.07.009.
82. Cancer Genome Atlas Research Network, Ley TJ, Miller C, Ding L, Raphael BJ, Mungall AJ, et al. Genomic and epigenomic landscapes of adult de novo acute myeloid leukemia. N Engl J Med. 2013;368(22):2059–74. https://doi.org/10.1056/NEJMoa1301689.
83. Kuiper JL, Heideman DA, Thunnissen E, Paul MA, van Wijk AW, Postmus PE, et al. Incidence of T790M mutation in (sequential) rebiopsies in EGFR-mutated NSCLC-patients. Lung Cancer. 2014;85(1):19–24. https://doi.org/10.1016/j.lungcan.2014.03.016.
84. Park C, Lee IJ, Jang SH, Lee JW. Factors affecting tumor recurrence after curative surgery for NSCLC: impacts of lymphovascular invasion on early tumor recurrence. J Thorac Dis. 2014;6(10):1420–8. https://doi.org/10.3978/j.issn.2072-1439.2014.09.31.
85. Topper MJ, Vaz M, Chiappinelli KB, DeStefano Shields CE, Niknafs N, Yen RC, et al. Epigenetic therapy ties MYC depletion to reversing immune evasion and treating lung cancer. Cell. 2017;171(6):1284–300 e21. https://doi.org/10.1016/j.cell.2017.10.022.
86. Zhang S, Wu K, Feng J, Wu Z, Deng Q, Guo C, et al. Epigenetic therapy potential of suberoylanilide hydroxamic acid on invasive human non-small cell lung cancer cells. Oncotarget. 2016;7(42):68768–80. https://doi.org/10.18632/oncotarget.11967.
87. Taguchi YH, Iwadate M, Umeyama H. SFRP1 is a possible candidate for epigenetic therapy in non-small cell lung cancer. BMC Med Genomics. 2016;9(Suppl 1):28. https://doi.org/10.1186/s12920-016-0196-3.
88. Duruisseaux M, Esteller M. Lung cancer epigenetics: from knowledge to applications. Semin Cancer Biol. 2018;51:116–28. https://doi.org/10.1016/j.semcancer.2017.09.005.
89. Armas-Lopez L, Pina-Sanchez P, Arrieta O, de Alba EG, Ortiz-Quintero B, Santillan-Doherty P, et al. Epigenomic study identifies a novel mesenchyme homeobox2-GLI1 transcription axis involved in cancer drug resistance, overall survival and therapy prognosis in lung cancer patients. Oncotarget. 2017;8(40):67056–81. https://doi.org/10.18632/oncotarget.17715.
90. Zakharia Y, Monga V, Swami U, Bossler AD, Freesmeier M, Frees M, et al. Targeting epigenetics for treatment of BRAF mutated metastatic melanoma with decitabine in combination with vemurafenib: a phase lb study. Oncotarget. 2017;8(51):89182–93. https://doi.org/10.18632/oncotarget.21269.
91. Fu S, Wu H, Zhang H, Lian CG, Lu Q. DNA methylation/hydroxymethylation in melanoma. Oncotarget. 2017;8(44):78163–73. https://doi.org/10.18632/oncotarget.18293.
92. Kapoor A, Goldberg MS, Cumberland LK, Ratnakumar K, Segura MF, Emanuel PO, et al. The histone variant macroH2A suppresses melanoma progression through regulation of CDK8. Nature. 2010;468(7327):1105–9. https://doi.org/10.1038/nature09590.
93. Issa ME, Takhsha FS, Chirumamilla CS, Perez-Novo C, Vanden Berghe W, Cuendet M. Epigenetic strategies to reverse drug resistance in heterogeneous multiple myeloma. Clin Epigenetics. 2017;9:17. https://doi.org/10.1186/s13148-017-0319-5.
94. Lapinska K, Faria G, McGonagle S, Macumber KM, Heerboth S, Sarkar S. Cancer progenitor cells: the result of an epigenetic event? Anticancer Res. 2018;38(1):1–6. https://doi.org/10.21873/anticanres.12184.
95. Lapinskas T, Pedrizzetti G, Stoiber L, Dungen HD, Edelmann F, Pieske B, et al. The intraventricular hemodynamic forces estimated using routine CMR cine images: a new marker of the failing heart. JACC Cardiovasc Imaging. 2019;12(2):377–9. https://doi.org/10.1016/j.jcmg.2018.08.012.
96. Leary M, Heerboth S, Lapinska K, Sarkar S. Sensitization of drug resistant cancer cells: a matter of combination therapy. Cancers (Basel). 2018;10(12) https://doi.org/10.3390/cancers10120483.
97. Abdul QA, Yu BP, Chung HY, Jung HA, Choi JS. Epigenetic modifications of gene expression by lifestyle and environment. Arch Pharm Res. 2017;40(11):1219–37. https://doi.org/10.1007/s12272-017-0973-3.
98. Chung H, Sidhu KS. Epigenetic modifications of embryonic stem cells: current trends and relevance in developing regenerative medicine. Stem Cells Cloning. 2008;1:11–21.

99. Bayat S, Shekari Khaniani M, Choupani J, Alivand MR, Mansoori Derakhshan S. HDACis (class I), cancer stem cell, and phytochemicals: cancer therapy and prevention implications. Biomed Pharmacother. 2018;97:1445–53. https://doi.org/10.1016/j.biopha.2017.11.065.

100. Munoz P, Iliou MS, Esteller M. Epigenetic alterations involved in cancer stem cell reprogramming. Mol Oncol. 2012;6(6):620–36. https://doi.org/10.1016/j.molonc.2012.10.006.

101. Sui H, Fan ZZ, Li Q. Signal transduction pathways and transcriptional mechanisms of ABCB1/Pgp-mediated multiple drug resistance in human cancer cells. J Int Med Res. 2012;40(2):426–35. https://doi.org/10.1177/147323001204000204.

102. McIntosh K, Balch C, Tiwari AK. Tackling multidrug resistance mediated by efflux transporters in tumor-initiating cells. Expert Opin Drug Metab Toxicol. 2016;12(6):633–44. https://doi.org/10.1080/17425255.2016.1179280.

103. Geng S, Guo Y, Wang Q, Li L, Wang J. Cancer stem-like cells enriched with CD29 and CD44 markers exhibit molecular characteristics with epithelial-mesenchymal transition in squamous cell carcinoma. Arch Dermatol Res. 2013;305(1):35–47. https://doi.org/10.1007/s00403-012-1260-2.

104. Piao JH, Wang Y, Duncan ID. CD44 is required for the migration of transplanted oligodendrocyte progenitor cells to focal inflammatory demyelinating lesions in the spinal cord. Glia. 2013;61(3):361–7. https://doi.org/10.1002/glia.22438.

105. Wang C, Xie J, Guo J, Manning HC, Gore JC, Guo N. Evaluation of CD44 and CD133 as cancer stem cell markers for colorectal cancer. Oncol Rep. 2012;28(4):1301–8. https://doi.org/10.3892/or.2012.1951.

106. Kaiser MF, Johnson DC, Wu P, Walker BA, Brioli A, Mirabella F, et al. Global methylation analysis identifies prognostically important epigenetically inactivated tumor suppressor genes in multiple myeloma. Blood. 2013;122(2):219–26. https://doi.org/10.1182/blood-2013-03-487884.

107. Fernández de Larrea C, Martin-Antonio B, Cibeira MT, Navarro A, Tovar N, Diaz T, et al. Impact of global and gene-specific DNA methylation pattern in relapsed multiple myeloma patients treated with bortezomib. Leuk Res. 2013;37(6):641–6. https://doi.org/10.1016/j.leukres.2013.01.013.

108. Heuck CJ, Mehta J, Bhagat T, Gundabolu K, Yu Y, Khan S, et al. Myeloma is characterized by stage-specific alterations in DNA methylation that occur early during myelomagenesis. J Immunol. 2013;190(6):2966–75. https://doi.org/10.4049/jimmunol.1202493.

109. Boscolo-Rizzo P, Bussu F. Beware of the dangers along the path towards the diagnosis of HPV-driven oropharyngeal squamous cell carcinoma. Acta Otorhinolaryngol Ital. 2017;37(1):63–4. https://doi.org/10.14639/0392-100X-1323.

110. Boscolo-Rizzo P, Furlan C, Lupato V, Polesel J, Fratta E. Novel insights into epigenetic drivers of oropharyngeal squamous cell carcinoma: role of HPV and lifestyle factors. Clin Epigenetics. 2017;9:124. https://doi.org/10.1186/s13148-017-0424-5.

111. Schroeder L, Boscolo-Rizzo P, Dal Cin E, Romeo S, Baboci L, Dyckhoff G, et al. Human papillomavirus as prognostic marker with rising prevalence in neck squamous cell carcinoma of unknown primary: a retrospective multicentre study. Eur J Cancer. 2017;74:73–81. https://doi.org/10.1016/j.ejca.2016.12.020.

112. Anderson KS, Dahlstrom KR, Cheng JN, Alam R, Li G, Wei Q, et al. HPV16 antibodies as risk factors for oropharyngeal cancer and their association with tumor HPV and smoking status. Oral Oncol. 2015;51(7):662–7. https://doi.org/10.1016/j.oraloncology.2015.04.011.

113. Dahlstrom KR, Bell D, Hanby D, Li G, Wang LE, Wei Q, et al. Socioeconomic characteristics of patients with oropharyngeal carcinoma according to tumor HPV status, patient smoking status, and sexual behavior. Oral Oncol. 2015;51(9):832–8. https://doi.org/10.1016/j.oraloncology.2015.06.005.

114. Dahlstrom KR, Li G, Hussey CS, Vo JT, Wei Q, Zhao C, et al. Circulating human papillomavirus DNA as a marker for disease extent and recurrence among patients with oropharyngeal cancer. Cancer. 2015;121(19):3455–64. https://doi.org/10.1002/cncr.29538.

115. Chen X, Liu L, Mims J, Punska EC, Williams KE, Zhao W, et al. Analysis of DNA methylation and gene expression in radiation-resistant head and neck tumors. Epigenetics. 2015;10(6):545–61. https://doi.org/10.1080/15592294.2015.1048953.
116. Lin HY, Huang TH, Chan MW. Aberrant epigenetic modifications in radiation-resistant head and neck cancers. Methods Mol Biol. 2015;1238:321–32. https://doi.org/10.1007/978-1-4939-1804-1_17.
117. Furlan C, Polesel J, Barzan L, Franchin G, Sulfaro S, Romeo S, et al. Prognostic significance of LINE-1 hypomethylation in oropharyngeal squamous cell carcinoma. Clin Epigenetics. 2017;9:58. https://doi.org/10.1186/s13148-017-0357-z.
118. Stephen JK, Worsham MJ. Human papilloma virus (HPV) modulation of the HNSCC epigenome. Methods Mol Biol. 2015;1238:369–79. https://doi.org/10.1007/978-1-4939-1804-1_20.
119. Idris S, Lindsay C, Kostiuk M, Andrews C, Cote DW, O'Connell DA, et al. Investigation of EZH2 pathways for novel epigenetic treatment strategies in oropharyngeal cancer. J Otolaryngol Head Neck Surg. 2016;45(1):54. https://doi.org/10.1186/s40463-016-0168-9.
120. Lindsay CD, Kostiuk MA, Harris J, O'Connell DA, Seikaly H, Biron VL. Efficacy of EZH2 inhibitory drugs in human papillomavirus-positive and human papillomavirus-negative oropharyngeal squamous cell carcinomas. Clin Epigenetics. 2017;9:95. https://doi.org/10.1186/s13148-017-0390-y.
121. Balch C, Huang TH, Brown R, Nephew KP. The epigenetics of ovarian cancer drug resistance and resensitization. Am J Obstet Gynecol. 2004;191(5):1552–72. https://doi.org/10.1016/j.ajog.2004.05.025.
122. Enuka Y, Feldman ME, Chowdhury A, Srivastava S, Lindzen M, Sas-Chen A, et al. Epigenetic mechanisms underlie the crosstalk between growth factors and a steroid hormone. Nucleic Acids Res. 2017;45(22):12681–99. https://doi.org/10.1093/nar/gkx865.
123. Klymenko Y, Nephew KP. Epigenetic crosstalk between the tumor microenvironment and ovarian cancer cells: a therapeutic road less traveled. Cancers (Basel). 2018;10(9) https://doi.org/10.3390/cancers10090295.
124. Latcheva NK, Viveiros JM, Waddell EA, Nguyen PTT, Liebl FLW, Marenda DR. Epigenetic crosstalk: pharmacological inhibition of HDACs can rescue defective synaptic morphology and neurotransmission phenotypes associated with loss of the chromatin reader Kismet. Mol Cell Neurosci. 2018;87:77–85. https://doi.org/10.1016/j.mcn.2017.11.007.
125. Liu D, Zhang XX, Li MC, Cao CH, Wan DY, Xi BX, et al. C/EBPbeta enhances platinum resistance of ovarian cancer cells by reprogramming H3K79 methylation. Nat Commun. 2018;9(1):1739. https://doi.org/10.1038/s41467-018-03590-5.
126. Cacan E. Epigenetic-mediated immune suppression of positive co-stimulatory molecules in chemoresistant ovarian cancer cells. Cell Biol Int. 2017;41(3):328–39. https://doi.org/10.1002/cbin.10729.
127. Kandel P, Wallace MB, Stauffer J, Bolan C, Raimondo M, Woodward TA, et al. Survival of patients with oligometastatic pancreatic ductal adenocarcinoma treated with combined modality treatment including surgical resection: a pilot study. J Pancreat Cancer. 2018;4(1):88–94. https://doi.org/10.1089/pancan.2018.0011.
128. Cai MH, Xu XG, Yan SL, Sun Z, Ying Y, Wang BK, et al. Depletion of HDAC1, 7 and 8 by histone deacetylase inhibition confers elimination of pancreatic cancer stem cells in combination with gemcitabine. Sci Rep. 2018;8(1):1621. https://doi.org/10.1038/s41598-018-20004-0.
129. Ma YT, Leonard SM, Gordon N, Anderton J, James C, Huen D, et al. Use of a genome-wide haploid genetic screen to identify treatment predicting factors: a proof-of-principle study in pancreatic cancer. Oncotarget. 2017;8(38):63635–45. https://doi.org/10.18632/oncotarget.18879.
130. Kwon HM, Kang EJ, Kang K, Kim SD, Yang K, Yi JM. Combinatorial effects of an epigenetic inhibitor and ionizing radiation contribute to targeted elimination of pancreatic cancer stem cell. Oncotarget. 2017;8(51):89005–20. https://doi.org/10.18632/oncotarget.21642.

131. Stangelberger A, Waldert M, Djavan B. Prostate cancer in elderly men. Rev Urol. 2008;10(2):111–9.
132. Vatandoust S, Kichenadasse G, O'Callaghan M, Vincent AD, Kopsaftis T, Walsh S, et al. Localised prostate cancer in elderly men aged 80-89 years, findings from a population-based registry. BJU Int. 2018;121 Suppl 3:48–54. https://doi.org/10.1111/bju.14228.
133. Sun Y, Wang BE, Leong KG, Yue P, Li L, Jhunjhunwala S, et al. Androgen deprivation causes epithelial-mesenchymal transition in the prostate: implications for androgen-deprivation therapy. Cancer Res. 2012;72(2):527–36. https://doi.org/10.1158/0008-5472.CAN-11-3004.
134. Gu P, Chen X, Xie R, Han J, Xie W, Wang B, et al. lncRNA HOXD-AS1 regulates proliferation and chemo-resistance of castration-resistant prostate cancer via recruiting WDR5. Mol Ther. 2017;25(8):1959–73. https://doi.org/10.1016/j.ymthe.2017.04.016.
135. Katzenwadel A, Wolf P. Androgen deprivation of prostate cancer: leading to a therapeutic dead end. Cancer Lett. 2015;367(1):12–7. https://doi.org/10.1016/j.canlet.2015.06.021.
136. Yarmishyn AA, Batagov AO, Tan JZ, Sundaram GM, Sampath P, Kuznetsov VA, et al. HOXD-AS1 is a novel lncRNA encoded in HOXD cluster and a marker of neuroblastoma progression revealed via integrative analysis of noncoding transcriptome. BMC Genomics. 2014;15(Suppl 9):S7. https://doi.org/10.1186/1471-2164-15-S9-S7.
137. Yang YW, Flynn RA, Chen Y, Qu K, Wan B, Wang KC, et al. Essential role of lncRNA binding for WDR5 maintenance of active chromatin and embryonic stem cell pluripotency. Elife. 2014;3:e02046. https://doi.org/10.7554/eLife.02046.
138. Kim JY, Banerjee T, Vinckevicius A, Luo Q, Parker JB, Baker MR, et al. A role for WDR5 in integrating threonine 11 phosphorylation to lysine 4 methylation on histone H3 during androgen signaling and in prostate cancer. Mol Cell. 2014;54(4):613–25. https://doi.org/10.1016/j.molcel.2014.03.043.
139. Brikun I, Nusskern D, Decatus A, Harvey E, Li L, Freije D. A panel of DNA methylation markers for the detection of prostate cancer from FV and DRE urine DNA. Clin Epigenetics. 2018;10:91. https://doi.org/10.1186/s13148-018-0524-x.
140. Kuusk T, De Bruijn R, Brouwer OR, De Jong J, Donswijk M, Hendricksen K, et al. Outcome of sentinel lymph node biopsy in patients with clinically non-metastatic renal cell carcinoma. Scand J Urol. 2018;52(5–6):411–8. https://doi.org/10.1080/21681805.2018.1531057.
141. Santoni M, Piva F, De Giorgi U, Mosca A, Basso U, Santini D, et al. Autophagic gene polymorphisms in liquid biopsies and outcome of patients with metastatic clear cell renal cell carcinoma. Anticancer Res. 2018;38(10):5773–82. https://doi.org/10.21873/anticanres.12916.
142. Saeednejad Zanjani L, Madjd Z, Abolhasani M, Rasti A, Shariftabrizi A, Mehrazma M, et al. Human telomerase reverse transcriptase protein expression predicts tumour aggressiveness and survival in patients with clear cell renal cell carcinoma. Pathology. 2019;51(1):21–31. https://doi.org/10.1016/j.pathol.2018.08.019.
143. Winter S, Fisel P, Buttner F, Nies AT, Stenzl A, Bedke J, et al. Comment on "Epigenetic activation of the drug transporter OCT2 sensitizes renal cell carcinoma to oxaliplatin". Sci Transl Med. 2017;9(391) https://doi.org/10.1126/scitranslmed.aal2439.
144. Zheng X, Liu Y, Yu Q, Wang H, Tan F, Zhu Q, et al. Response to comment on "Epigenetic activation of the drug transporter OCT2 sensitizes renal cell carcinoma to oxaliplatin". Sci Transl Med. 2017;9(391) https://doi.org/10.1126/scitranslmed.aam6298.
145. Liu Y, Zheng X, Yu Q, Wang H, Tan F, Zhu Q, et al. Epigenetic activation of the drug transporter OCT2 sensitizes renal cell carcinoma to oxaliplatin. Sci Transl Med. 2016;8(348):348ra97. https://doi.org/10.1126/scitranslmed.aaf3124.
146. Balasubramanian D, Akhtar-Zaidi B, Song L, Bartels CF, Veigl M, Beard L, et al. H3K4me3 inversely correlates with DNA methylation at a large class of non-CpG-island-containing start sites. Genome Med. 2012;4(5):47. https://doi.org/10.1186/gm346.
147. Perini G, Diolaiti D, Porro A, Della Valle G. In vivo transcriptional regulation of N-Myc target genes is controlled by E-box methylation. Proc Natl Acad Sci U S A. 2005;102(34):12117–22. https://doi.org/10.1073/pnas.0409097102.

148. Xi W, Chen X, Sun J, Wang W, Huo Y, Zheng G, et al. Combined treatment with valproic acid and 5-Aza-2′-deoxycytidine synergistically inhibits human clear cell renal cell carcinoma growth and migration. Med Sci Monit. 2018;24:1034–43.
149. Bodnar L, Stec R, Cierniak S, Synowiec A, Wcislo G, Jesiotr M, et al. Role of WNT/beta-catenin pathway as potential prognostic and predictive factors in renal cell cancer patients treated with everolimus in the second and subsequent lines. Clin Genitourin Cancer. 2018;16(4):257–65. https://doi.org/10.1016/j.clgc.2018.01.008.
150. Li YL, Jin YF, Liu XX, Li HJ. A comprehensive analysis of Wnt/beta-catenin signaling pathway-related genes and crosstalk pathways in the treatment of As2O3 in renal cancer. Ren Fail. 2018;40(1):331–9. https://doi.org/10.1080/0886022X.2018.1456461.
151. Schodel J, Grampp S, Maher ER, Moch H, Ratcliffe PJ, Russo P, et al. Hypoxia, hypoxia-inducible transcription factors, and renal cancer. Eur Urol. 2016;69(4):646–57. https://doi.org/10.1016/j.eururo.2015.08.007.
152. Lin HW, Fu CF, Chang MC, Lu TP, Lin HP, Chiang YC, et al. CDH1, DLEC1 and SFRP5 methylation panel as a prognostic marker for advanced epithelial ovarian cancer. Epigenomics. 2018;10(11):1397–413. https://doi.org/10.2217/epi-2018-0035.
153. Ge G, Peng D, Xu Z, Guan B, Xin Z, He Q, et al. Restoration of 5-hydroxymethylcytosine by ascorbate blocks kidney tumour growth. EMBO Rep. 2018;19(8) https://doi.org/10.15252/embr.201745401.
154. Yeon A, You S, Kim M, Gupta A, Park MH, Weisenberger DJ, et al. Rewiring of cisplatin-resistant bladder cancer cells through epigenetic regulation of genes involved in amino acid metabolism. Theranostics. 2018;8(16):4520–34. https://doi.org/10.7150/thno.25130.
155. Khandelwal M, Anand V, Appunni S, Seth A, Singh P, Mathur S, et al. Decitabine augments cytotoxicity of cisplatin and doxorubicin to bladder cancer cells by activating hippo pathway through RASSF1A. Mol Cell Biochem. 2018;446(1–2):105–14. https://doi.org/10.1007/s11010-018-3278-z.
156. Szablewski V, Bret C, Kassambara A, Devin J, Cartron G, Costes-Martineau V, et al. An epigenetic regulator-related score (EpiScore) predicts survival in patients with diffuse large B cell lymphoma and identifies patients who may benefit from epigenetic therapy. Oncotarget. 2018;9(27):19079–99. https://doi.org/10.18632/oncotarget.24901.
157. Wilson S, Filipp FV. A network of epigenomic and transcriptional cooperation encompassing an epigenomic master regulator in cancer. NPJ Syst Biol Appl. 2018;4:24. https://doi.org/10.1038/s41540-018-0061-4.
158. Liu B, Wang T, Wang H, Zhang L, Xu F, Fang R, et al. Oncoprotein HBXIP enhances HOXB13 acetylation and co-activates HOXB13 to confer tamoxifen resistance in breast cancer. J Hematol Oncol. 2018;11(1):26. https://doi.org/10.1186/s13045-018-0577-5.
159. Ojo D, Lin X, Wu Y, Cockburn J, Bane A, Tang D. Polycomb complex protein BMI1 confers resistance to tamoxifen in estrogen receptor positive breast cancer. Cancer Lett. 2018;426:4–13. https://doi.org/10.1016/j.canlet.2018.03.048.
160. Wu Y, Zhang Z, Cenciarini ME, Proietti CJ, Amasino M, Hong T, et al. Tamoxifen resistance in breast cancer is regulated by the EZH2-ERalpha-GREB1 transcriptional axis. Cancer Res. 2018;78(3):671–84. https://doi.org/10.1158/0008-5472.CAN-17-1327.
161. Yang H, Bueso-Ramos C, DiNardo C, Estecio MR, Davanlou M, Geng QR, et al. Expression of PD-L1, PD-L2, PD-1 and CTLA4 in myelodysplastic syndromes is enhanced by treatment with hypomethylating agents. Leukemia. 2014;28(6):1280–8. https://doi.org/10.1038/leu.2013.355.
162. Hogg SJ, Vervoort SJ, Deswal S, Ott CJ, Li J, Cluse LA, et al. BET-bromodomain inhibitors engage the host immune system and regulate expression of the immune checkpoint ligand PD-L1. Cell Rep. 2017;18(9):2162–74. https://doi.org/10.1016/j.celrep.2017.02.011.
163. Lee HZ, Kwitkowski VE, Del Valle PL, Ricci MS, Saber H, Habtemariam BA, et al. FDA approval: belinostat for the treatment of patients with relapsed or refractory peripheral T-cell lymphoma. Clin Cancer Res. 2015;21(12):2666–70. https://doi.org/10.1158/1078-0432.CCR-14-3119.

164. Raynal NJ, Da Costa EM, Lee JT, Gharibyan V, Ahmed S, Zhang H, et al. Repositioning FDA-approved drugs in combination with epigenetic drugs to reprogram colon cancer epigenome. Mol Cancer Ther. 2017;16(2):397–407. https://doi.org/10.1158/1535-7163.MCT-16-0588.
165. Abdelfatah E, Kerner Z, Nanda N, Ahuja N. Epigenetic therapy in gastrointestinal cancer: the right combination. Therap Adv Gastroenterol. 2016;9(4):560–79. https://doi.org/10.1177/17 56283X16644247.
166. Conte M, De Palma R, Altucci L. HDAC inhibitors as epigenetic regulators for cancer immunotherapy. Int J Biochem Cell Biol. 2018;98:65–74. https://doi.org/10.1016/j.biocel.2018.03.004.
167. Zhao L, Duan YT, Lu P, Zhang ZJ, Zheng XK, Wang JL, et al. Epigenetic targets and their inhibitors in cancer therapy. Curr Top Med Chem. 2018;18(28):2395–419. https://doi.org/10.2174/1568026619666181224095449.
168. Verma M, Banerjee HN. Epigenetic inhibitors. Methods Mol Biol. 2015;1238:469–85. https://doi.org/10.1007/978-1-4939-1804-1_24.
169. Verma SK. Recent progress in the discovery of epigenetic inhibitors for the treatment of cancer. Methods Mol Biol. 2015;1238:677–88. https://doi.org/10.1007/978-1-4939-1804-1_35.

Chapter 10
Nanomedicine and Drug Delivery Systems in Overcoming Resistance to Targeted Therapy

Matt McTaggart and Cecile Malardier-Jugroot

Abstract The first nanomedicine was approved for clinical use over 20 years ago. In the intervening time, our ability to engineer materials at the nanoscale has advanced immensely, yet a revolution in targeted drug delivery remains elusive. Nowhere is this more keenly felt than in the treatment of multi-drug resistant cancers, where nanotechnology's fine control over drug release rate, location, and sequence promises a suite of tools for the effective long-term management of disease. This chapter provides a survey of the current knowledge and trajectory of nanomaterial drug delivery systems for avoiding or overcoming multiple drug resistance in cancer treatment. Existing nanocarriers in development incorporate a variety of materials and properties designed to transit through the circulatory system, concentrate at tumor sites, selectively bind to cancerous cells, and release their drug payloads. However, a greater understanding of the biological barriers to achieving each of those steps is still needed for drug delivery systems to successfully translate into clinical treatment. Greater attention on the interactions between specific delivery systems and their specific target cells *in vivo* might be achieved through a 'disease-first' design strategy and closer integration of materials and physiology during training.

Keywords Drug delivery systems · Nanocarriers · Enhanced permeability and retention · Active targeting

M. McTaggart · C. Malardier-Jugroot (✉)
Department of Chemistry and Chemical Engineering, Royal Military College of Canada, Kingston, ON, Canada
e-mail: Matt.McTaggart@rmc.ca; Cecile.Malardier-Jugroot@rmc.ca

© Springer Nature Switzerland AG 2019
M. R. Szewczuk et al. (eds.), *Current Applications for Overcoming Resistance to Targeted Therapies*, Resistance to Targeted Anti-Cancer Therapeutics 20, https://doi.org/10.1007/978-3-030-21477-7_10

Abbreviations

ECM   Extracellular matrix
EPR   Enhanced permeability and retention
FDA   United States Food and Drug Administration
MDR   Multiple drug resistant
NP   Nanoparticle
PEG   Polyethylene glycol
TME   Tumour microenvironment

10.1 Introduction

The ability to view and manipulate matter on the smallest scale has influenced the direction of research across all fields, and medical technology is no exception [1, 2]. Regulatory bodies vary in their definitions of medical nanotechnology but in general the term comprises materials or material components designed to perform some medicinal function with at least one dimension between 1 and 100 nm. Nanoscale objects are small enough that they can interact with biological structures, yet large enough that they may exert a level of control over their surroundings and, often, encapsulate a payload [3]. Microsilica particles, for instance, often extend to 400 nm but are included in this category because it is the nanoscale pores dotting their highly textured exterior, and not their overall diameter, that provide the advantage [4]. However, most nanoparticles (NPs) under investigation for use as targeted drug delivery vehicles described in this chapter do maintain at least one dimension below 100 nm.

10.1.1 Nanoparticles as a Vector

It would be misleading to describe the medical nanotechnology presented here as a drug in and of itself. While its structure or one of its components may impart some therapeutic effect, it is better to consider these nanomaterials as vectors or delivery vehicles for the therapeutic agents they contain. Just as the spread of vector-borne disease is determined by the physiology and mobility of its host, so the fate of a drug payload vehicles is a function of the behaviour of its carrier within the body. Encapsulation of a drug by a nanocarrier provides a means to control the direction, duration, concentration, and destination of chemotherapeutic agents with far greater accuracy than the systemic release of the free drug [5].

   In addition to precise control of the location of payload release, targeted delivery by nanoparticle may permit co-delivery of treatments whose timing or concentrations would be difficult to coordinate without a common carrier. For example, if a chemotherapeutic drug acts on a pathway for which two or more phenotypes exist, tumour cells may circumvent the drug by up-regulating expression of a compensatory pathway, developing heterogeneity and possibly drug resistance. A well-designed nanoparticle could carry and release a variety of drugs to address each possible pathway without the need to recharacterize a tumour or produce toxic concentrations or interactions at the systemic level [4]. Adjuvants may also be loaded and released at the optimum time, place, and concentration to maximize their effects. Finally, the carrier itself may incorporate a physical treatment modality which could act in concert with the chemical it carries. For example, the use of gold nanoparticles as a thermogenic treatment might carry a drug that makes local cells more susceptible to heat stress.

This chapter will address the common nanomaterials under investigation for application in targeted treatment and the potential methods they may employ to avoid or overcome drug resistance in tumour cells. First, the existing classes of nanomaterials under investigation for application in targeted delivery of therapeutic or imaging agents will be described. A survey of the physiological barriers to precise targeting will help justify why some of the promises of medical nanotechnology remain unfulfilled. This survey will be followed by a discussion of the real motivations for continued effort towards the successful translation of tumour-targeted nanocarriers for combating multiple drug resistant (MDR) cancers. We will conclude by offering some considerations for future directions in the design of materials and policies.

10.2   Current Systems

Several classes of nanoparticles are being developed for medical applications [6–8]. Liposomes and polymeric structures are the most common, followed in no particular order by micelles, dendrites, and inorganic nanoparticles.

Liposomes Liposomes are simple self-assembling spheres of fatty acids. The surface forces that drive assembly draw the hydrophobic tail groups towards each other, aligning the hydrophilic head group towards the aqueous exterior, giving liposomes a spherical shape. They have the virtues of being biocompatible, self-assembling, and easily characterized. Liposomes were the first type of nano-medical drug delivery system approved by the United States Food and Drug Administration (FDA) [9]. While liposomes are susceptible to capture and breakdown by the immune system, their surface chemistry makes it possible to decorate them with molecules such as polyethylene glycol (PEG) that disrupt the body's defenses.

Micelles Micelles share numerous similarities and limitations with liposomes. They do, however, have more versatility in chemical composition and accessible shapes. Indeed, micelles formed by self-assembly of amphiphilic copolymers can generate exact shapes ranging from spheres to rods or lamellae as seen in Fig. 10.1. The shape of the self-assembled structures is often dictated by solvent composition

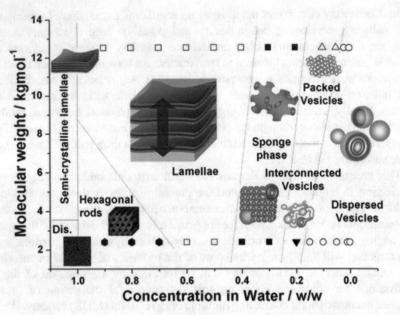

Fig. 10.1 Characteristics of micelles. Like many polymeric materials, the shape and size of the self-assembling nanostructure of this block copolymer can be simply controlled by small alterations in the molecular mass and concentration. Isothermal phase diagrams of poly(ethylene oxide)-co-poly(butylene oxide)/water reproduced with permission from ACS Publications [16]

and the ratio between water and an organic solvent. The shape of the drug carrier or the prodrug has been shown to influence the internalization pathway, blood circulation, cellular uptake, and observed cytotoxicity [10]. The influence of the shape of the nanocarriers on the release of the drug has also been highlighted in a review by Venkataraman and colleagues [11]. They found that changing the shape from a spherical to a filamentous micelle increased circulation time from 2 days to a week and resulted in a significant relative decrease in tumour size given an identical initial drug concentration [12]. The diverse chemical composition of the amphiphilic molecules permits different functional groups on the surface of micelles and allows for great versatility of the nanocarriers produced. Such facile functionalization opens direct and active targeting of the cancer cells to reduce side effects linked to the chemotherapeutic drug [13].

Polymeric Nanoparticles Polymeric structures offer much more physical and chemical versatility, forming anything from a amorphous gels to rigid crystalline structures [14]. Generally, polymers present a much more complicated toxicity profile but size, shape, inner and outer chemistry may each be tailored according to the application. Due to their easily-altered physical properties, polymers are the most investigated nanostructured material [15].

Dendrites Dendrites are polymers that branch from a common point to form fractal volumes with well-defined interior cavities and are another class of poly-

Dendritic Family

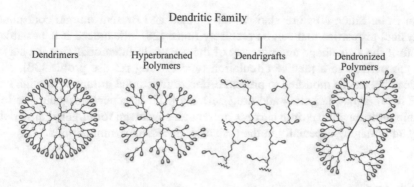

Dendrimers   Hyperbranched   Dendrigrafts   Dendronized
              Polymers   Polymers

Fig. 10.2 Polymeric dendrimers—regularly branching polymer nanoparticles—can be designed to take on a variety of shapes and sizes. The size and number of internal spaces or pores, which act as containers for drug payloads, are separately controllable. Reproduced with permission from RSC Publishing [25]

meric structure that shows promise for drug delivery applications as seen in Fig. 10.2 [17, 18]. Dendritic cavities can provide physical entrapment of guest molecules, a property that could be translated into drug capture and delivery, although this delivery system has not yet been clinically observed. Indeed, dendrites are sought for applications in drug delivery as well as gene transfection [19], bioimaging [20, 21], and tissue engineering [22, 23]. Like other polymeric structure, dendritic structures could potentially undergo chemical functionalization of the interior and exterior structure for an increased range or specialization of biological applications. However, the cost of production can be prohibitive, and problems with scalability, biocompatibility, and biodegradability, have limited the number of *in vivo* studies [24].

Inorganic Nanoparticles Inorganic nanoparticles include a broad range of materials from relatively large and porous silica to small metallic gold nanoparticles [26]. Most inorganic particles are non-reactive and rarely introduce challenges in toxicity. Inorganic nanoparticles such as quantum dots (CdTe or CdSe/ZnS), iron oxide, silver (Ag), zinc oxide (ZnO) or gold (Au) NPs are often functionalized to improve solubility and reduce aggregation. Cellular intake via endocytosis and combination with a lysosome exposes the NPs to a low pH environment. This change in pH, combined with low-specific enzymes, degrades the organic coating and induces NP aggregation and degradation [13]. While these may be detrimental to performance during transport or delivery, degradation of CdSe, Ag, or ZnO has also been associated with the production of cytotoxic ions [27]. Cytotoxicity linked to degradation has not been observed with Au NPs which can be used for both diagnostic and therapeutic purposes. The therapeutic effect of these nanoparticles can be fine-tuned and adapted to drug-resistant tumours. However, some challenges in the development of Au NPs remain. For instance, surface plasmon resonance is a function of NP size and surface coating, factors which are limited in range by their impact on cellular intake and circulation time. Silica NPs are also widely studied and present unique controllable physical properties that can be precisely tuned [28, 29]. Indeed it is possible to control the size, shape and porosity of the NP while functionalizing the surface of the particle to a precise circulation time or drug release profile [30]. Also, silica NPs can be modified to present different functional groups within the same NP for imaging, targeting and drug delivery [31]. In general, organic and inorganic multifunctional drug carriers present an advantage for targeted drug delivery and imaging especially in the case of drug-resistant tumour cells.

10.3 Mechanisms of Delivery

Nanocarriers promise to increase the efficacy of traditional chemical, biological, and radiological treatments by creating a platform for the rational design of an accurate and precise targeting system. Despite the robust research activity in the decades following the first FDA approved nanomedical cancer treatment, all currently approved therapies remain limited to relatively low-precision, passive targeting [32]. Arguably, nanotechnology's most significant impact on therapy has come from relatively simple materials that stabilize their drug payload during systemic circulation, reduce the exposure of healthy cells to cytotoxic agents, and tailor particle size to accumulate in a tumour preferentially. The following sections provide an overview of characteristics currently under study, which future nanocarriers may incorporate either individually or in combination.

10.3.1 Enhanced Pharmacokinetics and Stability in Circulation

Many chemotherapeutic drugs are small molecules with low water solubility and are subject to rapid renal clearance. Nanocarriers are used to increase circulation time and total exposure [33]. For example, doxorubicin is an effective anti-cancer drug used to treat a variety of cancer types. However, due to rapid clearance and non-specific uptake by healthy cells, a high dose is required to achieve an effect on a tumour. Encapsulation within a liposome, micelle, or polymer structure creates a nanocarrier system with a diameter large enough to avoid the renal clearance pathways that affect particles under 5 nm while also remaining small enough to passively accumulate in the tumour microenvironment due to the enhanced permeability and retention (EPR) effect depicted in Fig. 10.3 [34]. EPR arises because the vasculature that feeds rapidly growing tumours may be poorly formed and so suffer a higher rate of seepage between their endothelial cells. Particles in the 30–400 nm range are more likely to exit the bloodstream through the fenestrations (enhanced

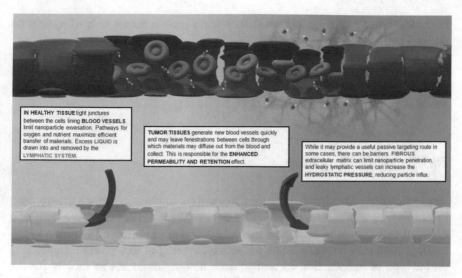

IN HEALTHY TISSUE tight junctures between the cells lining BLOOD VESSELS limit nanoparticle exvasation. Pathways for oxygen and nutrient maximize efficient transfer of materials. Excess LIQUID is drawn into and removed by the LYMPHATIC SYSTEM.

TUMOR TISSUES generate new blood vessels quickly and may leave fenestrations between cells through which materials may diffuse out from the blood and collect. This is responsible for the ENHANCED PERMEABILITY AND RETENTION effect.

While it may provide a useful passive targeting route in some cases, there can be barriers. FIBROUS extracellular matrix can limit nanoparticle penetration, and leaky lymphatic vessels can increase the HYDROSTATIC PRESSURE, reducing particle influx.

Fig. 10.3 Schematic of the Enhanced Permeability and Retention (EPR) effect in leaky tumour vasculature. Rapid tumour growth may lead to poorly-constructed blood and lymph vessels which permit nanoparticles to be preferentially deposited in the tumour microenvironment

permeability) and less likely to be carried into the lymphatic system, again due to the underdeveloped support system (retention) [35–37].

Passive targeting by EPR is often the only method incorporated into a nanocarrier's design. However, it is important to remember that there exist significant differences between cancers and heterogeneity within a given type of cancer [38]. Not all tumour vasculature produces the EPR effect to the same degree, and some tumours may not present the effect at all [39]. Low tumour drainage is itself a double-edged sword; while treatment carriers that manage to enter the tumour extracellular fluid are retained for a longer time, the pressure gradient works to resist particle inflow from the blood. Furthermore, longer exposure times do not improve outcomes in-and-of themselves but must be paired with a reliable method for extravasation and drug release [40]. Regardless of the method of encapsulation, some fraction of the drug payload is released in the bloodstream due to non-specific interactions, mechanical disruption, or another rare and randomly-occurring event [38]. Prolonged circulation time therefore increases the risk of exposure to a low concentration of the free drug and the likelihood that tumors can develop drug resistance before receiving an effective dose [41].

In addition to the diameter, the exterior chemistry can be tailored to promote or avoid interactions with colloidal proteins found in the bloodstream [42, 43]. Aggregation of proteins on the nanoparticle's surface will change the solubility and hemodynamic profile and may also mark it for removal by macrophages in the blood vessels, liver, or spleen. Protein aggregation reduces systemic availability and increases non-specific accumulation in the organs [44]. Liposomes are typically subject to protein interactions, but conjugation with a short polymer chain, such as

PEG, or another surface group sterically hinders protein access to binding sites on the lipid surface [45].

Drug encapsulation can, therefore, increase the circulation half-life from minutes to hours and the total exposure by orders of magnitude while eliminating the initial spike in serum concentration, allowing for the administration of dose amounts that would otherwise be toxic to patients [33, 34, 46, 47].

10.3.2 Active Targeting

Active targeting of tumour cells by nanocarriers implies that the delivery shell incorporates a mechanism to recognize the treatment target [48]. For example, a diseased cell known to express a much higher concentration of a certain membrane protein may be a candidate for active targeting of that protein. Depending on the type of nanocarrier, an antagonistic binding molecule or moiety for the membrane protein can be incorporated onto the exterior surface. Of course, the presence of reactive surface features complicates the task of unimpeded systemic transport. Recent work by Jin and colleagues addresses the need to protect or 'camouflage' the binding ligands until in proximity to the target receptors [49]. Once the nanocarrier reaches the cell, the targeting ligand will recognize and bind to the target receptor. This interaction could be made to initiate payload release in the ECM next to the cell membrane or to induce endocytosis and have the drug-loaded carrier into the cell interior [1, 50]. Once the drug delivery system is encapsulated within the cell, intracellular targeting of specific organelles may be possible [51].

10.4 Challenges to Delivery

The challenges faced in drug delivery are described below and summarized in Fig. 10.4.

10.4.1 Vascular Kinetics

Systemic travel from the point of injection to the target site poses numerous challenges to the drug-loaded nanosystem [52]. Clinical trials of unsuccessful carriers have nevertheless helped identify unknown or underappreciated challenges associated with effective delivery of chemotherapeutic agents to their intended targets. The following summarizes some of the pharmacokinetic issues posed by systemic circulation, navigating the tumour microenvironment and extracellular matrix,

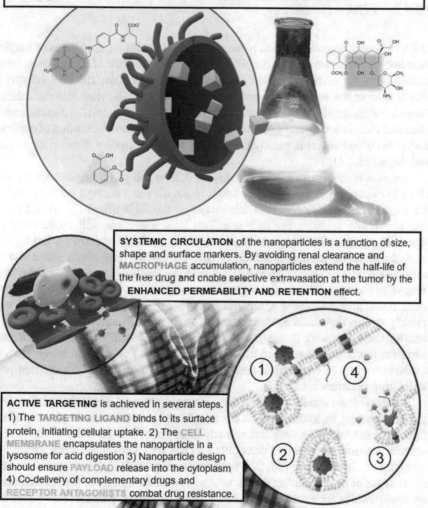

NANOPARTICLE PRODUCTION varies widely depending on the materials involved but commonly includes the assembly of a SHELL with internal dimensions and chemistry appropriate for the loading and stable storage of the ANTI-CANCER PAYLOAD, polymer SURFACE COATINGS that tailor the hydrodynamic radius and biological interactions and allow for conjugation with TARGETING LIGANDS and/or RECEPTOR ANTAGONISTS.

SYSTEMIC CIRCULATION of the nanoparticles is a function of size, shape and surface markers. By avoiding renal clearance and MACROPHAGE accumulation, nanoparticles extend the half-life of the free drug and enable selective extravasation at the tumor by the ENHANCED PERMEABILITY AND RETENTION effect.

ACTIVE TARGETING is achieved in several steps. 1) The TARGETING LIGAND binds to its surface protein, initiating cellular uptake. 2) The CELL MEMBRANE encapsulates the nanoparticle in a lysosome for acid digestion 3) Nanoparticle design should ensure PAYLOAD release into the cytoplasm 4) Co-delivery of complementary drugs and RECEPTOR ANTAGONISTS combat drug resistance.

Fig. 10.4 Schematized life of an archetypal nanocarrier from synthesis to drug delivery. Nanocarriers incorporate a number of design considerations including encapsulation method for the drug payload; shell material, size, shape, and chemistry; surface coatings; and targeting ligands. These design characteristics must be optimized for transport through systemic circulation and selective payload delivery at the diseased cells. Once the drug is released, the carrier can contribute to overcoming drug resistance by acting as a transport antagonist or be enhancing complimentary physical therapeutic methods

gaining access to the cell and drug release. The concordant considerations for the design of nanocarriers are discussed for each segment of the journey.

10.4.2 Hydrodynamics

In the first approximation, blood is merely a liquid medium inside tubes of varying diameter and pressure. In this simplified model, the behavior of nanocarriers when carried along by the blood flow is a matter of fluid dynamics. The flow velocity is slower against the vessel walls and faster in the center. Particles that concentrate towards the center of the vessel have less contact time with the walls, demonstrating increased circulation times but decreased extravasation. The distribution of particles within the blood vessel is mainly determined by their physical dimensions of size and shape [53, 54].

Size is a biologically relevant measure due to the physiological systems in place to ensure rapid clearance of small molecules and foreign cells as well as the nanocarrier's ability to take advantage of the EPR effect [37, 40]. Size is also physically relevant because it affects how a particle will move within a liquid. The proper size of a particle in a liquid is not its hard diameter but instead its hydrodynamic diameter, which is determined by how much water moves with the particle inflow. Fluid in contact with the walls of the vessel will be slow relative to the center due to the higher resistance to flow [55]. The faster moving inner molecules will have more influence on smaller nanoparticles and will quickly sweep them along, concentrating them in the center of the vessel and limiting their exposure to the vessel walls. This approach will increase circulation time but restrict access to their target tumours. The gradual breakdown of the nanocarriers in circulation creates the extended low-dose release that may incite drug resistance.

The shape is an equally vital but less discussed physical dimension of the nanocarrier regarding its hydrodynamic impact [11, 12]. Just as the shape of a falling object will determine its path and velocity through the air (consider the difference between a closed and opened parachute), so too will a particle's shape determine how it travels in the blood [56, 57]. Spherical nanoparticles are common due to the relative ease of their manufacture but tend to flow in the middle of the vessel, reducing opportunities for extravasation. Rod-shaped or fibrous particles fare better due to their higher aspect ratio. Disc-shaped particles spend the most time in contact with the vessel walls and therefore are the fastest to discover fenestrations large enough to escape the bloodstream [53]. It is perhaps unsurprising given that disc-shaped particles mimic the shape of platelets, blood components whose purpose is to find and block leakage from vessels. Liposomes are primarily limited to their spherical shape because of the radially symmetrical self-assembly of their phospholipid subunits. Polymers may be designed to take on an array of shapes, or in some cases to change shape in response to chemical or physical signals in their surroundings.

10.4.3 Extravasation

Extended circulation times are a good outcome only insofar as they promote extravasation of the nanoparticles at the targeted sites. For example, if the target tumour's vasculature is relatively well-constructed and EPR effect is moderate, then the longer circulation time provides opportunities to interact with the target site and therefore a greater chance that the carrier will enter a tumour. One must also recognize that the more extended circulation period equally enhances the opportunity for non-specific accumulation or other system clearance methods to take effect. If the probability of all other methods of exit for the drug-delivery system remains lower than the one that delivers the drug to the target, then the longer circulation time is understandable and desirable. Better still are methods to increase the probability of the desired outcome, such as those that include adjuvants that attack the tumour vasculature itself.

Tumour heterogeneity is a complex problem that is often ignored during the design phase of nanoparticles [58, 59]. Oversimplification or generalization of the physiological characteristics of diseased areas has failed when otherwise promising delivery strategies are translated to the clinic. To minimize this risk, Hare and colleagues suggest four changes of focus during the development process:

1. Begin with a greater understanding of nanomaterial interactions with tumour tissues,
2. Develop more representative animal models and testing protocols,
3. Pre-select patients with a higher likelihood of response, and
4. The shift from material-driven to disease-driven development [58].

The tendency to develop nanomaterials based on a general delivery strategy before considering which disease it might suitably address has led to many new materials but few effective treatments. This may be symptomatic of the scientific backgrounds of those leading the search for formulations. Training programs that straddle the nanomaterial-pathophysiological divide may realign nanomaterial innovation with the patient- and disease-focused development and improve rates of clinical translation.

10.4.4 Penetrating the Tumor Microenvironment

Size and shape are just as, if not more, important with regard to penetrating the tumour microenvironment (TME) as they are in contending with systemic circulation. The extracellular matrix (ECM) may be far more closely packed than healthy tissue, limiting incursion by particles optimized for relatively free-flowing blood vessels. Furthermore, poor vasculature is can restrict fluid drainage, increasing the local hydrostatic pressure [60]. Under these conditions, smaller particles or filament-shaped nanocarriers are likely the most effective. A larger particle that degrades into or releases smaller particles in response to environmental cues at the edge of the TME may also prove to be more effective at reaching its target [61].

The tumour microenvironment is often moderately acidic, so pH-sensitive release mechanisms are likely to begin to deposit their payload here [62]. If the drug reaches its effective concentration in the ECM as well as inside the cells, then drug release before cell entry is acceptable and may even be preferred. In this case, cancer cells have a reduced capacity for developing resistance since the target is the general tumour environment and not a specific marker on the surface of the cell. Other environmental cues that could trigger drug release include light, magnetic field, ultrasound, and heat [63]. Nanocarriers can be engineered to generate or enhance these conditions in concert with external stimulation.

10.4.5 Entering the Cell

Another targeting strategy is to decorate the surface of the nanocarrier with ligands that recognize and bond with a receptor on the cellular membrane which then initiates endocytosis [55]. Precise delivery is therefore dependent on the relative overexpression of the target molecule on cancer cells as compared to healthy cells. For example, both healthy and diseased cells may express folic acid receptors on their surface [13]. However, some cancers are known to significantly overexpress the receptor. When coupled to the EPR effect, the target cells will internalize the nanocarrier in a proportionally greater frequency than healthy cells [53]. While this strategy does allow for more precise targeting than passive collection and drug release by the EPR effect or the acidic tumour ECM, it also presents the potential for cells to develop resistance to it by downregulating expression of the target protein. Strategies to avoid this undesirable side-effect are discussed in more detail below.

10.4.6 Defeating the Lysosome

Once the targeting ligand binds to a receptor protein on the cancer cell's surface, the nanocarrier may be transported through the membrane via endosome [15]. The cell may then begin to pump protons into the endosome or combine it with lysosomes to reduce the internal pH and degrade the endosomal contents. The nanocarrier can be designed to remain stable in the slightly acidic tumour ECM but respond to stronger acidity, ensuring preferential drug release inside the target cells. The nanosystem must also be able to protect the payload from acid damage and incorporate some mechanism to free the drug from endosomal encapsulation. An elegant solution to accomplish both is to use a proton absorbing polymer that expands as it collects a positive charge on its surface [55]. The proton sponge ensures that the payload is not subjected to an acid attack while the build-up of repulsive electrostatic forces causes the polymer to push against the endosomal envelope until it bursts, freeing the intact drug. Other strategies include the inclusion of cationic polymers to induce membrane inversion or membrane-destabilizing peptides [53].

10.5   Applications in Multidrug-Resistant Cancers

As a fundamental design concept, nanocarriers for cancer treatment should be engineered to avoid or overcome the possible triggers for drug resistance concurrent to their release of the payload. Strategies include co-delivery and staged deployment of complementary drugs and adjuvants, the use of the nanocarrier itself as a sensitizer to a physical treatment method, and incorporation of drug efflux pump antagonists or disruptors. The application of any, or better yet all, of these methods in a targeted drug-delivery system should act to reduce the incidence and impact of drug resistance in tumours.

First, nanocarriers are ideal for the accurate delivery of precisely dosed cytotoxic drugs and their adjuvants, ideally those with complementary target pathways [64–66]. By creating contemporary challenges to the cell, co-delivery designs overwhelm possible routes for the rise of resistance and increase the probability of cell death [67–69]. To fully realize the potential of this approach, ongoing efforts address two significant challenges: loading drugs with reliable and repeatable stoichiometric ratios and loading molecules with significantly different solubility profiles into a single carrier. While polymeric structures are attractive carriers due to their relatively well-controlled size, shape, and chemistry, non-covalent encapsulation leads to relatively high variance in drug loading [53]. Prodrug-polymer covalent conjugation is one solution to improve reproducibility, though the introduction of a linker and the requirement for hydrolysis to activate the payload at the release site increases system complexity. Microfluidic methods that measure and coat droplets to generate synthetic vesicles may be another avenue for a reliable polymer or liposome drug encapsulation. The second challenge is to combine different drugs in a single delivery vehicle or set of vehicles [70]. For example, liposomes tend to have a hydrophilic interior while polymeric micelles and dendrites tend to be hydrophobic. Block- or alternating- copolymers that self-assemble into ordered structures that incorporate regions of different solvation properties present a potentially viable solution that accommodates both hydrophilic and hydrophobic species [13].

Staged drug release is a challenging but potentially powerful strategy to defeat the rise of resistance in cancer cells. Zhang and colleagues reported the co-encapsulation of pro-apoptotic drug doxorubicin with antiangiogenic curcumin in a pH-sensitive copolymer delivery vehicle [71]. The antiangiogenic action of the curcumin targets the tumour vasculature to entrap the cytotoxic drug with its target, increasing uptake and decreasing cell migration from the tumour site. Similarly, a multi-component staged release nanocarrier first releases the antiangiogenic factor combretastatin followed by cellular uptake of polymer-linked paclitaxel [72]. Lastly, Hu et al. note in their review that the timing of dose delivery against the cell cycle can have a significant impact on drug efficacy [65]. Sequentially timed release functions could present a mechanism to control for this previously uncontrollable factor [73].

Second, inorganic nanocarriers concentrated in the proximity of the diseased tissue could also act as sensitizing agents to physical therapies once they have released their chemotherapeutic payloads. For example, gold nanoparticles and nanoshells are already employed for imaging and light-induced hyperthermia [74, 75]. By modifying the gold nanoparticles for targeted drug delivery, they incorporate two distinct treatment modalities, and the combination is more effective than either alone [5]. Other nanocarriers built around an inorganic nanostructure sensitive to light, magnetic fields, or ultrasound can fulfill the same function [76, 77]. Nanocarriers that simultaneously deliver complimentary treatment agents and modalities to their targets demonstrate a significantly lower risk of multiple drug resistance in tumours [78, 79].

Third, nanocarriers, especially polymeric structures, can be engineered to incorporate efflux pump inhibitors whose antagonistic interaction disrupts the cell's ability to decrease its drug loading. Because more of the drug remains in the target cell, efflux inhibitors allow for lower total dosing, faster tumour shrinkage, and decreased cytotoxicity of surrounding healthy tissues. This strategy may also prove to be fertile grounds for the application of biological agents such as short interfering RNA for silencing efflux pump expression [80].

In summary, by offering a path towards delivering the right dose of the right therapies at the right time in the right place, nanoscale drug delivery vehicles present an undeniably promising mechanism for cancer treatment that avoids or overcomes drug resistance.

10.6 Concepts for Future Development

The fact that much of the potential of nanomedicine remains unrealized may be at least partly explained by a large number of previously unknown physiological encumbrances discovered by the research program over its 30-year history [81]. Figure 10.5 highlights the progress of studies relating to nanotechnology and cancer. Cell, animal, and clinical trials of nanosystems for diagnostics and therapy have succeeded in probing the complexities of the path that a drug must follow from insertion into systemic circulation to its target inside the cell [50]. Past challenges suggest some measures that can be taken to hasten the future development of drug delivery systems.

First, the overall carrier structure should be optimized according to what is known about nanoparticle distribution in the body. Size, shape, and surface coating are particularly important factors for effective systemic transport. Second, co-delivery of multiple drugs and adjuvants reduce the likelihood of resistance by simultaneously attacking multiple response channels. Third, after delivering its payload, the carrier shell itself should be pressed into service as a sensitizing agent in the tumour environment to external therapy sources. Moreover, finally, more

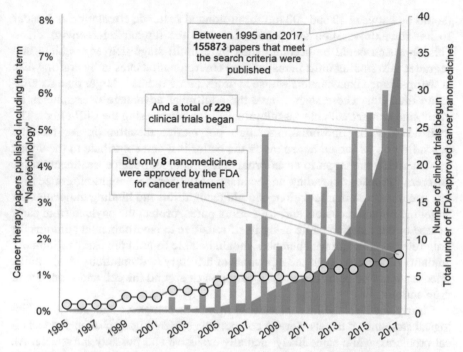

Fig. 10.5 Total number of papers published that contain the terms "nanotechnology AND cancer AND treatment" as a fraction of "cancer AND treatment" [Google Scholar] (left-hand scale, blue curve), the number of clinical trials begun per year [Interventional trial for the treatment of "cancer", "tumor", "neoplasm", or "malignancy" containing the search term "nanoparticle" 2002–2017; National Institutes of Health, clinicaltrials.gov] (right-hand scale, grey bars), and the total number of FDA cancer nanomedicines approved, [32] (right-hand scale, orange dots) from 1995 to 2017

specialized training is necessary to ensure sufficient knowledge of both nanoscience and physiology as well as practical experience with the regulatory process and standards a delivery system would be expected to surpass before approval for widespread use.

10.6.1 Material Properties

Designing a single self-assembling, biocompatible and degradable material that can self-tailor its size and shape according to the environment and conduct a targeted, staged, multimodal attack on the tumour site must, for now, only be imagined as a theoretical ideal [82]. Reality still falls short of this goal.

Twenty years of advances in nanomaterials and their dispersion characteristics in the body have left us with a set of general principles. In summary of the findings cited above, the maximum cross-sectional size of the nanocarrier should lie between 40 and 200 nm for prolonged systemic circulation and under 20 nm for extravasation and penetration into the tumour microenvironment. This approach could be accomplished by a multi-stage delivery vehicle that degrades into smaller units in response to environmental cues or by crafting disc or worm-shaped nanocarriers whose hydrodynamic radius is larger than its minimum diameter. These shapes have the additional advantage over spheres by increasing contact with the vasculature walls and increasing the EPR effect. The scaffold may be liposomal, micellar, polymeric, metallic or non-metallic depending on its target, but so much the better if it can contribute to the attack by sensitizing the target to an external energy source. Surface treatments serve different purposes depending on the stage of delivery: it should minimize protein accumulation in circulation, contain recognition and binding molecules for target membrane receptors and drug efflux pores, protect the payload from early release or degradation while being itself sensitive to environmental stimulus for drug release. The storage chambers should be able to hold precisely ratiometric amounts of various drugs and adjuvants of arbitrary hydrophilicity. And finally, release should be coordinated for location in or around the cell and sequence of drug action.

Clearly, the ideal hybrid nanomaterial may be as complex a structure as the biological structures it targets. Several components present highly challenging technical problems, while some likely mutually-exclusive and possibly intractable. All evidence suggests that material science will continue to press incrementally closer to the goal above. If we are to achieve higher rates of success in the treatment of patients, which is, ultimately, the goal of the material design programme, the field must look past the material formulation and place more focus on the disease targets. While materials scientists cite general tumour properties to evaluate the 'promise' of their formulation, nanomedicines currently in clinical use are approved for specific pathologies, and the specific target cell should be taken into account earlier in the design process [58].

10.6.2 Training

In that same vein, dedicated bio-nanoengineering graduate-level training programs are increasingly necessary to connect the disparate fields of material chemistry and physiology [32, 83]. Increased rates of success in the translation of nanocarriers into clinical cancer treatment will depend on a greater understanding of the complex interactions of complex nanostructures and complex pathophysiologies. Materials-driven development has made remarkable advances, but the disease-driven clinical application requires a level of biological expertise lacking in most chemistry and material science programs, nor do regular medical and microbiology programs teach chemical synthesis or characterization. The interleaving properties of hybrid nanomaterials and their potential to prevent or overcome drug resistance in tumours presents enormous potential for innovation to those able to approach the problem equally well from both sides of the interaction.

10.6.3 Regulation

Nanocarriers present a new class of treatment tool, lying between drug and device. Regulators may be challenged to adapt existing rules to control the testing and promote the safe manufacture of emerging materials and technologies [84, 85]. If a nanocarrier is to be responsive to the differences between cancers, patient physiologies, and heterogeneity within a tumour cell population, then bolt-on targeting ligands may be the key. However, considering the number of materials, targeting mechanisms, and payloads available it is evident that separate trials for each possible combination are impractical.

Optimally, medical adaptation would be as rapid as cellular adaptation, although this would be a daunting standard to achieve. First, it would require affordable and rapid access to genetic testing to allow monitoring of the tumour phenotype and rise of resistance [86, 87]. Second, the nanocarrier would have to be conceived to permit rapid exchange of its surface decoration with minimal impact to its assembly, stability, or pharmacokinetic profile. This would be the synthetic equivalent of the influenza virus and its ability to rapidly exchange its surface markers for staying ahead of vaccinations. Lastly, a regulatory framework would have to be flexible enough that each of the possible nanocarrier surfaces could be approved without the need to test each combination in a clinical trial. Not only would the sheer number of combinations be an insurmountable challenge, but it would also prove impossible to recruit a sufficient number of patients in any single combination to achieve statistically significant results. Of course, cancer nanotherapeutics are not the only field edging toward personalized medicine so policy may yet lead innovation in this case.

10.7 Conclusion

In this chapter, we described the most popular nanomaterials under consideration for application as targeted drug delivery vectors for cancer treatment. These same nanocarriers are being engineered to avoid or overcome multiple drug resistance in tumour cells through co-delivery of concerted physical, chemical, or immunological therapies. The ability to design reliable and precisely assembled medical devices no larger than some cellular organelles presents an enormous potential, though much of it has yet to be realized. For improved translation from lab bench to bedside, we suggest a greater emphasis on disease-driven development, training programs to include equal weighting of materials synthesis and characterization with microbiology and pathophysiology, and for regulatory bodies to begin considering their approach to the expanded applications of medical nanotechnology on the horizon.

References

1. Bertrand N, Wu J, Xu X, Kamaly N, Farokhzad OC. Cancer nanotechnology: the impact of passive and active targeting in the era of modern cancer biology. Adv Drug Deliv Rev. 2014;66:2–25.. https://doi.org/10.1016/j.addr.2013.11.009
2. Wicki A, Witzigmann D, Balasubramanian V, Huwyler J. Nanomedicine in cancer therapy: challenges, opportunities, and clinical applications. J Control Release. 2015;200:138–57. https://doi.org/10.1016/j.jconrel.2014.12.030.
3. Ventola CL. Progress in nanomedicine: approved and investigational nanodrugs. P T. 2017;42(12):742–55.
4. Castillo RR, Colilla M, Vallet-Regí M. Advances in mesoporous silica-based nanocarriers for co-delivery and combination therapy against cancer. Expert Opin Drug Deliv. 2017;14(2):229–43. https://doi.org/10.1080/17425247.2016.1211637.
5. Gao Z, Zhang L, Sun Y. Nanotechnology applied to overcome tumor drug resistance. J Control Release. 2012;162(1):45–55. https://doi.org/10.1016/j.jconrel.2012.05.051.
6. Bobo D, Robinson KJ, Islam J, Thurecht KJ, Corrie SR. Nanoparticle-based medicines: a review of FDA-approved materials and clinical trials to date. Pharm Res. 2016;33(10):2373–87. https://doi.org/10.1007/s11095-016-1958-5.
7. Caster JM, Patel AN, Zhang T, Wang A. Investigational nanomedicines in 2016: a review of nanotherapeutics currently undergoing clinical trials. Wiley Interdiscip Rev Nanomed Nanobiotechnol. 2017;9(1). https://doi.org/10.1002/wnan.1416.
8. Markman JL, Rekechenetskiy A, Holler E, Ljubimova JY. Nanomedicine therapeutic approaches to overcome cancer drug resistance. Adv Drug Deliv Rev. 2013;65(13–14):1866–79. https://doi.org/10.1016/j.addr.2013.09.019.
9. Barenholz Y. Doxil®—the first FDA-approved nano-drug: lessons learned. J Control Release. 2012;160(2):117–34. https://doi.org/10.1016/j.jconrel.2012.03.020.
10. Hu X, Hu J, Tian J, Ge Z, Zhang G, Luo K, Liu S. Polyprodrug amphiphiles: hierarchical assemblies for shape-regulated cellular internalization, trafficking, and drug delivery. J Am Chem Soc. 2013;135(46):17617–29. https://doi.org/10.1021/ja409686x.
11. Venkataraman S, Hedrick JL, Ong ZY, Yang C, Ee PLR, Hammond PT, Yang YY. The effects of polymeric nanostructure shape on drug delivery. Adv Drug Deliv Rev. 2011;63(14–15):1228–46. https://doi.org/10.1016/j.addr.2011.06.016.
12. Geng Y, Dalhaimer P, Cai S, Tsai R, Tewari M, Minko T, Discher DE. Shape effects of filaments versus spherical particles in flow and drug delivery. Nat Nanotechnol. 2007;2(4):249–55. https://doi.org/10.1038/nnano.2007.70.
13. Li X, McTaggart M, Malardier-Jugroot C. Synthesis and characterization of a pH responsive folic acid functionalized polymeric drug delivery system. Biophys Chem. 2016;214–215:17–26. https://doi.org/10.1016/j.bpc.2016.04.002.
14. Livney YD, Assaraf YG. Rationally designed nanovehicles to overcome cancer chemoresistance. Adv Drug Deliv Rev. 2013;65(13–14):1716–30. https://doi.org/10.1016/j.addr.2013.08.006.
15. Peer D, Karp JM, Hong S, Farokhzad OC, Margalit R, Langer R. Nanocarriers as an emerging platform for cancer therapy. Nat Nanotechnol. 2007;2:751–60. https://doi.org/10.1038/nnano.2007.387.
16. Battaglia G, Ryan AJ. Effect of amphiphile size on the transformation from a lyotropic gel to a vesicular dispersion. Macromolecules. 2006;39(2):798–805. https://doi.org/10.1021/ma052108a.
17. Du X, Zhao C, Zhou M, Ma T, Huang H, Jaroniec M, Zhang X, Qiao SZ. Hollow carbon nanospheres with tunable hierarchical pores for drug, gene, and photothermal synergistic treatment. Small. 2017;13(6):1–11. https://doi.org/10.1002/smll.201602592.
18. Wei T, Chen C, Liu J, Liu C, Posocco P, Liu X, Cheng Q, Huo S, Liang Z, Fermeglia M, et al. Anticancer Drug Nanomicelles formed by self-assembling amphiphilic dendrimer to combat cancer drug resistance. Proc Natl Acad Sci. 2015;112(10):2978–83. https://doi.org/10.1073/pnas.1418494112.

19. Guillot-Nieckowski M, Eisler S, Diederich F. Dendritic vectors for gene transfection. New J Chem. 2007:1111–27. https://doi.org/10.1039/b614877h.
20. Wu X, Zhang Y, Takle K, Bilsel O, Li Z, Lee H, Zhang Z, Li D, Fan W, Duan C, et al. Dye-sensitized core/active shell upconversion nanoparticles for optogenetics and bioimaging applications. ACS Nano. 2016;10(1):1060–6. https://doi.org/10.1021/acsnano.5b06383.
21. Jeyaraman J, Malecka A, Billimoria P, Shukla A, Marandi B, Patel PM, Jackson AM, Sivakumar S. Immuno-silent polymer capsules encapsulating nanoparticles for bioimaging applications. J Mater Chem B. 2017;5(26):5251–8. https://doi.org/10.1039/c7tb01044c.
22. Yang J, Zhang Q, Chang H, Cheng Y. Surface-engineered dendrimers in gene delivery. Chem Rev. 2015;115(11):5274–300. https://doi.org/10.1021/cr500542t.
23. Thompson JMT. Basic principles in the general theory of elastic stability. J Mech Phys Solids. 1963;11(1):13–20. https://doi.org/10.1016/j.drudis.2016.12.007.
24. Wang D, Zhao T, Zhu X, Yan D, Wang W. Bioapplications of hyperbranched polymers. Chem Soc Rev. 2015;44(12):4023–71. https://doi.org/10.1039/c4cs00229f.
25. Svenson S. The dendrimer paradox-high medical expectations but poor clinical translation. Chem Soc Rev. 2015;44(12):4131–44. https://doi.org/10.1039/c5cs00288e.
26. He Q, Shi J. MSN anti-cancer nanomedicines: chemotherapy enhancement, overcoming of drug resistance, and metastasis inhibition. Adv Mater. 2014;26(3):391–411. https://doi.org/10.1002/adma.201303123.
27. Soenen SJ, Parak WJ, Rejman J, Manshian B. (Intra) cellular stability of inorganic nanoparticles: effects on cytotoxicity, particle functionality, and biomedical applications. Chem Rev. 2015;115(5):2109–35. https://doi.org/10.1021/cr400714j.
28. Anselmo AC, Mitragotri S. A review of clinical translation of inorganic nanoparticles. AAPS J. 2015;17(5):1041–54. https://doi.org/10.1208/s12248-015-9780-2.
29. Manzano M, Vallet-regi M. Mesoporous silica nanoparticles in nanomedicine applications. J Mater Sci Mater Med. 2018;29:65. https://doi.org/10.1007/s10856-018-6069-x.
30. Klose D, Siepmann F, Elkharraz K, Krenzlin S, Siepmann J. How porosity and size affect the drug release mechanisms from PLGA-based microparticles. Int J Pharm. 2006;314(2):198–206. https://doi.org/10.1016/j.ijpharm.2005.07.031.
31. Liong M, Lu J, Kovochich M, Xia T, Ruehm SG, Nel AE, Tamanoi F, Zink JI. Multifunctional inorganic nanoparticles for imaging, targeting, and drug delivery. ACS Nano. 2008;2(5):889–96. https://doi.org/10.1021/nn800072t.
32. Shi J, Kantoff PW, Wooster R, Farokhzad OC. Cancer nanomedicine: progress, challenges and opportunities. Nat Rev Cancer. 2017;17(1):20–37. https://doi.org/10.1038/nrc.2016.108.
33. Gabizon A, Catane R, Uziely B, Kaufman B, Safra T, Cohen R, Martin F, Huang A. Prolonged circulating time and enhanced accumulation in malignant exudates of doxorubicin encapsulated in polyethylene-glycol coated liposomes. Cancer Res. 1994;54:987–92.
34. Gabizon A, Shmeeda H, Barenholz Y. Pharmacokinetics of pegylated liposomal doxorubicin: review of animal and human studies. Clin Pharmacokinet. 2003;42(5):419–36. https://doi.org/10.2165/00003088-200342050-00002.
35. Iyer AK, Khaled G, Fang J, Maeda H. Exploiting the enhanced permeability and retention effect for tumor targeting. Drug Discov Today. 2006;11(17–18):812–8. https://doi.org/10.1016/j.drudis.2006.07.005.
36. Maeda H. Tumor-selective delivery of macromolecular drugs via the EPR effect: background and future prospects. Bioconjug Chem. 2010;21:797–802. https://doi.org/10.1021/bc100070g.
37. Maeda H, Tsukigawa K, Fang J. A retrospective 30 years after discovery of the enhanced permeability and retention effect of solid tumors: next-generation chemotherapeutics and photodynamic therapy—problems, solutions, and prospects. Microcirculation. 2016;23(3):173–82. https://doi.org/10.1111/micc.12228.
38. Maeda H. Toward a full understanding of the EPR effect in primary and metastatic tumors as well as issues related to its heterogeneity. Adv Drug Deliv Rev. 2015;91:3–6. https://doi.org/10.1016/j.addr.2015.01.002.
39. Hollis CP, Weiss HL, Leggas M, Evers BM, Gemeinhart RA, Li T. Biodistribution and bioimaging studies of hybrid paclitaxel nanocrystals: lessons learned of the EPR effect and

image-guided drug delivery. J Control Release. 2013;172(1):12–21. https://doi.org/10.1016/j. jconrel.2013.06.039.

40. Nichols JW, Han Y. EPR: evidence and fallacy. J Control Release. 2014;190:451–64. https:// doi.org/10.1016/j.jconrel.2014.03.057.

41. Gao C, Bhattarai P, Chen M, Zhang N, Hameed S, Yue X, Dai Z. Amphiphilic drug conjugates as nanomedicines for combined cancer therapy. Bioconjug Chem. 2018;29(12):3967–81. https://doi.org/10.1021/acs.bioconjchem.8b00692.

42. Choi HS, Liu W, Liu F, Nasr K, Misra P, Bawendi MG, Frangioni JV. Design considerations for tumour-targeted nanoparticles. Nat Nanotechnol. 2009;5(1):42–7. https://doi.org/10.1038/nnano.2009.314.

43. Bradley AJ, Devine DV, Ansell SM, Janzen J, Brooks DE. Inhibition of liposome-induced complement activation by incorporated poly (ethylene glycol)-lipids. Arch Biochem Biophys. 1998;357(2):185–94. https://doi.org/10.1006/abbi.1998.0798.

44. Choi HS, Ipe BI, Misra P, Lee JH, Bawendi MG, Frangioni JV. Tissue- and organ-selective biodistribution of NIR fluorescent quantum dots. Nano Lett. 2009;9(6):2354–9. https://doi.org/10.1021/nl900872r.

45. Gabizon A, Martin F. Polyethylene glycol-coated (pegylated) liposomal doxorubicin. rationale for use in solid tumours. Drugs. 1997;54(Suppl 4):15–21.

46. Harris JM, Chess RB. Effect of pegylation on pharmaceuticals. Nat Rev Drug Discov. 2003;2(3):214–21. https://doi.org/10.1038/nrd1033.

47. Gabizon AA, Patil Y, La-Beck NM. New insights and evolving role of pegylated liposomal doxorubicin in cancer therapy. Drug Resist Updat. 2016;29:90–106. https://doi.org/10.1016/j. drup.2016.10.003.

48. Shi J, Kantoff PW, Wooster R, Farokhzad OC. Cancer nanomedicine: progress, challenges and opportunities. Nat Rev Cancer. 2016;17(1):20–37. https://doi.org/10.1038/nrc.2016.108.

49. Jin Q, Deng Y, Chen X, Ji J. Rational design of cancer nanomedicine for simultaneous stealth surface and enhanced cellular uptake. ACS Nano. 2019;13:954–77. https://doi.org/10.1021/acsnano.8b07746.

50. Pérez-Herrero E, Fernández-Medarde A. Advanced targeted therapies in cancer: drug nanocarriers, the future of chemotherapy. Eur J Pharm Biopharm. 2015;93(March):52–79. https://doi.org/10.1016/j.ejpb.2015.03.018.

51. Ma P, Chen J, Bi X, Li Z, Gao X, Li H, Zhu H, Huang Y, Qi J, Zhang Y. Overcoming multidrug resistance through the GLUT1-mediated and enzyme-triggered mitochondrial targeting conjugate with redox-sensitive paclitaxel release. ACS Appl Mater Interfaces. 2018;10(15):12351–63. https://doi.org/10.1021/acsami.7b18437.

52. Kirtane AR, Kalscheuer SM, Panyam J. Exploiting nanotechnology to overcome tumor drug resistance: challenges and opportunities. Adv Drug Deliv Rev. 2013;65(13–14):1731–47. https://doi.org/10.1016/j.addr.2013.09.001.

53. Blanco E, Shen H, Ferrari M. Principles of nanoparticle design for overcoming biological barriers to drug delivery. Nat Biotechnol. 2015;33(9):941–51. https://doi.org/10.1038/nbt.3330.

54. Wong C, Stylianopoulos T, Cui J, Martin J, Chauhan VP, Jiang W, Popovic Z, Jain RK, Bawendi MG, Fukumura D. Multistage nanoparticle delivery system for deep penetration into tumor tissue. Proc Natl Acad Sci U S A. 2011;108(6):2426–31. https://doi.org/10.1073/pnas.1018382108.

55. Chou LYT, Ming K, Chan WCW. Strategies for the intracellular delivery of nanoparticles. Chem Soc Rev. 2011;40(1):233–45. https://doi.org/10.1039/C0CS00003E.

56. Decuzzi P, Lee S, Bhushan B, Ferrari M. A theoretical model for the margination of particles within blood vessels. Ann Biomed Eng. 2005;33(2):179–90. https://doi.org/10.1007/s10439-005-8976-5.

57. Shah S, Liu Y, Hu W, Gao J. Modeling particle shape-dependent dynamics in nanomedicine. J Nanosci Nanotechnol. 2011;11(2):919–28. https://doi.org/10.1166/jnn.2011.3536.Modeling.

58. Hare JI, Lammers T, Ashford MB, Puri S, Storm G, Barry ST. Challenges and strategies in anti-cancer nanomedicine development: an industry perspective. Adv Drug Deliv Rev. 2017;108:25–38. https://doi.org/10.1016/j.addr.2016.04.025.

59. von Roemeling C, Jiang W, Chan CK, Weissman IL, Kim BYS. Breaking down the barriers to precision cancer nanomedicine. Trends Biotechnol. 2017;35(2):159–71. https://doi.org/10.1016/j.tibtech.2016.07.006.

60. Patel NR, Pattni BS, Abouzeid AH, Torchilin VP. Nanopreparations to overcome multidrug resistance in cancer. Adv Drug Deliv Rev. 2013;65(13–14):1748–62. https://doi.org/10.1016/j.addr.2013.08.004.

61. Li HJ, Du JZ, Liu J, Du XJ, Shen S, Zhu YH, Wang X, Ye X, Nie S, Wang J. Smart superstructures with ultrahigh pH-sensitivity for targeting acidic tumor microenvironment: instantaneous size switching and improved tumor penetration. ACS Nano. 2016;10(7):6753–61. https://doi.org/10.1021/acsnano.6b02326.

62. Binauld S, Stenzel MH. Acid-degradable polymers for drug delivery: a decade of innovation. Chem Commun. 2013;49(21):2082. https://doi.org/10.1039/c2cc36589h.

63. Yin Q, Shen J, Zhang Z, Yu H, Li Y. Reversal of multidrug resistance by stimuli-responsive drug delivery systems for therapy of tumor. Adv Drug Deliv Rev. 2013;65(13–14):1699–715. https://doi.org/10.1016/j.addr.2013.04.011.

64. Fontana F, Liu D, Hirvonen J, Santos HA. Delivery of therapeutics with nanoparticles: what's new in cancer immunotherapy? Wiley Interdisc Rev Nanomed Nanobiotechnol. 2017;9(1). https://doi.org/10.1002/wnan.1421.

65. Hu CMJ, Zhang L. Nanoparticle-based combination therapy toward overcoming drug resistance in cancer. Biochem Pharmacol. 2012;83(8):1104–11. https://doi.org/10.1016/j.bcp.2012.01.008.

66. Iyer AK, Singh A, Ganta S, Amiji MM. Role of integrated cancer nanomedicine in overcoming drug resistance. Adv Drug Deliv Rev. 2013;65:1784–802. https://doi.org/10.1016/j.addr.2013.07.012.

67. Parhi P, Mohanty C, Sahoo SK. Nanotechnology-based combinational drug delivery: an emerging approach for cancer therapy. Drug Discov Today. 2012;17(17–18):1044–52. https://doi.org/10.1016/j.drudis.2012.05.010.

68. Scarano W, de Souza P, Stenzel MH. Dual-drug delivery of curcumin and platinum drugs in polymeric micelles enhances the synergistic effects: a double act for the treatment of multidrug-resistant cancer. Biomater Sci. 2015;3(1):163–74. https://doi.org/10.1039/C4BM00272E.

69. Sun R, Liu Y, Li SY, Shen S, Du XJ, Xu CF, Cao ZT, Bao Y, Zhu YH, Li YP, et al. Co-delivery of all-trans-retinoic acid and doxorubicin for cancer therapy with synergistic inhibition of cancer stem cells. Biomaterials. 2015;37:405–14. https://doi.org/10.1016/j.biomaterials.2014.10.018.

70. Meng F, Wang J, Ping Q, Yeo Y. Camouflaging nanoparticles for ratiometric delivery of therapeutic combinations. Nano Lett. 2019;19(3):1479–87. https://doi.org/10.1021/acs.nanolett.8b04017.

71. Zhang J, Li J, Shi Z, Yang Y, Xie X, Lee SMY, Wang Y, Leong KW, Chen M. pH-sensitive polymeric nanoparticles for co-delivery of doxorubicin and curcumin to treat cancer via enhanced pro-apoptotic and anti-angiogenic activities. Acta Biomater. 2017;58:349–64. https://doi.org/10.1016/j.actbio.2017.04.029.

72. Wang Z, Ho PC. A nanocapsular combinatorial sequential drug delivery system for anti-angiogenesis and anticancer activities. Biomaterials. 2010;31(27):7115–23. https://doi.org/10.1016/j.biomaterials.2010.05.075.

73. Cai Y, Shen H, Zhan J, Lin M, Dai L, Ren C, Shi Y, Liu J, Gao J, Yang Z. Supramolecular "Trojan Horse" for nuclear delivery of dual anticancer drugs. J Am Chem Soc. 2017;139(8):2876–9. https://doi.org/10.1021/jacs.6b12322.

74. Haume K, Rosa S, Grellet S, Śmiałek MA, Butterworth KT, Solov'yov AV, Prise KM, Golding J, Mason NJ. Gold nanoparticles for cancer radiotherapy: a review. Cancer Nanotechnol. 2016;7(1):8. https://doi.org/10.1186/s12645-016-0021-x.

75. Li N, Zhao P, Astruc D. Anisotropic gold nanoparticles: synthesis, properties, applications, and toxicity. Angew Chem Int Ed. 2014;53(7):1756–89. https://doi.org/10.1002/anie.201300441.

76. Elumalai R, Patil S, Maliyakkal N, Rangarajan A, Kondaiah P, Raichur AM. Protamine-carboxymethyl cellulose magnetic nanocapsules for enhanced delivery of anticancer drugs

against drug resistant cancers. Nanomed Nanotechnol Biol Med. 2015;11(4):969–81. https://doi.org/10.1016/j.nano.2015.01.005.

77. Shapira A, Livney YD, Broxterman HJ, Assaraf YG. Nanomedicine for targeted cancer therapy: towards the overcoming of drug resistance. Drug Resist Updat. 2011;14(3):150–63. https://doi.org/10.1016/j.drup.2011.01.003.

78. Jabr-Milane LS, van Vlerken LE, Yadav S, Amiji MM. Multi-functional nanocarriers to overcome tumor drug resistance. Cancer Treat Rev. 2008;34(7):592–602. https://doi.org/10.1016/j.ctrv.2008.04.003.

79. Kemp JA, Shim MS, Heo CY, Kwon YJ. "Combo" nanomedicine: co-delivery of multi-modal therapeutics for efficient, targeted, and safe cancer therapy. Adv Drug Deliv Rev. 2016;98:3–18. https://doi.org/10.1016/j.addr.2015.10.019.

80. Xiong XB, Lavasanifar A. Traceable multifunctional micellar nanocarriers for cancer-targeted co-delivery of MDR-1 SiRNA and doxorubicin. ACS Nano. 2011;5(6):5202–13. https://doi.org/10.1021/nn2013707.

81. Kunjachan S, Rychlik B, Storm G, Kiessling F, Lammers T. Multidrug resistance: physiological principles and nanomedical solutions. Adv Drug Deliv Rev. 2013;65(13–14):1852–65. https://doi.org/10.1016/j.addr.2013.09.018.

82. Xu X, Ho W, Zhang X, Bertrand N, Farokhzad O. Cancer nanomedicine: from targeted delivery to combination therapy. Trends Mol Med. 2015;21(4):223–32. https://doi.org/10.1016/j.molmed.2015.01.001.

83. Bregoli L, Movia D, Gavigan-Imedio JD, Lysaght J, Reynolds J, Prina-Mello A. Nanomedicine applied to translational oncology: a future perspective on cancer treatment. Nanomed Nanotechnol Biol Med. 2016;12(1):81–103. https://doi.org/10.1016/j.nano.2015.08.006.

84. Havel H, Finch G, Strode P, Wolfgang M, Zale S, Bobe I, Youssoufian H, Peterson M, Liu M. Nanomedicines: from bench to bedside and beyond. AAPS J. 2016;18(6):1373–8. https://doi.org/10.1208/s12248-016-9961-7.

85. Sainz V, Conniot J, Matos AI, Peres C, Zupančič E, Moura L, Silva LC, Florindo HF, Gaspar RS. Regulatory aspects on nanomedicines. Biochem Biophys Res Commun. 2015;468(3):504–10. https://doi.org/10.1016/j.bbrc.2015.08.023.

86. Ellis LM, Hicklin DJ. Resistance to targeted therapies: refining anticancer therapy in the era of molecular oncology. Clin Cancer Res. 2009;15(24):7471–8. https://doi.org/10.1158/1078-0432.CCR-09-1070.

87. Linnekamp JF, Wang X, Medema JP, Vermeulen L. Colorectal cancer heterogeneity and targeted therapy: a case for molecular disease subtypes. Cancer Res. 2015;75(2):245–9. https://doi.org/10.1158/0008-5472.CAN-14-2240.

Index

© Springer Nature Switzerland AG 2019
M. R. Szewczuk et al. (eds.), *Current Applications for Overcoming Resistance to Targeted Therapies*, Resistance to Targeted Anti-Cancer Therapeutics 20, https://doi.org/10.1007/978-3-030-21477-7

Printed in the United States
By Bookmasters